Surgical Oncology

Cancer Treatment and Research

Steven T Rosen, M.D., *Series Editor*

Hansen HH (ed): Basic and Clinical Concepts of Lung Cancer. 1989. ISBN 0-7923-0153-6
Lepor H, Ratliff TL (eds): Urologic Oncology. 1989. ISBN 0-7923-0161-7
Benz C, Liu E (eds): Oncogenes. 1989. ISBN 0-7923-0237-0
Ozols RF (ed): Drug Resistance in Cancer Therapy. 1989. ISBN 0-7923-0244-3
Surwit EA, Alberts DS (eds): Endometrial Cancer. 1989. ISBN 0-7923-0286-9
Champlin R (ed): Bone Marrow Transplantation. 1990. ISBN 0-7923-0612-0
Goldenberg D (ed): Cancer Imaging with Radiolabeled Antibodies. 1990. ISBN 0-7923-0631-7
Jacobs C (ed): Carcinomas of the Head and Neck. 1990. ISBN 0-7923-0668-6
Lippman ME, Dickson R (eds): Règulatory Mechanisms in Breast Cancer: Advances in Cellular and
    Molecular Biology of Breast Cancer. 1990. ISBN 0-7923-0868-9
Nathanson L (ed): Malignant Melanoma: Genetics, Growth Factors, Metastases, and Antigens. 1991.
    ISBN 0-7923-0895-6
Sugarbaker PH (ed): Management of Gastric Cancer. 1991. ISBN 0-7923-1102-7
Pinedo HM, Verweij J, Suit HD (eds): Soft Tissue Sarcomas: New Developments in the Multidisciplinary
    Approach to Treatment. 1991. ISBN 0-7923-1139-6
Ozols RF (ed): Molecular and Clinical Advances in Anticancer Drug Resistance. 1991. ISBN 0-7923-1212-0
Muggia FM (ed): New Drugs, Concepts and Results in Cancer Chemotherapy 1991. ISBN 0-7923-1253-8
Dickson RB, Lippman ME (eds): Genes, Oncogenes and Hormones: Advances in Cellular and Molecular
    Biology of Breast Cancer. 1992. ISBN 0-7923-1748-3
Humphrey G, Bennett, Schraffordt Koops H, Molenaar WM, Postma A (eds): Osteosarcoma in Adolescents
    and Young Adults: New Developments and Controversies. 1993. ISBN 0-7923-1905-2
Benz CC, Liu ET (eds): Oncogenes and Tumor Suppressor Genes in Human Malignancies. 1993.
    ISBN 0-7923-1960-5
Freireich EJ, Kantarjian H, (eds): Leukemia: Advances in Research and Treatment. 1993.
    ISBN 0-7923-1967-2
Dana BW (ed): Malignant Lymphomas, Including Hodgkin's Disease: Diagnosis, Management, and Special
    Problems. 1993. ISBN 0-7923-2171-5
Nathanson L (ed): Current Research and Clinical Management of Melanoma. 1993. ISBN 0-7923-2152-9
Verweij J, Pinedo HM, Suit HD (eds): Multidisciplinary Treatment of Soft Tissue Sarcomas. 1993.
    ISBN 0-7923-2183-9
Rosen ST, Kuzel TM (eds): Immunoconjugate Therapy of Hematologic Malignancies. 1993.
    ISBN 0-7923-2270-3
Sugarbaker PH (ed): Hepatobiliary Cancer. 1994. ISBN 0-7923-2501-X
Rothenberg ML (ed): Gynecologic Oncology: Controversies and New Developments. 1994.
    ISBN 0-7923-2634-2
Dickson RB, Lippman ME (eds): Mammary Tumorigenesis and Malignant Progression. 1994.
    ISBN 0-7923-2647-4
Hansen HH, (ed): Lung Cancer, Advances in Basic and Clinical Research. 1994. ISBN 0-7923-2835-3
Goldstein LJ, Ozols RF (eds): Anticancer Drug Resistance. Advances in Molecular and Clinical Research.
    1994. ISBN 0-7923-2836-1
Hong WK, Weber RS (eds): Head and Neck Cancer. Basic and Clinical Aspects. 1994. ISBN 0-7923-3015-3
Thall PF (ed): Recent Advances in Clinical Trial Design and Analysis. 1995. ISBN 0-7923-3235-0
Buckner CD (ed): Technical and Biological Components of Marrow Transplantation. 1995.
    ISBN 0-7923-3394-2
Muggia FM (ed): Concepts, Mechanisms, and New Targets for Chemotherapy. 1995. ISBN 0-7923-3525-2
Klastersky J (ed): Infectious Complications of Cancer. 1995. ISBN 0-7923-3598-8
Kurzrock R, Talpaz M (eds): Cytokines: Interleukins and Their Receptors. 1995. ISBN 0-7923-3636-4
Sugarbaker P (ed): Peritoneal Carcinomatosis: Drugs and Diseases. 1995. ISBN 0-7923-3726-3
Sugarbaker P (ed): Peritoneal Carcinomatosis: Principles of Management. 1995. ISBN 0-7923-3727-1
Dickson RB, Lippman ME (eds): Mammary Tumor Cell Cycle, Differentiation and Metastasis. 1995.
    ISBN 0-7923-3905-3
Freireich EJ, Kantarjian H (eds): Molecular Genetics and Therapy of Leukemia. 1995. ISBN 0-7923-3912-6
Cabanillas F, Rodriguez MA (eds): Advances in Lymphoma Research. 1996. ISBN 0-7923-3929-0
Miller AB (ed): Advances in Cancer Screening. 1996. ISBN 0-7923-4019-1
Hait WN (ed): Drug Resistance. 1996. ISBN 0-7923-4022-1
Pienta KJ (ed): Diagnosis and Treatment of Genitourinary Malignancies. 1996. 0-7923-4164-3

Surgical Oncology

edited by

RAPHAEL E POLLOCK, M.D., Ph.D.
The University of Texas
M.D. Anderson Cancer Center
Houston, Texas

1997 **KLUWER ACADEMIC PUBLISHERS**
BOSTON / DORDRECHT / LONDON

Distributors for North America:
Kluwer Academic Publishers
101 Philip Drive
Assinippi Park
Norwell, Massachusetts 02061 USA

Distributor for all other countries:
Kluwer Academic Publishers Group
Distribution Centre
Post Office Box 322
3300 AH Dordrecht, THE NETHERLANDS

Library of Congress Cataloging-in-Publication Data
Surgical oncology / edited by Raphael E. Pollock.
     p. cm. — (Cancer treatment and research)
    Includes bibliographical references and index.
    ISBN 0–7923–9900–5 (alk. paper)
    1. Cancer—Surgery. 2. Cancer—Diagnosis. 3. Cancer—Treatment.
I. Pollock, Raphael E. II. Series.
    [DNLM: 1. Neoplasms—surgery. 2. Neoplasms—diagnosis.
W1 CA693   1997 / QZ 268 S961101 1997]
RD651.S883   1997
616.99′4059—dc21
DNLM/DLC
for Library of Congress   97–5016
                                                      CIP

Printed on acid-free paper.

PRINTED IN THE UNITED STATES OF AMERICA

Contents

Contributors

ABBRUZZESE, James L., M.D., M.D. Anderson Cancer Center, 1515 Holcombe Blvd., Houston, TX 77030

ANDRASSAY, Richard J., M.D., 6431 Fannin, Ste. 6.264, Houston, TX 77030

BRENNAN, Murray F., M.D., Memorial Sloan-Kettering Cancer Center, 1275 York Ave., New York, NY 10021

CADY, Blake M.D., New England Deaconess Hospital, 110 Francis St., Boston, MA 02215

CHARNSANGAVEJ, Chusilp M.D., M.D. Anderson Cancer Center, 1515 Holcombe Blvd., Houston, TX 77030

CHIAO, Paul J., M.D., M.D. Anderson Cancer Center, 1515 Holcombe Blvd., Houston, TX 77030

CORPRON, Cynthia A., M.D., M.D. Anderson Cancer Center, 1515 Holcombe Blvd., Houston, TX 77030

CURLEY, Steven A., M.D., M.D. Anderson Cancer Center, 1515 Holcombe Blvd., Houston, TX 77030

DHINGRA, Kapil M.D., M.D. Anderson Cancer Center, 1515 Holcombe Blvd., Houston, TX 77030

ELLIS, Lee M., M.D., M.D. Anderson Cancer Center, 1515 Holcombe Blvd., Houston, TX 77030

EVANS, Douglas B., M.D., M.D. Anderson Cancer Center, 1515 Holcombe Blvd., Houston, TX 77030

FEIG, Barry W., M.D., M.D. Anderson Cancer Center, 1515 Holcombe Blvd., Houston, TX 77030

GILLENWATER, Ann M., M.D., M.D. Anderson Cancer Center, 1515 Holcombe Blvd., Houston, TX 77030

HUNT, Kelly K., M.D., M.D. Anderson Cancer Center, 1515 Holcombe Blvd., Houston, TX 77030

JOHNSON, Mark E., M.D., M.D. Anderson Cancer Center, 1515 Holcombe Blvd., Houston, TX 77030

LEE, Jeffrey E., M.D., M.D. Anderson Cancer Center, 1515 Holcombe Blvd., Houston, TX 77030

LENZI, Renato, M.D., M.D. Anderson Cancer Center, 1515 Holcombe Blvd., Houston, TX 77030

LEUNG, Denis H.Y., Ph.D., Memorial Sloan-Kettering Cancer Center, 1275 York Ave., New York, NY 10021

MANSFIELD, Paul F., M.D., M.D. Anderson Cancer Center, 1515 Holcombe Blvd., Houston, TX 77030

MARCHESA, Pienrenrico M.D., Cleveland Clinic Foundation, 9500 Euclid Ave., Cleveland, OH 44195-5044

MILLER, Julie A., M.D., Washington University Medical School, 660 S. Euclid Ave., St. Louis, MO 63110

MILSOM, Jeffrey W., M.D., Cleveland Cl. Foundation, C & R Surg., 9500 Euclid Ave., Desk A111, Cleveland, OH 44195-5044

NORTON, Jeffrey A., M.D., Washington University Medical School, Department of Surgery, Box 8120, 660 S, Euclid Ave., St. Louis, MO 63110

OTA, David M., M.D., University of Missouri, Ellis Fischel Cancer Center, 115 Business Loop 70 West, Columbia, MO 65203

PISTERS, Peter W.T., M.D., M.D. Anderson Cancer Center, 1515 Holcombe Blvd., Houston, TX 77030

POLLOCK, Raphael E., M.D., Ph.D., M.D. Anderson Cancer Center, 1515 Holcombe Blvd., Houston, TX 77030

ROBB, Geoffrey L., M.D., M.D. Anderson Cancer Center, 1515 Holcombe Blvd., Houston, TX 77030

ROH, Mark S., M.D., M.D. Anderson Cancer Center, 1515 Holcombe Blvd., Houston, TX 77030

ROSEMAN, Barry M.D., M.D. Anderson Cancer Center, 1515 Holcombe Blvd., Houston, TX 77030

ROSS, Merrick I., M.D., M.D. Anderson Cancer Center, 1515 Holcombe Blvd., Houston, TX 77030

SCHUSTERMAN, Mark A., M.D., M.D. Anderson Cancer Center, 1515 Holcombe Blvd., Houston, TX 77030

SINGLETARY, S. Eva, M.D., M.D. Anderson Cancer Center, 1515 Holcombe Blvd., Houston, TX 77030

SKIBBER, John M., M.D., M.D. Anderson Cancer Center, 1515 Holcombe Blvd., Houston, TX 77030

TADJALLI, Helen E., M.D., M.D. Anderson Cancer Center, 1515 Holcombe Blvd., Houston, TX 77030

VIGNALI, Andrea M.D., Cleveland Clinic Foundation, 9500 Euclid Ave., Cleveland, OH 44195-5044

WEBER, Randal S., M.D., M.D. Anderson Cancer Center, 1515 Holcombe Blvd., Houston, TX 77030

YASKO, Alan M., M.D., M.D. Anderson Cancer Center, 1515 Holcombe Blvd., Houston, TX 77030

YU, Di-Hua, M.D., Ph.D., M.D. Anderson Cancer Center, 1515 Holcombe Blvd., Houston, TX 77030

Preface

Among the standard oncology modalities, surgical oncology is singular in that it lacks a separate board certification or even an added qualification mechanism. 'Card-carrying' surgical oncologists are certified by the American Board of Surgery, as are all other general surgeons. What distinguishes the surgical oncologist is a set of cognitive skills rather than a specific armamentarium of surgical techniques. This different conceptual framework is derived from extensive additional training that leads to an in-depth understanding of the natural history and biologic behavior of the various solid tumor systems. Equipped with this perspective, the surgical oncologist is particularly well positioned to integrate the various available therapeutic modalities into a coherent care program for the solid tumor patient.

As a central theme, the chapters of this book demonstrate that increasingly sophisticated diagnostic and staging approaches are helping to move chemotherapy and radiotherapy into the preoperative neoadjuvant setting. This fundamental alteration is based on the awareness that even early-stage solid tumor disease is frequently systemic at the time of presentation, at least on a subclinical level. And although the primary tumor may be controllable by surgery with radiotherapy, the uncontrolled (and initially clinically unapparent) distant disease ultimately determines patient survival. The other perspective driving the neoadjuvant approach is an emerging awareness that for most solid tumor systems, neoadjuvant treatment responses can facilitate less mutilating surgery with comparable levels of local disease control. These unifying concepts have reached increasing acceptance and are being extended via the crucible of clinical trials.

The chapters of this book collectively seek to impart a sense of what is pertinent in the rapidly evolving field of surgical oncology. By identifying new developments in each solid tumor site, the reader may gain an anticipatory sense of where the discipline of surgical oncology is headed. The next several years will almost certainly witness the introduction of molecular-based regional treatment of solid tumors. These exciting advancements will of necessity involve surgeons at both the translational and clinical research levels. The dawning of this new era is already upon us, as is clear from the innovative efforts discussed in this book; on behalf of my coauthors, I would like to thank you for your interest in this effort.

Surgical Oncology

1. Prospective randomized trials in melanoma: Defining contemporary surgical roles

Merrick I. Ross

Introduction

Some of the most important advances in the management of patients with melanoma have taken place in the past 5 years. The completion of well-designed prospective clinical trials is responsible for much of this progress, and the recent initiation of new trials will lead to continued refinements of the standard of care. Critical surgical issues, such as appropriate excision margins for primary melanomas and the respective roles for elective lymph node dissection (ELND) and adjuvant limb perfusion in the management of high-risk stage I and II patients, have now been properly addressed in prospective/randomized settings.

The emergence of lymphatic mapping and sentinel node biopsy offers a more selective approach to regional lymphadenectomy as well as a minimally invasive method of nodal staging [1–4]. Modifications to this novel technique have already evolved improving the ability to localize the sentinel node. However, the long-term accuracy of sentinel node biopsies and any survival advantage that may be achieved with selective lymphadenectomy has yet to be established. These latter issues are presently being investigated in a multicenter randomized trial.

Dramatic tumor responses produced by the addition of tumor necrosis factor (TNF) to melphalan in a perfusion circuit for the treatment of advanced local extremity recurrences and in-transit limb metastases was recently reported in a study from Europe [5–6]. This experience has generated renewed interest in limb perfusion in the United States, leading to the genesis of a prospective randomized trial of melphalan alone versus melphalan plus in patients with measurable disease.

Data have recently been published demonstrating a modest but statistically significant survival benefit with the use of high-dose adjuvant interferon-alpha administered to patients for 1 year following lymphadenectomy for regional nodal metastases [7]. This publication provided the basis for the first drug to be licensed for adjuvant use in melanoma patients and has provided the impetus to pursue subsequent randomized trials attempting to identify more efficacious systemic adjuvant approaches. This chapter reviews the aforementioned

Raphael E. Pollock (ed.), SURGICAL ONCOLOGY. Copyright © 1997. Kluwer Academic Publishers. ISBN 0-7923-9900-5. All rights reserved.

developments and focuses on how these clinical research accomplishments will be integrated into the contemporary management of the various stages of melanoma.

Surgical management of stages I and II patients

Although the incidence of melanoma continues to climb, the vast majority of newly diagnosed melanoma patients fortunately present with disease that is clinically confined to the primary site (American Joint Committee on Cancer [AJCC] stages I and II) [8,9]. Defining standards of care for this heterogeneous group of patients has been a challenge. Optimal excision margins of the primary tumor and the role for ELND and adjuvant limb perfusion have represented the major surgical issues needing resolution. The appreciation of tumor thickness as the single most important prognostic factor predicting the natural history of early stage melanoma [10] was a critical advance aiding in the design of large prospective randomized trials.

Margins of excision

Historical surgical dogma has advocated an aggressive approach to all primary melanomas that has included a 5 cm margin of excision followed by skin grafting. Earlier diagnosis; the identification of important prognostic factors, in particular tumor thickness; the completion of clinical trials; and advances in surgical techniques have all contributed to the evolution of more rational and less morbid surgical guidelines in which the extent of surgery is tailored to the predicted aggressiveness of disease. The issue of excision margins for primary tumors has been addressed in a careful stepwise fashion, resulting in fairly straightforward recommendations.

A prospective randomized trial conducted by the World Health Organization (WHO), published in 1991, clearly demonstrated that a 1 cm surgical excision margin was oncologically safe for lesions that were ≤1 mm in thickness [11]. The published results by Balch et al. from the Intergroup Melanoma Committee Trial demonstrated that a 2 cm excision margin is preferable to a wider 4 cm excision for patients with intermediate thickness melanomas (1–4 mm in thickness) [12]. The narrower (2 cm) excision margin resulted in a significantly reduced need for skin grafting and a shorter hospital stay without impacting negatively on local recurrence rates or survival. In 90% of the patients undergoing a 2 cm excision, primary closure could be accomplished [12].

These two well-conducted prospective randomized trials are complimentary to each other and provide the basis for the contemporary recommendations for primary melanomas of different thickness ranges (Table 1). Although

2

Table 1. Recommendations for margins of excision

Tumor thickness	Margin
In situ	0.5–1 cm
≤1 mm	1 cm
1–4 mm[a]	2 cm[a]
>4 mm	≥2 cm

[a]For subset of patients between 1 and 2 mm, a 1 cm margin is appropriate for lesions in anatomic locations where a 2 cm margin would compromise vital structures or local available skin is inadequate to allow primary closure.

the guidelines are relatively straightforward, there are some gray areas worthy of discussion.

Those patients with melanomas between the thickness of 1 and 2 mm represent an overlap area between the WHO and Intergroup melanoma trials, as this group of patients was included in both studies. The WHO trial randomized patients with melanomas ≤2 mm to a 1 cm versus a 3 cm margin of excision [11]. The survival data show that, regardless of the extent of excision, survival rates were the same. However, the incidence of local recurrence for patients with lesions between 1 and 2 mm was greater in the patients who underwent the narrow excision margins. The actual number of events is small, six versus one, and therefore no statistically significant differences were noted [11]. These data do raise the concern of an increased local recurrence rate in this group of patients, which may be, in part, related to the extent of surgical margin. However, since no survival disadvantage was demonstrated for this subset, it is not unreasonable to offer these patients a 1 cm excision margin. This is particularly prudent when the primary lesion is located in an anatomically restrictive area, such as the head-and-neck region, where the primary melanoma may be adjacent to vital structures, or for some in the distal extremities, where the available skin needed to accomplish primary closure is limited. In the absence of the aforementioned limitations, a 2 cm margin is preferred for this subset of patients.

Approach to the clinically negative regional lymph node basin

Although the percentage of melanoma patients diagnosed at an early stage is increasing, many patients, particularly those with primary tumors thicker than 1 mm, harbor occult metastases in regional nodes and therefore are at a high risk for subsequent relapse [10,13,14]. These patients may derive benefit from a regional lymphadenectomy as part of their primary management. The role for ELND in the management of clinically localized melanoma continues to be a controversial issue. With the recent publication of effective adjuvant inter-feron therapy after lymphadenectomy in patients with positive nodes [7], histologic staging of clinically negative nodal basins becomes important. This can be accomplished with ELND but may be better achieved with the less morbid approach of lymphatic mapping and sentinel node biopsy.

Elective lymph node dissection controversy

A better understanding of the natural history of patients with melanoma and the appreciation of the predictive value of tumor-related factors, such as tumor thickness and ulceration, has allowed us to identify subsets of patients at high risk for harboring occult regional lymph node metastases. Relative risk groups for the development of clinically detectable nodal metastases as the first site of failure have been defined mainly according to primary tumor thickness: <1 m, 1–4 mm, and >4 mm as low, intermediate, and high risk, re-spectively [10,13,14]. It has been suggested that the intermediate-thickness group of patients could potentially benefit by the complete removal of micro-scopic nodal disease as a way to prevent future distant failure [10,13,14]. It is this contention that represents the center of the controversy.

The usefulness of ELND has been debated for decades. Surgeons, reporting data from a variety of retrospective analyses, have been equally divided be-tween those who support earlier removal of regional lymph nodes and those who believe that lymphadenectomy should only be performed when regional disease becomes clinically apparent or histologically confirmed [15–24]. The latter practice, referred to as a therapeutic lymph node dissection, reduces the number of unnecessary lymphadenectomies and may not jeopardize the chance for cure. Table 2 lists the various series supporting and opposing the ELND approach. Of note are two institutions (Duke University and the Sydney Melanoma Unit) reversing their stand based on a second retro-spective analysis performed after longer follow-up [20,21]. This underscores the difficulty in establishing definitive recommendations for surgical therapy based on data obtained in a retrospective fashion. The results of these series, however, do support the previous contentions that the intermediate-thickness group of patients could potentially benefit. As a result, the appropri-ate subsets of patients to accrue in a prospective and randomized fashion were identified.

The long-term results of the first prospective randomized trial addressing the ELND issue was conducted by the WHO Melanoma Program and failed to demonstrate a survival benefit with ELND for primary melanoma patients [25]. Although this trial, involving almost 600 patients, was a well-designed, randomized approach to a surgical issue, it was conducted prior to the estab-lishment of the critical prognostic primary tumor factors, and therefore the specific aforementioned subgroups were not delineated for stratification. The patient population was comprised mainly of females with distal extremity

4

Table 2. Results of ELND trials

Trial	Design	Results
Memorial Sloan Kettering, 1975	Retrospective	Benefit for intermediate thickness
WHO, 1977	Prospective/randomized (n = 553)	No benefit
University of Alabama, 1982	Retrospective	Benefit for intermediate thickness
Duke University, 1983	Retrospective	Benefit for intermediate thickness
Sydney Melanoma Unit, 1985	Retrospective	Benefit for intermediate thickness
University of Pennsylvania, 1985	Retrospective	No benefit for intermediate thickness
Mayo Clinic, 1986	Prospective/randomized (n = 171)	No benefit
Drepper et al., 1993	Retrospective (multicenter)	Survival benefit for intermediate thickness
Duke University, 1994	Retrospective	No benefit
Rompel et al., 1995	Retrospective (matched pair)	Survival benefit for intermediate thickness
Sydney Melanoma Unit, 1995	Retrospective	No benefit
WHO trial (>1.5 mm, trunk)	Prospective/randomized (n = 257)	Pending
Intergroup Melanoma (1–4 mm, all sites)	Prospective/randomized (n = 740)	Benefit for 1–2 mm subset and patients <60 years of age

lesions of all tumor thickness (predominantly thin). Although long-term follow-up revealed identical survival rates for patients receiving ELND compared with patients treated with wide local excision alone, it is conceivable that benefits afforded to higher risk subsets could have been masked by the overwhelming majority of low-risk patients. Indeed, a separate subset analysis, performed retrospectively, identified a small group of patients with intermediate-thickness tumors as the beneficiaries of improved survival [26].

A subsequent prospective randomized trial conducted by the Mayo Clinic also failed to reveal any survival benefit using ELND [27]. This trial, similar to the WHO study, did not address specific high-risk subsets and was also limited by a small sample size.

Recently two contemporary randomized trials have been completed. The design of these trials was influenced by the limitations mentioned earlier that existed in previous randomized trials, as well as by the retrospective data demonstrating that patients with higher risk primaries (intermediate-thickness groups) could potentially benefit from ELND. The WHO Trunk Trial has accrued only patients with melanomas thicker than 1.5 mm to receive ELND versus wide local excision alone. These patients were stratified according to gender and ranges of tumor thickness (1.5–4 mm vs. >4 mm). Long-term follow-up of this trial is not available. The more recently concluded trial, conducted by the Intergroup Melanoma Committee headed by Dr. Charles Balch, included patients only with melanomas between 1 and 4 mm in thickness from any anatomic subsite. The patients with trunk melanomas underwent preoperative lymphoscintigraphy to identify nodal basins at risk. In addition, patients were prospectively stratified according to ranges of tumor thickness (1–2 mm, 2–3 mm, and 3–4 mm), the presence or absence of ulceration, and anatomic subsite (extremity vs. trunk vs. head and neck). Long-term results of this study have been anxiously awaited, and the first interim analysis has been recently published. This first analysis does identify specific subsets of patients (1–2 mm groups) benefitting from ELND [28].

Selective lymphadenectomy using lymphatic mapping

Amidst the above-mentioned ongoing controversy, a rational alternative to ELND emerged. The technique of lymphatic mapping and sentinel node biopsy, introduced by Don Morton [1], relies on the concept that finite regions of the skin drain specifically to an initial node within the regional nodal basin via an organized array of specific afferent lymphatic channels. In theory, each lymph node within a nodal basin represents a sentinel node draining different regions of the skin, and the sentinal node is the first one encountered by metastatic cells. The identification of the sentinel node, followed by its biopsy, may accurately determine whether melanoma cells have metastasized to that specific lymph node basin. This would allow surgeons, using a minimally invasive procedure, to identify those patients who harbor occult lymph node disease and to apply a complete lymphadenectomy only for those patients (selective lymphadenectomy). This would spare the remaining patients the cost and morbidity of an unnecessary procedure. Over the last 4–5 years the technique, using a vital blue dye (Lymphazurin or Patent Blue-V) to localize the sentinel node, has been extensively examined.

The initial series, reported by Morton et al., demonstrated that the sentinel node could be confidently identified at least 80% of the time [1,2]. Two subsequent series, one as a collaboration between the M. D. Anderson Cancer Canter and the Moffitt Cancer Center, and the other from the Sydney Melanoma Unit in Australia, confirmed the results of the initial trial, with sentinel node identification rates greater than 85% [3,4,29]. Patients eligible for lymphatic mapping in these series were stage I and II patients with melanomas greater than 0.76 mm in thickness. The percentage of patients with occult nodal metastases was in the 20% range [1–4,29]. To determine the accuracy of the sentinel node biopsy in terms of identifying occult disease, it was necessary to perform complete lymphadenectomies in conjunction with the sentinel node biopsy. A false-negative event is defined as finding disease within a nonsentinel node when the biopsied sentinel node was determined to be histologically negative for metastatic melanoma. In the three aforementioned studies, the percentage of false-negative events was in single digits, thus establishing this technique as an accurate mechanism for staging the regional lymph node basin [1–4,29].

Improving sentinel node identification

The initial promising results with this technique elicited significant interest within the surgical oncology community. Efforts were made to improve the sentinel lymph node localization, particularly in the axilla. Although identification rates using the blue dye alone were very good, the learning curve within the axillary region was relatively long compared with the inguinal basin, and identification rates were hovering in the 85–90% range. The first maneuver attempting to enhance sentinel node localization was the use of preoperative dynamic cutaneous lymphoscintigraphy.

Prior to performing ELND, it is critical to obtain routine lymphoscintigraphy to determine nodal basins at risk in patients with primaries located in ambiguous drainage sites, such as on the trunk and the head-and-neck region. The use of anatomic proximity or historical lymphatic drainage guidelines established by Sappey [30] to accomplish this goal is oftentimes inaccurate [31]. Studies have demonstrated that an objective test, such as a lymphoscintigraphy, is the standard of care for describing lymphatic drainage patterns [31,32]. These lymphoscintigrams can be obtained using an intradermal injection of technetium-labeled sulfur colloid, antimony colloid, or human serum albumin followed by nodal scanning with a gamma counter.

In addition to obtaining only static views of nodal basins at specific time points after injection of the radiolabel, dynamic real-time studies of lymphatic flow can be performed at early time points [33–34]. The lymphatic flow can be described, and the specific region of initial entrance of the radiolabel into the nodal basin and localization of the sentinel node can be established. The sentinel node is always defined as the initial node concentrating the radiolabeled material. Therefore, lymphoscintigraphy can be used for two purposes: (1) to identify nodal basins at risk for melanomas in ambiguous drainage sites and (2) to help localize the sentinel node(s) from any cutaneous site. The group from the Sydney Melanoma Unit in Australia is a strong proponent of dynamic lymphoscintigraphy to help provide a preoperative road map. Lymphoscintigraphs obtained for lesions on the extremities distal to the elbow or the knee can determine if significant uptake occurs within the epitrochlear and/or popliteal nodal regions, respectively. In addition, lymphoscintigraphy obtained for trunk lesions can identify the occasional patient (about 5%) who has sentinel node drainage to a lymph node–bearing region outside of the normal anatomically described lymphatic basins, located either in transit to or just proximal to the formal nodal basin [34] (Fig. 1).

The second important technologic advance in sentinel node localization is the intraoperative use of a handheld gamma probe. Following the intradermal injection of a radiolabeled colloid, the gamma probe can be used to target the highest area of radioactive signal intensity, representing the area of the

7

sentinel node. This technology takes advantage of the fact that the colloid particles are large enough to be actively phagosotized by macrophages within the lymph node, therefore concentrating the radiolabel within the initial draining node and minimizing the passage to higher echelon nodes [35]. This allows for accurate preoperative localization of the node, resulting in a smaller and

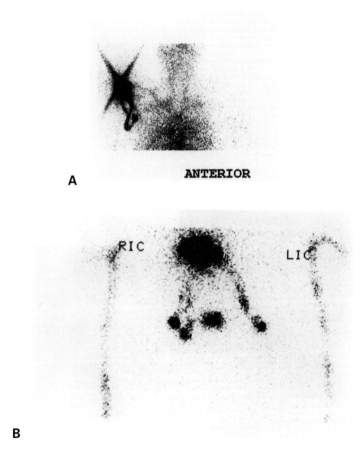

Figure 1. Lymphatic drainage patterns identified using lymphoscintigraphy of primary melanomas in ambiguous drainage sites. **A:** Primary melanoma on apex of right shoulder. Lymphoscintigraphy shows drainage exclusively to the right axilla with two afferent channels merging to one sentinel lymph node in the mid-axilla. **B:** Lymphatic drainage from an umbilical melanoma. No drainage to axillary regions but a bilateral inguinal drainage pattern is demonstrated. Two afferent channels are draining to two separate sentinel nodes on the right, and one sentinel node is identified on the left. The intense signal between the nodal basins represents uptake in the urinary bladder. **C:** Lymphoscintigram of primary melanoma of the back positioned in the midportion in the cranial-caudad plane and just to the left of the midline. Drainage patterns identifie intransit sentinel nodes on the left and the right, proximal to both axillary regions. No drainage is noted to the inguinal regions.

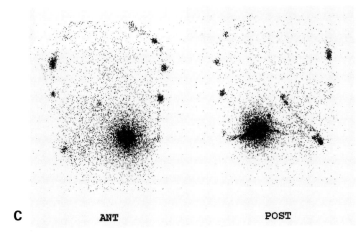

C   ANT   POST

Figure 1.1 (Continued).

more directed biopsy incision and rapid identification of the node. This technique was first introduced by a group from the University of Vermont and has subsequently been incorporated into practice at other centers [36,37]. Although this group used the colloid alone (did not use the vital blue dye), we feel that the two techniques are complimentary.

Studies demonstrate that, following injection of the colloid, it continues to be concentrated within the sentinel node, with the 4-hour time period providing the largest differential of radioactivity between the sentinel node and nonsentinel nodes [35–38]. Therefore, our practice includes an injection of the radiolabeled colloid in the nuclear medicine department followed by injection of the vital blue in the operating room. The patient is then appropriately prepped and draped, which provides ample time for the dye to travel through the afferent lymphatic channels to the sentinel node. The handheld gamma probe identifies the location of the sentinel node transcutaneously before making the incision. Assuming that the radiocolloid is injected in the same manner as the vital blue dye, the node containing the highest amount of radioactivity should also be stained blue. Following a small biopsy incision directed over the highest radioactive signal, the visual identification of the blue dye quickly identifies the lymph node that has the highest number of radioactive counts.

Occasionally, the first node encountered, although stained blue, may not necessarily represent the first or primary node of drainage, and therefore does not contain the highest level of radioactivity. The first node encountered may actually be a secondary echelon node that has received the blue dye through an efferent lymphatic channel attached in 'series' to the initial true sentinel node. More than one sentinel node from a particular primary site may be identified in a basin because lymphatic drainage may be accomplished through afferent channels arranged in 'parallel' (Fig. 2). These channels may converge to the node or may drain separately to two different nodes. It is also possible for one channel to split and drain to two separate nodes. The use of the handheld gamma probe can ensure that the sentinel node is ultimately identified. Following removal of what was assumed to be a sentinel node, the nodal basin can be scanned for residual radioactive activity. In our experience, we occasionally find a second blue-stained node with higher activity than the first node encountered that represents the true sentinel node, which may be deeper or a few centimeters removed.

Recurrence following sentinel lymph node biopsy alone

Subsequent to the publication of results documenting the identification rate and accuracy of sentinel lymph node biopsy, some centers adopted a selective lymphadenectomy approach as a current practice program for patients with stage I and II disease. In general, patients were offered lymphatic mapping and sentinel node biopsy as treatment for primary melanomas greater than 0.76 or 1mm. This approach was used to provide patients an opportunity to have an earlier therapeutic node dissection or to identify patients eligible for adjuvant therapy programs. The extensive experience at the M. D. Anderson Cancer Center and Moffitt Cancer Center with more than 600 patients undergoing

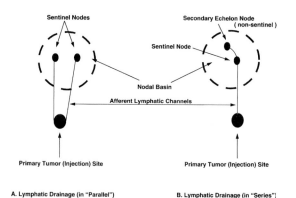

Figure 2. Conceptualized schematic of lymphatic drainage patterns from a primary melanoma site. Two afferent lymphatic channels are depicted in **A**, draining the primary site and leading to two separate sentinel nodes within the regional nodal basin. This type of drainage can be considered in 'parallel' and both nodes identified in the nodal basin are important in terms of staging the nodal basin for the presence or absence of metastases. The lymphatic drainage pattern depicted in **B** shows one channel draining from the injection site followed by identification of the sentinel node in the nodal basin with continued drainage in 'series' to a secondary echelon node. This node may be encountered first upon examining the lymph node basin. The second node in 'series' is a nonsentinel node and will not accurately stage the nodal basin. The hand-held gamma probe ensures that the first node, which is the true sentinel node, will be identified because it will have the highest number of radioactive counts.

lymphatic mapping and a median follow-up of 20 months was recently presented at the 1996 Annual Meeting of the Society of Surgical Oncology [39]. Using multivariate analyses, sentinel lymph node status was found to be the most important prognostic factor influencing disease-free and distant disease-free survival in stage I and II patients when evaluated along with the other known prognostic factors (Table 3).

Those patients who were found to have negative sentinel lymph nodes by routine histologic examination (n = 423) were then followed expectantly with the remaining lymph nodes intact. Twelve patients (2.8%) have subsequently developed nodal disease within a previously mapped lymph node basin as the first site of failure [39]. Three potential mechanisms can be offered to explain these false-negative events: (1) a technical failure — the true sentinel node was not identified; (2) pathologic failure — the appropriate lymph node was removed but routine histologic evaluations failed to unveil microscopic disease; and (3) biologic failure — recurrence in nodal basin secondary to residual microscopic satellites or intransits left behind after wide excision of the primary tumor. Paraffin blocks of the sentinel node previously removed were re-evaluated using serial sectioning as well as immunohistology (HMB-45 and S100). In all but 3 of these 12 patients, microscopic disease was subsequently identified using these more sensitive techniques. In actuality, by excluding those patients who were retrospectively identified to have positive sentinel nodes, the long-term false-negative rate with a median follow-up of 20 months is less than 1%, supporting the contention that lymphatic mapping and sentinel node biopsy accurately identifies the lymph node most likely to contain microscopic disease [39].

A multicenter international selective lymphadenectomy trial is presently actively accruing patients. Stage I and II patients with melanomas thicker than 1 mm are being randomized in a two-to-one fashion to sentinel lymph node biopsy versus wide local excision alone, respectively (Fig. 3). Patients with positive sentinel nodes will undergo a formal lymphadenectomy, and those with a negative sentinel node will have no further lymph node surgery at that time. This trial is designed to address two lymphatic mapping issues: (1) to

Table 3. Prognostic factors influencing distant disease-free survival after lymphatic mapping and SLN biopsy: 600 stage I & II patients

	Univariate p value	Multivariate p value
Age (>50)	n.s.	n.s.
Male gender	n.s.	n.s.
Tumor thickness	<0.001	n.s.
Clark's level >III	<0.001	n.s.
Axial location	<0.01	n.s.
Ulceration	<0.01	n.s.
Sentinel node positive	<0.001	<0.02

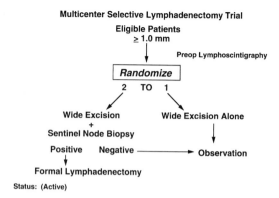

Multicenter Selective Lymphadenectomy Trial

Eligible Patients
≥ 1.0 mm

Preop Lymphoscintigraphy

Randomize

2   TO   1

Wide Excision
+
Sentinel Node Biopsy

Wide Excision Alone

Positive   Negative ───────→ Observation

Formal Lymphadenectomy

Status: (Active)

Figure 3. Treatment algorithm for multicenter selective lymphadenectomy trial. Patients with melanomas thicker than 1 mm are randomized, in a two-to-one fashion, to wide excision plus sentinel node biopsy versus wide excision alone, respectively.

determine whether or not an earlier lymph node dissection for patients with proven occult disease (selective lymphadenectomy) has a survival benefit, and (2) to determine the true failure rate in a previously mapped negative basin assessed in the context of a matched wide-local-excision control group.

Accurate staging

With the recent report of the use of high-dose interferon-alpha as an effective adjuvant after lymphadenectomy for patients with nodal disease, histologic assessment of nodal status for patients with stage I and II disease becomes very important. Therefore, the natural extension of lymphatic mapping and sentinel node biopsy is to provide accurate staging and thus to allow earlier entry into adjuvant therapy trials. Two components are required for accurate staging: (1) accurate localization of the sentinel node and (2) careful histologic evaluation. Routine histologic techniques for evaluating lymph nodes may underestimate disease, mainly because of sampling errors [40]. The combination of serial sectioning and immunostaining improves the detection of microscopic metastases [41–43].

Recent published data reporting on PCR techniques to detect tyrosinase messenger RNA have also increased the detection of microscopic disease [40–44]. The latter technique, molecular staging, requires clinical correlation to prove that patients with lymph nodes negative for metastasis based on routine histology (hematoxylin & eosin staining without serial sectioning) but positive by serial sectioning and immunostaining or PCR for tyrosinase predicts a poorer prognosis. The obvious advantage of PCR analysis is that it potentially allows for complete examination of the entire lymph node and therefore overcomes sampling error problems. A potential drawback is that finding disease at this submicroscopic level may not necessarily be clinically relevant.

Interest in these more sensitive pathologic techniques is growing, particularly in combination with lymphatic mapping and sentinel node biopsy. The combination of the two approaches provides a very attractive marriage of two technological advances. From a logistical and financial standpoint, it is certainly more feasible to apply these special techniques to one or two special nodes rather than to examine all lymph nodes removed within a formal lymphadenectomy specimen. Therefore, it may be more accurate, as well as less costly [45], to stage patients with sentinel node biopsies rather than with ELND.

Limb perfusion

Isolated limb perfusion for the treatment of extremity melanoma was first reported in 1950 [46]. During the past three decades, the perfusion procedure has been modified and refined to the point that this procedure has become routine practice in many oncologic centers. Regional perfusion with or without hyperthermia has been used for all stages of extremity melanoma, ranging from palliative treatment of bulky intransit disease to adjuvant treatment of high-risk primary melanoma patients. Unfortunately, up until recently the efficacy of this treatment has not been determined in controlled studies. Almost 40 years has elapsed since the initial application of perfusion, and the role for this procedure remains poorly defined.

The goal of isolated limb perfusion is to deliver a high concentration of a cytostatic agent to an extremity without systemic side effects. In theory, the effective treatment of either macroscopic or occult intransit disease could prevent the development of distant metastases, in addition to providing durable regional control. Melphalan has been the agent perfused most often worldwide [47]. There has been modest experience with other agents as well, such as dacarbazine (DTIC), cisplatin, actinomycin D, and nitrogen mustard, either in combination or alone, mainly because melphalan was not available for use in this setting in the United States for much of the past decade because controlled phase I toxicity studies had not previously been carried out.

A review of several studies using limb perfusion suggests that the response of melanoma to melphalan is substantial and provides useful palliation in the treatment of multiple intransit metastasis and locally recurrent disease; a melphalan perfusion is considered the treatment of choice in this situation, especially when the alternative surgical therapy is amputation [46–53]. More recently, a perfusion regimen of TNF and interferon gamma in combination with melphalan was reported to achieve a complete response in 90% and at least a partial response in 100% of patients treated for measurable extremity recurrences [5,6]. This magnitude of response initially reported by a group in Switzerland and subsequently confirmed in the Netherlands rekindled interest in perfusion in the United States [5,6]. These results have prompted the National Cancer Institute to embark on a multi-institutional trial to compare melphalan alone versus the above-described three-drug regimen in a prospective phase III clinical setting (Fig. 4). This is an actively accruing study that will address overall and durability of response and comparative toxicities of the regimens.

The more controversial issue is determining what role this procedure plays in the management of patients with clinically localized melanoma who are at high risk for recurrence following surgery. As with the debate centered around the role for elective lymph node dissection, similar questions arise: Can isolated limb perfusion eliminate microscopic metastatic cells trapped in dermal lymphatic not removed by surgery alone? Does this prevent locoregional recurrences and improve survival?

Several retrospective studies have included patients with clinically localized disease who were treated with perfusion on an adjuvant basis [54–58,60]. Literature or historical surgery-alone controls were used for comparison and did not fully take into account the influence of all possible prognostic factors. Although modest increases in survival were reported (84–96% 5-year survival with perfusion, compared with 60–94% 5-year survival with surgery-alone controls), the nature of the study designs limits the interpretation of the results. A modest number of studies have been carried out, however, that have targeted the presumed appropriate high-risk patient group, patients with clinically localized disease with more than 1.5-mm thick lesions (stage II). All of these studies were retrospective in nature, except the one by Ghussen et al. [59], which was prospective and randomized.

A retrospective study by Martijn et al. [60] compared the efficacy of wide local excision combined with regional perfusion performed entirely at one center (Groningen) with matched controls who received local excision only at a different center (Sidney). The study did show a significant disease-free and overall 10-year survival benefit and significantly fewer locoregional recurrences for the perfusion group. However, only a sufficient number of female

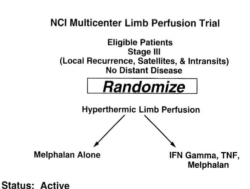

Figure 4. Treatment algorithm in patient eligibility for NCI multicenter limb perfusion trial. Patients are randomized to melphalan alone versus triple-drug therapy with melphalan plus interferon-gamma and tumor necrosis factor.

14

patients having tumors in the lower extremity were available to participate in the study. A later retrospective analysis compared a large group of patients treated with perfusion, again at the Groningen center, with matched groups of patient from five hospitals in the Netherlands and bordering areas of West Germany [61]. This study failed to show a benefit with perfusion in terms of limb recurrence, time to regional node metastasis, time to distant metastasis, or disease-free and overall survival.

A study by Edwards et al. [62] from the M. D. Anderson Cancer Center compared the adjuvant use of DTIC with melphalan (L-PAM). One hundred patients comprising each treatment group had primary tumor thickness greater than 1.5 mm. No patients underwent regional lymphadenectomy in conjunction with the perfusion. The patients treated with L-PAM had significantly fewer local and intransit recurrence at 2-year follow-up than the DTIC-treated group (4% vs. 12%). The recurrence rate in the DTIC-treated group approximates the expected incidence of local and intransit recurrences of patients with similar-thickness tumors and no adjuvant therapy. Interestingly, the recurrence rates in the regional nodal basins did not differ between the two treatment groups.

A prospective randomized trial comparing perfusion with surgery alone was published by Ghussen et al. [59] in 1988 and included stage II and III patients with high-risk primaries. All patients received regional node dissection, whether or not they were perfused. The method of perfusion implemented modifications that were identified to be beneficial in preclinical animal studies [63,64]. Of the patients who presented with clinically localized disease, the perfused group fared better in terms of 5-year disease-free survival (>90% vs. 60%) [59]. The overall survival data revealed a barely significant benefit for the entire perfused group but did not report overall survival data separately for the patients with clinically localized disease. The study is provocative but limited by its small numbers.

This experience, however, ultimately led to a large multi-institutional study conducted through a combined effort of the EORTC and the WHO that accrued nearly 800 stage II patients (>1.5 mm) to receive melphalan perfusion in addition to wide excision of the primary, versus wide excision alone (Fig. 5). The main endpoints were time to regional and distant failure. Interim analysis has failed to demonstrate any survival benefit. Although this is a well-designed trial, the patient population is probably overly inclusive, and any benefit afforded to the small minority of a highest risk subset could easily be obscured. The clinical entity of local recurrence and or in-transit disease as the first site of failure probably only represents 10% of the patient cohort. This differs from the issues concerning ELND, in which 40% of patients with intermediate-thickness primaries will develop nodal disease [14]. Therefore, the most recent randomized ELND trial targetted the appropriate patient population, while most efforts of the EORTC/WHO may not have.

The population most likely to benefit from 'adjuvant' perfusion is the subset with resectable local, satellite, or in-transit recurrences. This group clearly

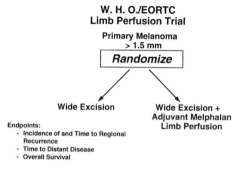

W. H. O./EORTC
Limb Perfusion Trial

Primary Melanoma
> 1.5 mm

Randomize

Wide Excision

Wide Excision +
Adjuvant Melphalan
Limb Perfusion

Endpoints:
- Incidence of and Time to Regional
  Recurrence
- Time to Distant Disease
- Overall Survival

Status: (Completed)

Figure 5. Treatment algorithm for combined WHO/EORTC limb perfusion trial for patients with higher risk primary melanomas.

harbors intralymphatic disease, which could lead to additional regional and subsequent distant failure. Results of a small randomized trial published by the Swedish Melanoma Study Group addressed this particular subset [65]. Patients were randomized to receive surgical excision of extremity recurrences alone versus excision plus melphalan perfusion. An improvement in tumor-free survival was attributed mainly to a decrease in locoregional failure after perfusion. The overall survival trended towards an improvement for the perfused patients [65]. Unfortunately, the sample size was small.

In summary, isolated limb perfusion is effective in reducing the incidence of in-transit disease in patients who are at a higher risk of developing regional recurrence. Few studies suggest that perfusion performed adjuvantly in the same patient populations may provide enhanced survival rates. At the present time, however, the routine use of adjuvant isolated hyperthermic perfusion for primary stage II patients (>1.5 mm) is not standard therapy and should only be employed as part of a clinical trial.

Adjuvant therapy for high-risk patients

Subsets of patients have been clearly defined as being high risk for distant failure following surgical resection of all measurable disease and, therefore, excellent candidates for adjuvant approaches. These subsets include patients with thick primary tumors (>4mm), nodal metastases, local recurrences, isolated in-transit disease satellites, and following resection of isolated distant metastases (stage IV no evidence of disease [NED]). Historically, we have been relatively unsuccessful in identifying a systemic regimen that could have an impact on reducing the risk for distant failure and therefore improving survival. Until recently there has been no adjuvant therapy sanctioned for the above-mentioned high-risk groups. The ECOG trial #1684, recently published by Kirkwood et al., is the first step in establishing an effective adjuvant approach for patients with melanoma [7]. This trial was a prospective random-ized evaluation of high-dose interferon for 1 year following surgery versus surgical resection alone for patients with synchronous or metachronous nodal metastases and high-risk primaries (T4 lesions) [7] (Fig. 6). The vast majority of the cohort were those with nodal metastases. A modest but statistically significant improvement in survival was obtained for the entire group who received interferon [7]. A subset analysis of those patients with nodal disease alone demonstrates an even stronger benefit with interferon. The small group of patients (n = 31) with T4 lesions did not show a benefit with interferon, but this group is too small to derive any conclusions.

The high-dose regimen includes a 1-month induction period administered intravenously at 20 million U/m^2 5 days a week. Subsequent to the induction, a maintenance high dose is administered 3 times a week subcutaneously at a dose of 10 million U/m^2. The survival benefits using this approach are clearly not without cost in terms of toxicity. Twenty-five percent of the patients who received interferon discontinued therapy because of adverse effects. The ma-jority of these patients withdrew from the study during the induction phase, and the remaining patients discontinued in the early portion of the mainte-nance period. Therefore, some evidence of tachyphylaxis occurred because very few patients discontinued therapy after 5 months into the regimen. Of the patients who did complete the regimen, >65% of the patients received >80% of the prescribed dose [7]. Therefore, significant numbers of patients under-went dose reduction during the therapy. Careful monitoring and appropriate dose reduction is critical to administer this therapy safely. Two patients died from hepatic toxicity early on because close monitoring of liver function was not initially mandated. Fever and chills are the most common side effects on a short-term basis, but chronic fatigue is the major obstacle for these patients [7].

It is not unreasonable to extrapolate this survival benefit to other high-risk groups [66]. In particular, those patients with resectable local recurrences,

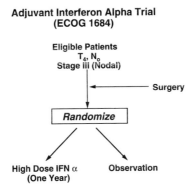

Figure 6. Treatment algorithm for completed adjuvant interferon trial — ECOG 1684.

intransits, and satellites could potentially benefit from this adjuvant therapy [66]. It is unlikely that enough patients in these particular subsets would ever be accrued in a subsequent study to address this issue specifically. Therefore, in the absence of a clinical trial, it is not unreasonable to treat these patients with adjuvant interferon for a year as prescribed by the ECOG group. A follow-up three-arm randomization study (ECOG 1690), addressing the same patient population as ECOG 1684, of high-dose interferon for 1 year versus low-dose interferon (3 million U three times a week) for 2 years versus surgery alone was completed in June 1995. This trial was performed to confirm the results of the initial study and to determine if the less toxic low-dose regimen was as effective as the high-dose regimen (Fig. 7).

Although the data on the high-dose interferon regimen are promising, this represents only the first in a series of advances yet to come in adjuvant therapy. Clinical trials are already planned for the near future to examine other therapies that may be as effective as interferon but less toxic. In addition, combination regimens may improve survival benefits over interferon alone. The next clinical trial sponsored by the ECOG group is set to examine the efficacy of a ganglioside vaccine (GM2) versus high-dose interferon (Fig. 8). The basis for this comparison was established by a relatively small prospective randomized trial at Memorial Sloan Kettering, directed by Phil Livingston [67]. This trial included 120 patients randomized to receive surgery alone versus surgery plus ganglioside vaccine. The patients who were eligible were primarily stage III patients, predominately with nodal metastasis, as well as some patients with resectable intransit disease. All patients were treated in an adjuvant setting. Overall, no significant survival difference was observed for the group as a whole, but a subset of patients who initially tested negative for the presence of antibodies to ganglioside received a benefit with ganglioside therapy compared with surgery alone [67]. Although this subset was not pro-

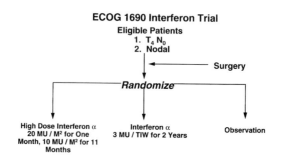

Figure 7. Treatment algorithm for follow-up prospective randomized interferon trial (ECOG 1690). High-dose interferon versus low-dose interferon versus observation alone for patients with thick primaries and nodal metastases.

18

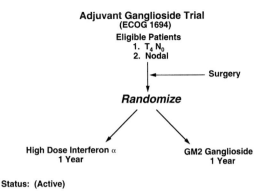

Adjuvant Ganglioside Trial
(ECOG 1694)
Eligible Patients
1. $T_4 N_0$
2. Nodal

Surgery

Randomize

High Dose Interferon α
1 Year

GM2 Ganglioside
1 Year

Status: (Active)

Figure 8. Treatment algorithm for adjuvant ganglioside trial. Randomization of high-dose interferon versus ganglioside vaccine.

spectively stratified, it did represent the bulk of the patients entered into the trial and provided some very interesting data.

Other similarly nontoxic approaches using vaccination have been spearheaded by Don Morton at the John Wayne Cancer Center [68]. Their allogeneic melanoma cell vaccine has shown some activity in patients with measurable stage IV disease and compelling survival data in patients following resection of distant metastases. Compared with historical controls, the patients who received vaccination have improved survival times [68]. There is a growing interests in examining this vaccine preparation in a prospective randomized setting in the following subsets of patients: (1) stage IV NED patients following resection of distant metastases and (2) in an adjuvant setting for stage III patients as well as for high-risk stage II patients.

At the M. D. Anderson Cancer Center significant interest has been cultivated in evaluating the efficacy of combination chemotherapy with biologic therapy. These regimens, termed *biochemotherapy*, have been examined extensively in patients with measurable stage IV disease. The highest response rates reported in the literature have been achieved with such combinations that include platinum-based regimens with IL-2 and alpha interferon. The specific regimen used at M. D. Anderson is the combination of cisplatin, vinblastine, and DTIC along with IL-2 and alpha interferon. The combination biochemotherapy is given on days 1–4, as is IL-2. The alpha-interferon is given daily on days 1–5. A complete cycle of biochemotherapy is thus completed in 5 days of hospitalization.

Because of the impressive response rates with stage IV patients, on the order of 60–70% [69], a phase II trial in patients with measurable local regional recurrences (stage III) was also completed at the M. D. Anderson Cancer Center, with the hope of eventually bringing these approaches into an adjuvant setting. Response rates of 50% were achieved, with 25% of the patients receiving either a complete or near-complete pathologic response [70]. In this phase II study, which included 65 patients and accrued over an 18-

month period, all but one of the patients completed all planned cycles of therapy. The treatment algorithm includes two cycles of therapy followed by assessment of the responses. If at least a minor response was achieved with the initial two cycles, the patients received two more cycles prior to surgery. A phase II adjuvant trial has now been initiated comparing 1 year of high-dose interferon with four cycles of adjuvant biochemotherapy for patients following lymphadenectomy (Fig. 9). Patients will be rerandomized within the interferon randomization to receive high-dose interferon as prescribed by ECOG versus the same high maintenance dose for 12 months, excluding the 1-month IV induction period. This protocol has the potential to answer two very important questions: (1) Is interferon or biochemotherapy more effective? (2) What is the importance of the induction phase in the high-dose interferon regimen?

Interest has also been generated in identifying a relatively nontoxic adjuvant therapy for intermediate-risk stage II patients (1.5–4.0 mm). A randomized trial of an allogeneic melanoma lysate vaccine versus surgery alone has recently been completed by the Southwestern Oncology Group (SWOG). Using the technique of lymphatic mapping and sentinel node biopsy, we can now more accurately identify the node-positive and -negative patients and assign more homogenous groups of patients in future adjuvant trials.

Surgical recommendations by stage

The results of completed prospective randomized trials, as well as ongoing trials, have significantly impacted the management of patients with melanoma. The following sections summarize the clinical management recommendations by stage (Tables 4 and 5).

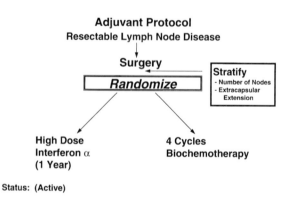

Figure 9. M.D. Anderson adjuvant protocol for patients with resectable lymph node metastases. Randomization is high-dose interferon for 1 year versus four cycles of biochemotherapy. Patients randomized to interferon will be rerandomized to interferon regimen with and without the 1-month induction period.

20

Table 4. Randomized clinical trials influencing management — stage I & II

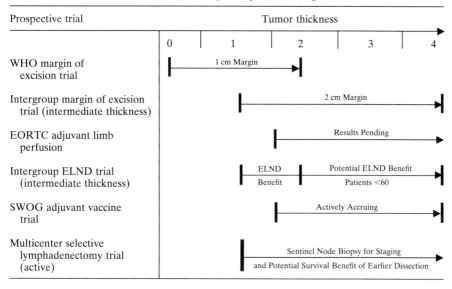

Prospective trial	Tumor thickness				
	0	1	2	3	4
WHO margin of excision trial		1 cm Margin			
Intergroup margin of excision trial (intermediate thickness)			2 cm Margin		
EORTC adjuvant limb perfusion			Results Pending		
Intergroup ELND trial (intermediate thickness)		ELND Benefit	Potential ELND Benefit Patients <60		
SWOG adjuvant vaccine trial			Actively Accruing		
Multicenter selective lymphadenectomy trial (active)			Sentinel Node Biopsy for Staging and Potential Survival Benefit of Earlier Dissection		

Table 5. Randomized clinical trials influencing management — stage III

Prospective trial	Nodal	Satellites/Intransits
ECOG #1684	Benefit with high-dose interferon for 1 yr	Consider interferon after surgical excision
ECOG #1690 (complete)	Results expected in fall 1998	
ECOG #1694 (active)	High-dose interferon vs. ganglioside vaccine	
M.D. Anderson adjuvant (active)	High-dose interferon vs. biochemotherapy	
Swedish Melanoma Study Group perfusion trial		Improved tumor-free survival with perfusion after excision of extremity recurrences
NCI Multicenter Limb Perfusion Trial (active)		Melphalan vs. melphalan + TNF

Stages I and II.

(1) ≤1 mm thickness primaries; 1 cm wide excision is the standard of care for these patients. The presence of Clark's level IV or ulceration within this tumor-thickness range predicts a higher risk for recurrence. Therefore, this particular subset of patients with thin melanomas should be considered for lymphatic mapping and sentinel node biopsy for staging of the nodal basin. (2) 1–4 mm in thickness; 2 cm margin of excision is the standard of care. Most of

these patients, especially with lesions on the trunk or the proximal extremity, can undergo a primary closure without difficulty. Those lesions on the head-and-neck region or the distal extremity may require closure with local flaps, advancement flaps, or skin grafts. These patients are also eligible for lymphatic mapping and sentinel node biopsy for staging purposes, and are also eligible for the Multicenter Selective Lymphadenectomy Trial (MSLT). (3) >4mm: At least a 2 cm margin of excision is required. These patients may also be eligible for sentinel lymph node biopsy for staging purposes. This would allow a more accurate stratification into postoperative adjuvant therapy trials. At the present time, the $T_4 N_0$ patients should probably not receive adjuvant interferon outside of a clinical protocol. These patients are excellent candidates for future adjuvant trials. The T_4 node-positive patients can receive an adjuvant interferon-off protocol as the standard of care but are also excellent candidates for future adjuvant trials in an attempt to identify more effective, and possibly less toxic, approaches.

Stage III.

(1) Patients who develop nodal disease require formal and complete lymphadenectomies in the involved nodal basin as standard surgical care. This includes all levels of the axillary region as well as superficial inguinal dissection and selective use of deep inguinal and iliac node dissections. Following surgical resection, all these patients should be considered for adjuvant approaches and a concentrated effort should be made to place these patients on phase III trials. In addition, those patients with bulky nodal disease with extracapsular extension or multiple nodes involved should be considered for adjuvant radiation therapy to the resected basin to help decrease local recurrence in the surgical field [71,72]. (2) Local recurrence/satellites/intransits: Those patients with locally advanced recurrences in the extremity are eligible for the NCI randomized isolated hypothermic limb perfusion trials, examining the efficacy of tumor necrosis factor added to melphalan. In the absence of access to a center participating in this trial, melphalan alone as the standard of care would be an appropriate alternative.

Those patients with isolated and limited in-transit disease in the extremity can undergo resection of measurable disease and be offered adjuvant interferon off protocol or other adjuvant therapies, such as vaccine, as well as 'adjuvant' perfusion.

Stage IV.

All of these patients are best treated with systemic therapies. There are subsets of patients who have resectable distant disease, either in soft tissue sites or visceral sites, who could benefit from surgical resection in a palliative or expectant palliation setting. Patients with symptomatic brain or gastrointestinal metastases are excellent candidates for surgical resection. After rendering these patients NED, consideration of adjuvant approaches is a reasonable next step.

The surgeon's role in the management of melanoma patients with different stages of diseases is of paramount importance. Surgical resection is the mainstay of therapy for patients with disease stages I–III. In addition, now that some adjuvant approaches have been proven to be effective, the roles of the surgeon have expanded to accurate staging for the earlier stage patients. It is critical that surgeons maintain their primary role in the care of these patients to accomplish cure when possible, local control for the more advanced-stage patients, and palliation when needed.

Conclusions

Prospective randomized trials over the last 5–10 years have provided the cornerstone for advances in the treatment of patients with all stages of melanoma. Appropriate margins of excision tailored to tumor thickness have been established. The role of elective node dissection in certain subsets of patients with earlier stage melanoma has been appropriately and definitively addressed in a prospective randomized setting. The lack of efficacy of adjuvant perfusion has been demonstrated in a large prospective randomized trial and, therefore, is now excluded in the management of patients with extremity primaries.

The ongoing multicenter sentinel lymph node trial is addressing critical issues related to lymphatic mapping and sentinel node biopsy. High-dose interferon alpha given adjuvantly to patients with nodal disease has now been established as the standard of care based on the results of a prospective randomized trial. Other trials are planned to help identify additional effective adjuvants that have less toxicity. The combination of surgery plus systemic therapy for patients with resectable stage IV disease is going to be tested in a multicenter fashion to help better define treatment options for patients with stage IV disease. The next 10 years are going to be a very exciting time for surgeons interested in melanoma. Surgeons should be familiar with the subsets of patients eligible for adjuvant studies and mindful of the systemic therapies available. In addition, they should participate in the design of future adjuvant trials and make sure that the surgical approaches are appropriate for the stage of disease so that their patients can be best positioned to receive benefit from these systemic therapies.

References

1. Morton DL, Wen DR, Wong JH, Economou JS, Cagel LA, Storm KS, Foshag LJ, Cochran AJ. Technical details of intraoperative lymphatic mapping for early stage melanoma. Arch Surg 127:392–399, 1992.

2. Morton DL, Wen DR, Cochran AJ. Management of early-stage melanoma by intraoperative lymphatic mapping and selective lymphadenectomy or 'watch and wait.' Surg Oncol Clin North Am 1:247–259, 1992.
3. Ross M, Reintgen DS, Balch C. Selective lymphadenectomy: Emerging role of lymphatic mapping and sentinel node biopsy in the management of early stage melanoma. Semin Surg Oncol 9:219–223, 1993.
4. Reintgen DS, Cruse CW, Berman C, Ross M, Rapaport D, Glass F, Fenske N, Messina J. An orderly progression of melanoma nodal metastases. Ann Surg 220:759–767, 1994.
5. Lienard D, Ewalenko P, Delmotte JJ, et al. High-dose recombinant tumor necrosis factor alpha in combination with interferon gamma and melphalan in isolation perfusion of the limbs for melanoma and sarcoma. J Clin Oncol 10:52–60, 1992.
6. Lejeune F, Lienard D, Eggermont A, Schnaffordt Goops H, Rosen F, Gerain J, Klaase J, Kroon B, Vandervekaw J, Schmitz P. Administration of high-dose tumor necrosis factor alpha by isolation perfusion of the limbs: Rationale and results. J Infusion Chemother 5:73–81, 1995.
7. Kirkwood JM, Strawderman MH, Ernstoff MS, Smith TJ, Borden EC, Blum RH. Adjuvant therapy of high-risk resected cutaneous melanoma: The Eastern Cooperative Oncology Group Trials EST 1684. J Clin Oncol, 1996.
8. Parker SL, Tong T, Bolden S, Wingo PA. Cancer statistics 1996. CA Cancer J Clin 46:5–25, 1996.
9. Grin CS, Riegel DS, Friedman FJ. Worldwide incidence of malignant melanoma. In Balch CM et al. (eds). Cutaneous Melanoma. Philadelphia: JB Lippincott, 1992.
10. Balch CM, Murad TM, Soong SJ, et al. Tumor thickness as a guide to surgical management of clinical stage I melanoma patients. Cancer 43:883–888, 1979.
11. Veronesi U, Cascinelli N. Narrow excision (1 cm margin): A safe procedure for thin cutaneous melanoma. Arch Surg 126:438–441, 1991.
12. Balch CM, Urist MM, Karakousis CP, Smith TJ, Temple WJ, Drzewiecki K, Jewell WR, Bartolucci AA, Mihm MC, Jr., Barnhill R, Wanebo HJ. Efficacy of 2-cm surgical margins for intermediate thickness melanomas (1–4 mm). Ann Surg 218:262–268, 1993.
13. Balch CM, Cascinelli N, Milton GW, et al. Elective node dissection: Pros and cons. In Balch CM, Milton GW (eds). Cutaneous Melanoma: Clinical Management and Treatment Results Worldwide. Philadelphia: JB Lippincott, 1985, pp 131–158.
14. Balch CM. The role of elective lymph node dissection in melanoma: Rationale, results and controversies. J Clin Oncol 6:163–172, 1988.
15. Reintgen DS, Cox EB, McCarty KM, Jr., et al. Efficacy of elective lymph node dissection in patients with intermediate thickness primary melanoma. Ann Surg 198:379–384, 1983.
16. Wanebo HJ, Woodruff J, Fortner JG. Malignant melanoma of the extremities: A clinico-pathologic study using levels of invasion (microstage). Cancer 35:666–676, 1975.
17. Elder DE, DuPont G, Van Horn M, et al. The role of lymph node dissection for clinical stage I malignant melanoma of intermediate thickness (1.51–3.99 mm). Cancer 56:413–418, 1985.
18. Drepper H, Kohler CO, Bastian B, Breuninger H, Brocker EB, Gohl J, Groth W, Hermanek P, Hohenberger W, Lippold A, Kolmel K, Landthaler M, Peters A, Tilgen W. Benefit of elective lymph node dissection in subgroups of melanoma patients. Cancer 3:741–749, 1993.
19. Rompel R, Garbe C, Buttner P, Teichelmann K, Petres J. Elective lymph node dissection in primary malignant melanoma: A matched-pair analysis. Melanoma Res 5:189–194, 1995.
20. Coates AS, Ingvar CI, Petersen-Schaefer K, Shaw HM, Milton GW, O'Brien CJ, Thompson JF, McCarthy WH. Elective lymph node dissection in patients with primary melanoma of the trunk and limbs treated at the Sydney Melanoma Unit from 1960–1991. J Am Colle Surg 180:402–409, 1995.
21. Slingluff CL, Stidham KR, Ricci WM, Stanley WE, Seigler HF. Surgical management of regional lymph nodes in patients with melanoma: Experience with 4682 patients. Ann Surg 219:120–130, 1994.
22. McCarthy WH, Shaw HM, Milton GW. Efficacy of elective lymph node dissection in 2347 patients with clinical stage I malignant melanoma. Surg Gynecol Obstet 161:575–580, 1985.
23. Milton GW, Shaw HM, McCarthy WH, et al. Prophylactic lymph node dissection in clinical

stage I cutaneous malignant melanoma: Results of surgical treatment in 1319 patients. Br J Surg 69:108–111, 1982.

24. Balch CM, Soong S-J, Milton GW, et al. A comparison of prognostic factors and surgical results in 1786 patients with localized (stage I) melanoma treated in Alabama, USA, and New South Wales, Australia. Ann Surg 196:677, 1982.

25. Veronesi U, Adamus J, Bandiera DC, et al. Inefficacy of immediate node dissection in stage I melanoma of the limbs. N Engl J Med 297:627–630, 1977.

26. Balch CM, Houghton AN, Milton GW, et al. (eds). Elective lymph node dissection: Pros and cons. Cutaneous Melanoma. Philadelphia: JB Lippincott, 1992, p 362.

27. Sin FH, Taylor WF, Pritchard DJ, et al. Lymphadenectomy in the management of stage I malignant melanoma: A prospective randomized study. Mayo Clin Proc 61:697–705, 1986.

28. Balch C, et al. A prospective randomized trial of 742 melanoma patients Comparing the efficacy of elective node dissection (immediate) versus observation (abstr). Am Acad Surg 1996.

29. Thompson JF, McCarthy WH, Bosch CMJ, O'Brien CJ, Quinn MJ, Paramaesvaran S, Crotty K, McCarthy SW, Uren RF, Howman-Giles R. Sentinel lymph node status as an indicator of the presence of metastatic melanoma in regional lymph nodes. Melanoma Res 5:255–260, 1995.

30. Sappey MPC. Injection, Preparationet Conservation Des Vaisseaux Lymphatique. These Pour Le Doctorat En Medecine, No. 241. Paris: Rignoux Imprimeur De La Factulte De Medecine, 1843.

31. Normal J, Cruse CW, Wells K, Berman C, Clark R, Reintgen DS. A redefinition of skin lymphatic drainage by lymphoscintigraphy for malignant melanoma. Am J Surg 162:432–437, 1991.

32. Meyer CM, Lecklitner ML, Logie JR, Balch C, Bessey PQ, Tauxe WN. Technetium-99m sulfur-colloid cutaneous lymphoscintigraphy in the management of truncal melanoma. Radiology 131:205–209, 1979.

33. Pijpers R, Collet GJ, Meijer S, Hoekstra OS. The impact of dynamic lymphoscintigraphy and gamma probe guidance on sentinel node biopsy in melanoma. Eur J Nucl Med 22:1238–1241, 1995.

34. Uren RF, Howman-Giles R, Thompson JF, Shaw HM, Quinn MJ, O'Brien CJ, McCarthy WH. Lymphoscintigraphy to identify sentinel lymph nodes in patients with melanoma. Melanoma Res 4:395–399, 1994.

35. Hung JC, Wiseman GA, Wahner HW, Mulla BP, Taggart TR, Dunn W. Filtered technetium-99m-sulfur colloid evaluated for lymphoscintigraphy. J Nucl Med 36:1895–1900, 1995.

36. Alex JC, Krag DN. Gamma-probe guided localization of lymph nodes. Surg Oncol 2:137–143, 1993.

37. Krag DN, Meijer SJ, Weaver DL, et al. Minimal-access surgery for staging of melanoma. Arch Surg 130:654–660, 1995.

38. Albertini JJ, Cruse CW, Rapaport D, Wells K, Ross MI, DeConti R, Berman CG, Jared K, Messina J, Lyman G, Glass F, Fenske N, Reintgen D. Intraoperative radiolymphoscintigraphy improves sentinel lymph node identification for patients with melanoma. Ann Surg ••.

39. Gershenwald J, Thompson W, Mansfield P, Lee J, Colome M, Balch C, Reintgen D, Ross M. Patterns of failure in melanoma patients after successful lymphatic mapping and negative sentinel node biopsy (abstr). Soc Surg Oncol, 1996.

40. Reintgen DS, Albertini J, Berman, et al. Accurate nodal staging of malignant melanoma. Cancer Control J Moffitt Cancer Center 2:405–414, 1995.

41. Robert MR, Wen DR, Cochran AJ. Pathological evaluation of the regional lymph nodes in malignant melanoma. Semin Diagnost Pathol 10:102–115, 1993.

42. Lane N, Lattes R, Malm J. Clinicopathological correlations in a series of 117 malignant melanomas of the skin of adults. Cancer 11:1025–1043, 1958.

43. Das Gupta TK. Results of treatment of 269 patients with primary cutaneous melanoma: a five-year prospective study. Ann Surg 186:201–209, 1977.

44. Wang X, Heller R, VanVoorhis N, et al. Detection of submicroscopic metastases with

polymerase chain reaction in patients with malignant melanoma. Ann Surg 220:768–774, 1994.

45. Reintgen DS, Einstein A. The role of research in cost containment. Cancer Control J Moffitt Cancer Center 2:429–431, 1995.

46. Krementz ET, Ryan RF. Chemotherapy of melanoma of the extremities by perfusion: Fourteen years of clinical experience. Ann Surg 175:900–917, 1972.

47. Cumberlin R, DeMoss E, Lassus M, et al. Isolation perfusion for malignant melanoma of the extremity: A review. J Clin Oncol 3:1022–1031, 1985.

48. Ryan RF. Chemotherapy perfusion techniques and problems. Surg Clin North Am 42:389–402, 1962.

49. Stehlin JS, Clark RL, Vickers WE, et al. Perfusion for malignant melanoma of the extremities. Am J Surg 105:607–614, 1963.

50. Bulman AS, Jamieson CW. Isolated limb perfusion with melphalan in the treatment of malignant melanoma. Br J Surg 67:660–662, 1980.

51. Rosin RD, Westburg G. Isolated limb perfusion for malignant melanoma. Practitioner 224:1031–1036, 1980.

52. Hafstrom L, Jonsson PE. Hyperthermia perfusion of recurrent malignant melanoma of the extremities. Acta Chir Scand 146:313–318, 1980.

53. Stehlin JS. Hyperthermic perfusion with chemotherapy for cancers of the extremity. Surg Gynecol Obstet 129:305–308, 1969.

54. Stehlin JS, Clark RL. Melanoma of the Extremities. Am J Surg 110:366–383, 1965.

55. Bulrnan AS, Jamieson CW. Isolated limb perfusion with melphalan in the treatment of malignant melanoma. Br J Surg 67:660–662, 1980.

56. Stehlin JS, Giovanelli BC, de Ipolyi PD, et al. Results of hyperthermic perfusion for melanoma of the extremities. Surg Gynecol Obstet 140:339–348, 1975.

57. Golomb FM, Bromberg J, Dubin N. A controlled study of the survival experience of patients with primary malignant melanoma of the distal extremities treated with adjuvant perfusion chemotherapy for stage I malignant melanoma of the extremity with literature review. Cancer 2:519–526, 1979.

58. Martijn H, Oldhoff J, Oesterhuis JW, et al. Indications for elective groin dissection in clinical stage I patients with malignant melanoma of the lower extremity treated by hyperthermic regional perfusion. Cancer 52:1526–1534, 1983.

59. Ghussen F, Kruger I, Groth W, et al. The role of regional hyperthermic cytostatic perfusion in the treatment of extremity melanoma. Cancer 6:654–659, 1988.

60. Martijn H, Koops HS, Milton GW, et al. Comparison of two methods of treating primary malignant melanomas Clark IV and V, thickness 1.5 mm and greater, localized on the extremities: Wide surgical excision with and without adjuvant regional perfusion. Cancer 57:1923–1930, 1986.

61. Franklin HR, Koops HS, Oldhoff J, et al. To perfuse or not to perfuse? A retrospective comparative study to evaluate the effect of adjuvant isolated regional perfusion in patients with stage I extremity melanoma with a thickness of 1.5 mm or greater. J Clin Oncol 6:701–708, 1988.

62. Edwards MJ, Boddie AW, Ames FC, et al. Isolated limb perfusion for stage I melanoma of the extremity: A comparison of mephalan and dacarbazine (DTTC). South Med J 82:985–989, 1989.

63. Ghussen F, Nagel K, Groth W, et al. A prospective randomized study of regional extremity perfusion in patients with malignant melanoma. Ann Surg 200:764–768, 1984.

64. Ghussen F, Isselford W. The limit of hyperthermic strain on skeletal muscle tissue during regional perfusion. Res Exp Med (Berl) 184:115–121, 1984.

65. Hafstrom L, Rudenstam C, Blomquist E, et al. Regional hyperthermic perfusion with melphalan after surgery for recurrent malignant melanoma. J Clin Oncol 9:2091–2094, 1991.

66. Balch CM, Buzaid AC. Finally a successful adjuvant therapy for high-risk melanoma [editorial]. J Clin Oncol 14:1–3, 1996.

67. Livingston PO, Wong GY, Adluri S, et al. Improved survival in stage III melanoma patients

with GN2 antibodies: A randomized trial of adjuvant vaccination with GM2 ganglioside. J Clin Oncol 12:1036–1044, 1994.

68. Morton DL, Foshag LJ, Moon DSB, Nizzie JF, Wanek LA, Chang C, Davtyan DG, Gupta RK, Elashoff R, Irie RF. Prolongation of survival in metastatic melanoma after active specific immunotherapy with a new polyvalent melanoma vaccine. Ann Surg 216:463–481, 1992.

69. Buzaid AC, Legha SS. Combination of chemotherapy with interleukin-2 and interferon-alfa for the treatment of advanced melanoma. Semin Oncol 21(Suppl 14):23–28, 1994.

70. Buzaid AC, Legha S, Bedikian A, Eton O, Papadopoulos N, Plager C, Ross M, Lee J, Mansfield PF, Strom E, Ring S, Rice J, Colome M, Benjamin R. Neoadjuvant biochemo-therapy in melanoma patients (PTS) with local regional metastases (LRM) (abstr). Proceed Am Soc Clin Oncol 15:1347, 1996.

71. Strom EA, Ross MI. Adjuvant radiation therapy after axillary lymphadenectomy for meta-static melanoma: Toxicity and local control. Ann Surg Oncol 2:455–449, 1995.

72. Ang KK, Peters LJ, Weber RS, Morrison WH, Frankenthaller RA, Garden AS, Geopfert H, Ha CS, Byers RM. Post-operative radiotherapy for cutaneous melanoma of the head and neck region. Int J Radiat Oncol Biol Physics 30:795–798, 1994.

2. Advances in rectal cancer treatment

John M. Skibber

Introduction

Attempts at improving our management of rectal cancer engender controversies. Advances are being made in parallel with the themes seen in much of modern solid tumor management. These are the optimization of patient outcomes by (1) a detailed understanding of the pathology of rectal cancer and its relation to surgical techniques; (2) multidisciplinary management; (3) organ and function conservation; and (4) analysis of outcomes based on quality of life as well as morbidity, recurrence, and survival; and (5) treatment selection based on biologic factors. These principles are being applied in the management of patients with all stages of rectal cancer. Selection of the best route to accomplish these goals is guided by the extent of disease at presentation. Advances in management involve both clinical and translational research issues.

Goals in the treatment of rectal carcinoma are local control of disease and cure, with maintenance of an acceptable quality of life. The biology of a particular patient's tumor is the most important factor in overall outcome. Adequate surgical removal of the tumor is the major treatment factor affecting local control and cure. The adequacy of the surgical removal of the tumor and overall outcome can be impacted by the use of adjuvant radiation and chemotherapy. The principles of the surgical management of rectal cancer are (1) removal of the primary tumor with adequate margins of normal tissue, (2) treatment of the draining lymphatics, and (3) restoration of function. Appropriate adjuvant therapies can enhance local control, reduce systemic recurrence, and increase organ preservation.

Clinical management issues

Our report will focus on the management advances and controversies at each stage of resectable rectal cancer. We describe the management controversies and advances in early localized rectal cancer and resectable locoregional disease. Scientific advances that are important pathways for future translational research are presented.

Raphael E. Pollock (ed.), SURGICAL ONCOLOGY. Copyright © 1997. Kluwer Academic Publishers. ISBN 0-7923-9900-5. All rights reserved.

Accomplishing the goals of rectal cancer management is easier for upper and middle rectal cancers than for low rectal cancers. In patients with low rectal cancer, abdominoperineal resection (APR) has been the gold standard of management. However, APR requires a permanent colostomy, which adversely affects the patient's quality of life. Advances in rectal cancer management and surgical techniques have improved our ability to achieve oncologic control and optimal patient function without APR, even in patients with low rectal cancers.

Local excision for rectal cancer

Full-thickness local excision is effective in the treatment of selected early low rectal cancers. Local excision is used as curative therapy for patients who have superficial tumors, and it is also used as alternative therapy in medically compromised patients and in those who refuse standard therapy.

The choice of technique for local excision is dictated by tumor characteristics and the surgeon's ability to have adequate exposure and control of the margins of excision. In general, the transanal approach has less morbidity. Posterior approaches can offer the advantage of better exposure for larger lesions. However, this entails a higher rate of fistula formation and the potential for tumor seeding of the posterior wound. Whichever method is selected, the surgeon must perform a full-thickness excision with at least 1 cm margins of normal tissue completely surrounding the tumor. Piecemeal or submucosal excision is not considered adequate surgical treatment of invasive rectal cancer. Fragmentation of the tumor is associated with an increased incidence of local recurrence. If the lesion cannot be adequately resected by local excision, then a more standard operative approach should be used.

The criteria used to select patients for local excision are intended to make make a negative-margin full-thickness local excision technically feasible and to ensure a low risk of lymph node metastases (Table 1). Physical assessment, computed tomography, and endorectal ultrasonography are helpful in the preoperative evaluation of those rectal cancer patients. Imaging findings can be used to select patients for local excision procedures by determining the depth of tumor penetration into the rectal wall and the presence of enlarged lymph nodes. Most patients with rectal cancer do not meet the criteria for

Table 1. Indications for the local excision of rectal cancer

Tumor <3 cm in greatest dimension
Invades only the submucosa or superficial muscularis
Favorable pathologic grade

From Nivatvongs S, Wolff BG. Technique of per anal excision for carcinoma of the low rectum. World J Surg 16:447–450, 1992, with permission.

treatment by local excision alone due to the size or extent of the tumor. Adjuvant therapy may expand the use of this technique.

The use of this approach is currently the focus of a national cooperative group registry in the United States. This study has enrolled patients who meet the usual criteria for the local excision of distal rectal cancer. These are mobile tumors confirmed to the rectal wall (T1/T2), which are less than 4 cm in size, are less than 40% of the bowel wall circumference, and are without evidence of lymph node involvement. Patients were registered after a negative margin full-thickness local excision. T1 rectal cancer patients received no further treatment, while T2 rectal cancer patients received adjuvant chemoradiation therapy. Accrual to this study has just closed. Outcomes will be compared with those of historical controls.

Curative surgical treatment for rectal cancer requires tumor excision with margins of normal tissue and treatment of the lymph nodes draining the tumor site. Local excision alone only achieves a negative margin excision. Factors that can help identify patients who are at low risk for lymphatic metastases include small tumor size, absence of lymphatic and vascular invasion, and absence of clinical or radiologic evidence of enlarged lymph nodes. This assumed low risk is then accepted in patients treated by local excision alone because such procedures do not resect the mesorectal lymph nodes. However, many of the classic criteria can be unreliable predictors of lymphatic involvement.

The major factor predicting patient survival and perirectal lymph node metastases is the depth of penetration of the primary tumor. Morson has reported that lymphatic metastases occur with 10% of tumors confined to the submucosa, 12% of tumors invading the muscularis propria, and 58% of tumors extending beyond the bowel wall [2]. Others have found a higher incidence of lymphatic metastases with T2 rectal carcinoma. A study of T1 and T2 tumors treated by radical resection showed an incidence of lymphatic metastasis of 12% for T1 tumors and 22% for T2 tumors [3]. The incidence of lymphatic metastasis was increased by lymphatic or blood vessel invasion and in poorly differentiated tumors. Nelson et al. reported that 29% of patients with lesions smaller than 2 cm in diameter had evidence of lymph node metastasis [4]. Thus, selection for local excision based on the classic indications will fail to adequately treat a significant number of patients with lymphatic involvement. This makes the addition of adjuvant therapy to local excision a logical choice.

The incidence of lymph node metastases in patients with T1 tumors approximates the recurrence rate for T1 cancers treated by local excision alone. Studies describe a 3–10% rate of local recurrence after excision alone [5]. Survival rates in patients with T1 rectal carcinomas treated with local excision alone or radical resection are 90–100% [6]. Local excision alone is a reasonable treatment for T1 carcinoma of the rectum if the tumor meets the previous selection criteria. A caveat is that blood vessel or lymphatic invasion is a significant predictor of lymph node involvement and poor survival. Either standard surgical therapy, or if it is refused or the patient is unable to tolerate standard surgical therapy, the use of adjuvant therapy after local excision, should be considered.

In patients with T2 rectal carcinomas, the risk of lymph node metastasis is 10–30 [2,3]. However, local excision procedures preclude lymph node excision. Studies show higher local recurrence rates for tumors involving the muscularis propria that are treated with local excision alone, possibly because of the failure to treat these lymphatic metastases. Recurrence rates may be 17–24% in patients with T2 tumors. Survival rates are 78–82% with excision alone. In patients with T2 carcinomas of the rectum, the risk of lymph node metastasis in the mesorectum must be addressed by either resection of the mesorectum during proctectomy or, if a local excision is done, the addition of chemotherapy and radiation therapy to reduce the incidence of pelvic recurrence.

A prospective series from The University of Texas M. D. Anderson Cancer Center reported excellent local control rates for 46 patients treated with local excision and postoperative chemotherapy/radiation therapy [7]. T3 tumors were also treated in medically compromised patients or in those who refused standard therapy.

Tumors were lesions less than 5 cm from the anal verge that were smaller than 4 cm in diameter. All patients had refused standard therapy, and all patients underwent negative-margin, full-thickness excisions via a transanal, trans-sphincteric, or posterior approach to the rectum. Postoperative radiation therapy (53 Gy) was given through posterior and two lateral fields. Concomitantly, fluorouracil was given during radiotherapy to eight patients with T3 lesions. Follow-up was complete on all patients and included standard clinical, endoscopic, and radiologic exams. The overall survival rate at 3 years was 93%. Table 2 shows the pattern of failure by the American Joint Committee on Cancer (AJCC) T stage. Local-recurrence-free survival at 3 years was 90%. None of the patients with T1 tumors demonstrated treatment failure. One of the patients with a T2 tumor and vascular and lymphatic invasion had simultaneous local and distant failure. Three of the 15 patients with T3 tumors had local failure as a component of their recurrence. T1 and T2 rectal carcinomas could be adequately controlled with this program of local excision and postoperative radiation, but T3 tumors were not well controlled by this program.

Other single institution reports are similar. Excellent control rates for T1 and T2 rectal cancers treated by local excision and postoperative adjuvant radiotherapy. We anticipate that the effect of adjuvant therapy will be verified in the national registry of patients undergoing local excision and adjuvant therapy. This study will be important to establish this treatment as an effective approach to T2 rectal cancer compared with the more standard approaches of low anterior resection or APR resection. In general, local excision cannot be recommended for T3 rectal cancer.

Patients with T3 carcinoma of the rectum are considered at high risk for local recurrence, lymph node metastasis, and distant metastasis. Reported series show that local excision alone for T3 carcinomas results in an unacceptably high recurrence rate. Trials of adjuvant chemotherapy and radiation therapy with radical surgical treatment for these high-risk tumors have demonstrated that patients benefit from the addition of chemotherapy and radiation therapy. The use of chemotherapy and radiation therapy in patients with T3 rectal cancers undergoing local excision improves local control compared with excision alone. However, this control is not equivalent to the control that can be obtained by more radical surgical procedures and adjuvant therapy. Patients with T3 tumors that are selected for local excision often are poor candidates for a more extensive surgical procedures, and their options are therefore limited. It would seem reasonable to add our best adjuvant chemotherapy and radiation therapy to the local excision when it is done for patients with T3 rectal cancer.

Neoadjuvant therapy in patients with T3 rectal carcinomas can decrease the size and penetration of these lesions and sterilize regional lymph nodes. Preoperative chemoradiation therapy can reduce the incidence of positive lymph nodes in rectal cancer resection specimens from patients with T3 carcinomas and result in a significant rate of complete pathologic responses. Despretz reported results in 25 with rectal cancer patients treated by preoperative external radiation therapy (35 Gy) followed by local excision and brachytherapy. Local recurrence developed in 5 of the 25 patients. Marks reported results in 14 patients who underwent preoperative radiation (45 Gy) followed by full-thickness excision; local recurrence developed in 3 patients. Complete response rates are higher in patients treated with preoperative chemotherapy and radiation therapy than in those treated with preoperative radiation therapy alone. We are examining our experience with patients undergoing chemoradiation therapy and subsequent local excision of T3 tumors. This approach appears to be technically feasible but should be considered only in patients with T3 tumors who are not candidates for a more standard surgical approach.

In summary, patients who undergo local excision of T1 low rectal cancers who have no adverse prognostic characteristics can avoid subsequent adjuvant therapy. For patients with T1 tumors with adverse pathologic characteristics or T2 tumors, the increased risk of lymph node metastasis may justify the use of adjuvant radiation therapy if local excision is used, although validation of these approaches will await the results of the current national registry. For patients with T3 carcinomas, it appears that postoperative chemotherapy and radiation are required after local excision. The preoperative use of chemotherapy and radiation therapy to downstage the disease and to permit a more satisfactory local excision may be feasible. Validation of such an approach is currently not available. It should only be considered in medically compromised patients with T3 rectal cancer.

Locoregional resection and multimodality treatment for rectal cancer

Patients with stage II and III rectal cancer have tumors that are large and biologically aggressive. They are at higher risk of local and systemic recurrence after treatment. Accordingly, strategies have been developed to address these issues through multimodality therapy. About 60–80% of patients with rectal cancer have stage II or III disease.

Advances in the surgical management of stage II and III tumors are based on several issues: (1) the importance of the lateral spread of rectal cancer in local tumor recurrence, (2) the need for total mesorectal excision to minimize pelvic recurrence, (3) restoration of function by coloanal anastomosis after resection of low rectal cancers, and (4) optimization of bowel function and quality of life after low rectal anastomosis. Surgical management cannot be separated from the use of preoperative or postoperative chemoradiation for most patients with stage II or III rectal cancer.

The risk of spread to local lymph nodes and the risk of local recurrence increase as tumor penetration of the rectal wall increases. This has led to the development of operations such as the APR that achieve tumor-free proximal and distal tissue margins, and remove the upward pathways of lymphatic spread from rectal cancer. The distal margin has been shown to be adequate when it is a distance of 2 cm from the edge of the tumor. However, more recently the work of Quirke and others has dramatically demonstrated the importance of lateral tumor spread in the local recurrence of resected rectal cancers.

The pelvis confines the rectum by its bony sidewalls with major blood vessels and nerves. It is filled with viscera that are important to functional well-being. This allows little room for obtaining wide margins of normal tissue around a transmural rectal tumor, especially when located anteriorly in males. Tumor involvement at the circumferential margin of resection has been associated with local recurrence in 85% of cases [8]. While distal margins are measured in centimeters, circumferential margins are often measured in millimeters. Because of problems in obtaining adequate exposure in the low pelvis and the surrounding structures, circumferential margins around rectal cancer can be highly variable and minimal. Controlled sharp dissection must be done with close attention to these margins. The mechanism for involvement of the circumferential margins can be direct spread, mesenteric implants, vascular or lymphatic invasion, or cancer-bearing lymph nodes [9]. Tumor involvement of the circumferential margins of resection is frequently due to spread in the mesorectum distal to the tumor (Table 2) [10]. This factor is an important cause of involvement of the radial margin. If resection margins are limited to 2 cm beyond the tumor, then it becomes critical to completely resect the mesorectum beyond this limit to eliminate this source of local recurrence. The long-term outcome is poor in the presence of a positive circumferential margin [10].

Understanding the importance of the circumferential clearance of rectal

Table 2. Patterns of failure by AJCC T stage of disease after local excision and adjuvant therapy

	T1 (n = 15)	T2 (n = 15)	T3 (n = 15)	Total (%) (n = 46)
Local recurrence only	0	0	2	2 (4%)
Distant recurrence only	0	0	4	4 (7%)
Combined recurrence	0	1	1	2 (4%)

From Ota DM, Skibber JM, Rich TA. M.D. Anderson Cancer Center experience with local excision and multimodality therapy for rectal cancer. Surg Clin North Am 1:147–152, 1992, with permission.

tumors has impacted the accepted surgical procedures for the management of rectal cancer. The mesorectum is the extension of the large bowel mesentery along the posterior wall of the rectum. This blood vessel– and lymph node–bearing structure is enveloped by the fascia propria of the rectum. Total mesorectal excision by full mobilization of the rectum along anatomic planes has been demonstrated to be effective in the surgical management of rectal cancer [11]. Dissection is carried out along areolar planes, which allow for hemostasis, identification of important nerves, and prevention of violation of the visceral fascia investing the mesorectum and rectum itself. This type of surgical resection for rectal cancer will minimize the potential for a circumferential radial margin and thereby reduce the possibility of local recurrence.

McAnena et al. have described the long-term outcome of 57 patients treated with this approach [11]. The mean follow-up was 4.8 years. Local recurrences were seen in only 3.5% of the patients, and overall 5-year survival was 81%. While these are commendable data, it should be noted that 31% of the patients had Dukes' A lesions, in which local and distant failure would be less common than in Dukes' B and C lesions. It should also be noted that 'serious' postoperative complications occurred in 17% of patients and that the diverting colostomies were not closed in six patients. In a subsequent larger review of their experience with total mesorectal excision for rectal cancer. MacFarlane et al. reported on 135 patients with Dukes' B and C rectal cancers treated over a 13-year period with a mean of follow-up of 7.5 years [12]. These patients did not have adjuvant radiation nor chemotherapy. Despite this fact, there was only a 5% local recurrence rate. This compares favorably with the results from the North Central Cancer Treatment Group study that forms the basis for current recommendations for adjuvant therapy in the United States.

In North America similar results have been obtained with high rates of local recurrence-free survival when a total mesorectal excision is done by meticulous sharp dissection along the pelvic sidewalls. Enker's report on this subject called for full rectal mobilization along anatomic planes to obtain complete mesorectal excision. In a series of 42 who men underwent sphincter-preserving surgery for low rectal cancer using this technique, there was only one local recurrence (median follow-up 20 months) [13]. This result was accomplished with preservation of potency in 86.7% of patients. In this study meticulous sharp dissection accomplished the goals of the total circumferential clearance of the tumor and preservation of sexual function.

Both Heald and Enker question the need for adjuvant radiation and chemotherapy when this type of surgery is performed for T3, N0, M0 rectal cancers. This controversial point may be answered through a proposed European-based trial involving surgeons trained in this technique. Fielding reported on a 1995 conference that discusses the application of the surgical techniques proposed by Heald [14]. They identify two issues that address the use of proper surgical technique to reduce the local recurrence of rectal cancer. Fielding states that it is 'abundantly clear that in Europe and North America only a minority of patients with rectal cancer are treated by surgeons highly skilled in total mesorectal excision.' The answer to this by Norwegian surgeons has been to remove rectal cancer surgery from routine surgical teaching and to concentrate training in total mesorectal excision among specialized 'gastrointestinal surgeons.' In addition, they propose that the surgical specimens obtained by such surgeons be audited. Both of these issues will be highly controversial in the United States, given concerns over the fragmentation of general surgical training and current practice patterns.

More controversial, however, is the assertion by Heald that systemic micrometastases in rectal cancer patients are from local recurrence occurring as a result of inadequate surgical clearance of the primary tumor. He proposes a reduction in the use of systemic adjuvant therapy based on this concept. This directly conflicts with the studies that form the basis for adjuvant therapy recommendations in the United States. It also conflicts with the concept of the early systemic spread of colorectal cancer producing micrometastases that are present at the time of the locoregional treatment of primary rectal cancers.

Current standards of care for high-risk (stage II and III) rectal cancer in the United States are based on a study conducted by the North Central Cancer Treatment Group [15]. Reported in 1991 by Krook et al., this large randomized trial for high-risk (stage II and III) rectal cancer patients compared postoperative fluorouracil combined with radiation to postoperative radiation alone. Reduced local recurrence, systemic recurrence, and cancer-related death, and improved overall survival compared with the effect of radiation alone, were seen. It appears that the improvement in local control could accrue from the direct cytotoxic effects of the chemotherapy as well as from fluorouracil's radiation-sensitizing effects on residual microscopic disease in the pelvis. Clearly, the reduction in distant metastases was the major factor in the overall improvement in survival; however, prevention of the impact of a pelvic recurrence on a patient's quality of life cannot be overlooked.

The next major step in adjuvant therapy for rectal cancer can be found in the report from an intergroup trial testing the role of protracted or continuous intravenous infusion of fluorouracil combined with radiation therapy as postoperative therapy. The rationale for this was based on in vitro studies indicating that optimal cytotoxicity was obtained by continuous exposure of tumor cells to fluorouracil after irradiation [16]. A pilot study by Rich et al. showed the regimen to be well tolerated during radiation therapy [17]. In a trial of 680 patients, significant reductions were seen in overall rates of tumor relapse and distant metastases [18]. Survival was significantly increased in those who received the protracted infusion of fluorouracil during irradiation. The protracted infusion did not appear to reduce local recurrence; however, analysis may have been hampered by the small number of local recurrences seen in the study.

For rectal cancer patients, a major component of quality of life is sphincter preservation. This is simple to accomplish in middle and upper rectal cancers, for which low anterior resection allows adequate removal of the tumor and surrounding lymphatics and end-to-end anastomosis. In patients with low rectal cancers that do not involve the levators or sphincters, the anus may still be spared by proctectomy and coloanal anastomosis. Preoperative chemoradiation may facilitate this. However, patients with levator or sphincter involvement are best managed by APR resection and permanent colostomy.

A recent review of 117 patients from the Mayo and Cleveland Clinics provides a perspective on its current utility of proctectomy and coloanal anastomosis in patients with low rectal cancer [19]. The patients were treated over a 10-year period (1981–1991). The median distance of the tumor from the anal verge was 6–7 cm. The technique used required complete mobilization of the rectum to the levators, transanal transection of the rectum, complete mobilization of the left colon, and endoanal anastomosis. The authors recommend loop ileostomy in most patients. The effectiveness of the a procedure in preventing local recurrence was demonstrated by the low local recurrence rate of 7%. However, it should be noted that 46% of the patients in this series had stage I disease. This point is important when assessing the wider applicability of this technique. Fecal continence was satisfactory in 78%, and overall bowel function appeared to be improved in patients who had a colonic J pouch reservoir created for the coloanal anastomosis. There were no surgery-related deaths. Early and late complications were related mainly to the anastomosis leaking (10%) and healing with a stricture (21%). The role of adjuvant therapy in the 43% of patients receiving radiation or chemotherapy could not be assessed.

Performance of a coloanal anastomosis is really an extension of a properly done low anterior resection. The proctectomy is extended down to the level of the upper anal canal and levators. Lateral ligaments are divided with attention to obtaining an adequate radial margin and to preserving the pelvic autonomic nerves. It seems helpful to perform the posterior aspect of the dissection initially to facilitate the more difficult anterior dissection. This dissection results in the complete exposure of the pelvic floor and complete excision of the mesorectum. The fully mobilized rectum can then be considered for amputation by a transanal technique or by transection at the upper end of the anal canal with a stapler.

The reconstruction consists of delivering the mobilized left colon to the anal canal and performing an anastomosis. An anastomosis is then performed with full-thickness stitches through the colon and internal sphincter. Alternatively, a stapled anastomosis may be done. A diverting stoma is then usually created. We tend to use a diverting ileostomy, which provides for adequate fecal division.

Several groups have reported on patients who have a 6- to 10-cm colonic J pouch reservoir constructed with no additional risk or compromise of the anastomosis [20]. This technique is done in hopes of increasing the volume of the neorectum and thereby decreasing stool frequency. Others have disputed these advantages. In general, we try to use such a pouch in most patients undergoing coloanal anastomosis. Its use may be limited in those with an inadequate length of colon or those with a small pelvis and a thick mesentery.

The results of a properly done coloanal anastomosis appear oncologically equivalent to APR resections in properly selected patients. Less than 5–10% of patients fail to resume normal anorectal function. Pelvic infection rates are about 6%. Anal sphincter tone is usually preserved, and sensation and reflex inhibition of the anal sphincters have been demonstrated to be retained.

Major long-term postoperative complaints of patients are related to rectal capacitance and compliance. These manifest as the problems of urgency and frequency in their bowel movements. This gradually improves over the 9–10 months after temporary stoma closure. Complete fecal continence is usually achieved in 85–100% of patients. Occasional soiling due to the inability to differentiate between gas and stool may occur in 10% of patients. In a series from the Mayo Clinic by Drake et al., patients who had a coloanal anastomosis for malignancies had a stool frequency of 2.6 per 24 hours, and only 1 of 19 patients were incontinent [21].

The Mayo and Cleveland Clinic study is similar to the reports of others in describing proctectomy and coloanal anastomosis for rectal cancers [22]. In the absence of cancer recurrence or gross incontinence, patients are usually satisfied with the results, and the need for conversion to a permanent colostomy is rare.

However, it is critical to avoid pelvic sepsis during the postoperative period to reduce the risk of anal stricture, which is often untreatable and results in unsatisfactory function. Thus, proctectomy and coloanal anastomosis can be done on selected patients with low local recurrence rates, acceptable functional results, and low mortality. While complication rates can be significant, the ability to achieve sphincter preservation when the only alternative is a permanent colostomy seems worthwhile in studies of long-term outcome.

In these series, however, this technique has been restricted to highly selected patients. Can or should it be applied to the more common cases of stage III low rectal cancer? Efforts to widen the role of such sphincter-preserving surgery to those previously requiring APR resection have used preoperative radiation and more recently concurrent chemoradiation.

Minsky et al. reported the efficacy and toxicity of preoperative radiation and proctectomy with coloanal anastomosis for low rectal cancer in patients who otherwise would have required an APR [22]. Twenty-two patients with a diagnosis of invasive, resectable T2/T3 primary adenocarcinoma of the distal rectum (median distance from anal verge, 4 cm) were treated. All were believed to require APR as a standard operative approach. External-beam radiation therapy was given to a total dose of 50.4 Gy. Four to 5 weeks later, resection was performed in 21 of the 22 patients. Ninety percent of those who had resection had a coloanal anastomosis performed. Ten percent of patients had a complete response. Therapy was well tolerated and the anastomic leak rate was only 6%. Eighty-nine percent had a good or excellent functional result. Local failure alone occurred in 5%. These data reveal acceptable local control, survival, and results in selected patients treated with preoperative radiation therapy and proctectomy with coloanal anastomosis as an alternative to APR.

Numerous other single-institution reports have described similar results. For example, outstanding sphincter-preserving results in the treatment of low rectal cancers after preoperative radiation have been described by Marks et al. at Thomas Jefferson University [23]. They demonstrated long-term adequate sphincter function in 91% of patients, with local recurrence rates of less than 13%.

Preoperative radiation therapy does not appear to increase the morbidity of sphincter-preservation procedures, and bowel habits and sphincter function after preoperative therapy and surgery are acceptable. This management approach to rectal carcinomas whose distal edge is located from 3 to 7 cm from the anal verge will be applicable to many more patients than will local excision techniques.

Considerable downstaging can occur after preoperative radiation or chemoradiation. With radiation alone, the complete pathologic response rate is reported to be 10–17%. With preoperative concurrent chemoradiation, complete response rates can be 20–30%. Obviously, a smaller tumor may allow achievement of acceptable negative margins and may facilitate sphincter preservation. However, it must be noted that at this time the impact of preoperative treatment on what are 'acceptable' margins is unclear. Indeed, it is unclear what a pathologic complete response means for a patient in long-term follow-up. It is clear that the absence of mucosal tumor does not assure a complete response (CR) because residual tumor may be found within or beyond the rectal wall, or within lymph nodes, in the absence of residual mucosal tumor [24]. The determination of adequate margins after preoperative treatment will require clinical trials.

It needs to be emphasized that this preoperative chemoradiation can be given on an outpatient basis with virtually no increase in operative complications. The use of preoperative therapy has been demonstrated to have lower treatment toxicity than the use of postoperative chemoradiation [25]. Minsky et al. reported that when identical chemoradiation regimens are given preoperatively or postoperatively, significantly fewer patients experience grade

3–4 toxicity when the adjuvant treatment is preoperative. In this study 13% of patients treated preoperatively experienced gastrointestinal toxicity, while 48% of the postoperatively treated patients had grade 3 or 4 gastrointestinal or genitourinary toxicity.

Rich et al. reported on the outcome of 77 patients treated with preoperative chemoradiation therapy who then underwent resection of low rectal T3 cancers staged by ultrasound [26]. The preoperative treatment was continuous infusion fluorouracil (300 mg/m^2/day) given with daily irradiation (45 Gy in 25 fractions over 5 weeks). Surgery was performed 6 weeks later. Sphincter preservation was accomplished in 67% of these patients, in whom the mean distance of the tumor from the anal verge was 5 cm. A complete pathologic response was found in 29% of patients. Local recurrence was seen in 4% of cases. Acute, perioperative, and late complications of treatment were not increased compared with historical data on the use of radiation alone.

Two other papers bring up issues that bear on the functional outcome of sphincter preservation and the use of adjuvant therapy. Quality of life after rectal cancer treatment can be greatly impacted by bowel function regardless of whether there is a stoma. If function is poor after sphincter-preserving surgery, the patient's quality of life may be impaired more than if a permanent colostomy is present [27]. This issue will need to be addressed in future clinical studies. Kollmorgen and coworkers have studied the long-term effects of chemoradiation therapy on bowel function when this adjuvant therapy is given postoperatively [28]. One hundred patients were studied after extensive exclusions were made to minimize confounding variables affecting outcomes. The group of patients who did not receive postoperative treatment uniformly had less problems with bowel function. They reported increased clustering of bowel movements, stool frequency, and fecal soiling when the reconstructed rectum was postoperatively irradiated (see Table 4). It is clear from this study that long-term detrimental effects on bowel function can result from postoperative chemoradiation.

Further support for this conclusion can be drawn from the results of a study by Paty et al. on the functional outcomes of coloanal anastomosis for rectal cancer [29]. Postoperative radiation significantly increased the frequency of

Table 3. Importance of distal mesorectal spread in producing an involved radial margin

Curative resection specimens (n = 20)	Distal mesorectal spread	Involvement of radial margin
16	Negative	2 (13%)
4	Positive	2 (50%)

From Adam IJ, Mohamdee MO, Martin IG, Scott N, Firan PJ, Johnston D, Dixon MF, Quirke P. Role of circumferential involvement in the local recurrence of rectal cancer. Lancet 344:707–711, 1994, with permission.

stools and significantly impaired the pattern of evacuation. These studies imply that for patients who need adjuvant chemoradiation, it may be advantageous to deliver this therapy preoperatively. By not irradiating the rectal pouch used for reconstruction, subsequent problems with rectal compliance, causing symptoms of urgency and frequency, may be avoided. This issue is being addressed in the current trials of preoperative and postoperative chemoradiation for low rectal cancer being done in the United States in which both quality of life and bowel function are being studied.

Sphincter preservation during multivisceral resections for locally advanced rectal cancer can be performed. These patients have involvement of adjacent pelvic organs from locally advanced cancers. Almost all patients who require multivisceral resections are treated preoperatively with radiation therapy or chemoradiation therapy. This is due to the limited ability to obtain negative margins in the confines of the pelvis, even with multivisceral resections. The use of neoadjuvant therapy has markedly reduced local recurrence rates and has improved sphincter preservation rates, even for fixed tumors. Selected patients may benefit from intraoperative radiation therapy or brachytherapy [30].

Data show that preoperative chemoradiotherapy does not appear to increase the morbidity of resections in patients with locally advanced rectal cancer [31]. It is reasonable to perform reconstruction of the rectum after multivisceral resections for rectal cancers without fear of compromising the oncologic outcome [32]. After resections of adjacent organs, such as the bladder or uterus, as well as a large portion of the rectum, the pelvis is quite empty. This added exposure is a double-edged sword: although the increased area to work with in the pelvis increases the ability to do a technically satisfactory anastomosis, it also creates a large empty space that may play a role in postoperative pelvic infection or subsequent small bowel obstructions. One of the ways to fill this pelvic space is to perform rectal reconstruction, either to a remaining rectal stump or with coloanal anastomosis. Additionally, well-vascularized non-irradiated tissues, such as the omentum or a rectus muscle flap, may be placed into the pelvis to further fill the space and to improve healing of the irradiated pelvic tissues. Such pelvic reconstruction can be performed with safety and good functional results [33].

Translational research issues

Advances in the basic science of cancer are likely to drive our next therapeutic advances in rectal cancer management. Better predictors of outcomes may allow us to more selectively treat patients for optimal results. Better predictors of response to therapies may identify those who may or may not require more intensive therapy than is considered standard. If more intensive therapies are clinically effective, they will result in improved oncologic results and a better quality of life for rectal cancer patients. A clinical example of this is

Table 4. Long-term effect of postoperative chemoradiation therapy on bowel function in rectal cancer patients

Postoperative therapy	Median bowel movement per day	Clustering of bowel movements	Fecal incontinence		
			Occasional	Frequent	Urgency
None	2	3%	7%	0%	19%
Chemoradiation	7	42%	39%	17%	17%

From Adam IJ, Mohamdee MO, Martin IG, Scott N, Firan PJ, Johnston D, Dixon MF, Quirke P. Role of circumferential involvement in the local recurrence of rectal cancer. Lancet 344:707–711, 1994, with permission.

the improvement in sphincter preservation rates brought about by the use of preoperative chemoradiation therapy and coloanal anastomosis. Molecular predictors of response to preoperative adjuvant therapies may be the next step in more effectively applying treatments. The application of molecular biologic advances may provide the rationale for the next advance in therapy.

Proliferating cell nuclear antigen (PCNA) is a 36kDa protein that is associated with a subunit of DNA polymerase. It serves as a marker for proliferation in cells that rapidly increase its expression during GI and it accumulates it through S phase. Detection of this accumulated protein in cells will describe the overall rate of proliferation for a population of cells. Its deregulated expression may also be a factor in helping to drive proliferation. There are a multitude of other markers of tumor proliferation, such as Ki-67, mitotic index, tumor doubling times, and the percentage of cells in S phase.

In an initial study of 90 patients, Willett described the association between the pretreatment proliferative state of a rectal cancer measured by PCNA staining and the tumor's response to preoperative irradiation [34]. Significant responses were seen in 37% of the patients. Eleven had no residual tumor in the operative specimen. Two features of the tumors correlated with the response. Tumor size and tumor proliferative activity were independently associated with the response to preoperative irradiation. Tumors that were less than 5 cm and had high proliferative activity had a marked tumor reduction in 90% of cases. Conversely, large tumors with a low proliferative activity showed no pathologic regression in eight cases studied. Intermediate tumor proliferative indices were correlated with a 26–44% marked regression rate.

The same authors describe a correlation between an elevated post-irradiation proliferative activity in a rectal tumor and an improved survival [35]. In this study 14 patients had complete responses, and all these had moderate to extensive pretreatment proliferation activity measured in biopsies by Ki-67 and PCNA staining. Preoperative irradiation significantly reduced tumor size and tumor proliferative activity indices from pretreatment measurements in these tumors with a high pretreatment proliferation activity.

Tumors that were reduced to being contained within the bowel wall demonstrated a high pretreatment and post-treatment proliferation activity.

The post-irradiation pathologic characteristics and proliferative activities were studied in regard to disease-free survival at 5 years after treatment. Post-treatment pathologic stage was found to be a highly significant predictor of survival. Indeed, tumors undergoing a complete response had a 100% 5-year actuarial survival. This is one of the few studies that have analyzed the utility of post-irradiation stage as a predictor of survival. This could have important implications for the use of postoperative adjuvant therapy in patients treated with neoadjuvant therapy for rectal cancer. If complete responders have a high survival without postoperative adjuvant chemotherapy, as in this study, is additional chemotherapy needed? This concept goes against the common notions about the spread of micrometastases being the major factor in survival. These data demonstrate a subset of patients with transmural tumors and high proliferation rates who may have prolonged survival without treatment for micrometastases. Does this post-treatment stage and measure of tumor biology (PCNA) tell us about the tumor's previous history of causing micrometastases? Post-irradiation PCNA staining was also shown to be a predictor of disease-free survival. High proliferative activity by PCNA staining of the post-treatment tumor was seen in 55 patients who had a 66% 5-year survival compared with a 24% survival seen in 40 patients with minimal post-treatment PCNA staining.

Might patients with relatively low-risk tumors have the potential to have less extensive (i.e., local excision) procedures after preoperative treatment? Conversely, are there patients with tumors unlikely to respond to such treatment who could be selected for immediate extensive surgery or innovative neoadjuvant treatment strategies? Terry and Peters have discussed this issue using more sophisticated measures of tumor proliferation, such as the calculation of tumor potential doubling time after bromodeoxyuridine incorporation [36]. They have previously demonstrated that the response of aneuploid rectal tumors to preoperative flourouracil and radiotherapy was positively correlated with the labeling index, demonstrating a higher proliferative rate. This supports the observations of Willett.

Progressive tumor growth is dependent upon the development of blood vessels to supply oxygen and nutrients. Angiogenesis is an important factor in sustaining the uncontrolled growth of a primary or metastatic tumor. There is substantial direct and indirect evidence for its importance in experimental tumor growth and metastasis [37,38]. The contribution of angiogenesis to tumor progression goes beyond tumor perfusion, however. Endothelial cells may secrete factors that drive tumor proliferation [39]. Angiogenesis may also correlate with metastatic risk by two mechanisms. Within a primary tumor, areas of angiogenesis are heterogenous. Areas of intense neovascularity may be a source of highly angiogenic cells. These cells may be more likely to disseminate because of the increased surface area of microvessels allowing entry into the lymphatic and vascular systems. Disseminated tumor cells from these areas of intense angiogenesis may also be more likely to develop into established distant metastases based on their increased angiogenic properties [40].

The clinical relevance of angiogenesis in colorectal cancer has been demonstrated by Takahashi et al. [41]. Immunohistochemical analysis was performed on paraffin-embedded primary tumor specimens from 52 patients with colorectal cancer or adenomas. Staining for vascular endothelial growth factor (VEGF) and microvessel counts in primary tumor specimens correlated with metastatic spread to lymph nodes or viscera. It is interesting to note that increased PCNA staining correlated with the presence of metastases and with vessel counts. Similar results were obtained in rectal cancer patients studied with angiogenesis 'scores' by Saclarides et al. [42]. Higher 'scores' correlated with failure to survive 5 years beyond diagnosis.

Aside from the overall prognostic value of angiogenesis measurements, what could the practical value be? The highly significant correlation between lymph node metastases and VEGF or microvessel density in the primary tumor seen in the studies of Ellis could be important in the selection of patients for local excision. Since local excision precludes adequate lymph node dissection and lymph node involvement is a contraindication to local excision, intense VEGF staining or high microvessel counts in biopsies of the primary tumor may be important in the selection of patients for this treatment. Prospective data acquisition and analysis will be required to determine this. In other tumor types, measurements of angiogenesis have been correlated with the response to radiation therapy [43]. If this is borne out in rectal cancer, it may be a selection factor for the use of adjuvant therapy.

p53 is a tumor suppressor gene that is central in understanding human carcinogenesis. Loss of p53 function is associated with many human cancers. It has a role in both hereditary cancers and sporadic tumor development. Its multiple functions include the activation of transcription, control of DNA synthesis, progression through the cell cycle, and the control of programmed cell death. These issues are extensively reviewed by Greenblatt et al. [44]. A complete review of this gene's important role is beyond the scope of this chapter; however, several issues of possibly relevance to future rectal cancer management are discussed.

Work from Vogelstein's group has demonstrated the role for the loss of p53 function in colorectal cancer development [45]. It was demonstrated that p53 mutations occurred in four highly conserved regions of the gene that code for important functional regions of the protein. These mutations occurred mainly as point mutations, resulting in nonsense codons or amino acid substitutions. These mutations were rare in adenomas. However, in carcinomas point mutations were common and correlated strongly with subsequent allelic loss. Loss of controls in cellular reproduction provided by abnormal p53 function will facilitate tumor progression by promoting the multiple other genetic alterations seen in colorectal cancer development.

An example of this is that abnormal p53 function can prevent programmed cell death in cells having DNA damage. This programmed cell death in response to DNA damage or genetic alteration is termed *apoptosis* The process is important in both the elimination of damaged cells from an organ and also in the response of tumor cells to antineoplastic therapy. Sinicrope et al. studied the relationship between the expression of *bcl-2*, a protooncogene inhibiting apoptosis, and *p53* in colorectal neoplasia [46]. Activation of *bcl-2* promotes escape from normal p53-triggered apoptosis and allows neoplastic progression in genetically damaged cells. An inverse relationship was demonstrated between *bcl-2* expression and *p53* expression in colorectal adenomas. The apoptotic activity of carcinomas was correlated with *bcl-2* expression. These data indicated that the inhibition of apoptosis by *bcl-2* overexpression in carcinomas produced low rates of spontaneous apoptosis.

How can these findings be brought to bear on our clinical management? Investigators have addressed the importance of *p53* in determining prognosis, in predicting lymph node involvement, and in predicting response to therapy. An example of the value of *p53* nuclear expression measured by immunohistochemical staining was demonstrated in a homogenous group of node-positive but resectable colorectal cancer patients by Zeng et al. [47]. They found that 46.7% of the 107 patients studied had tumors demonstrating *p53* nuclear staining. The intensity of staining did not correlate with any clinicopathologic variables, such as tumor differentiation, lymphatic invasion, or number of lymph node mestastases. However, 60% of the patients with tumors and *p53*-positive staining developed recurrent disease. Only 35% of patients with *p53*-negative tumors had recurrence. Survival was also significantly worse in those patients with *p53*-positive tumors. Upon analysis *p53* nuclear staining was an independent predictor of recurrence and survival.

Goh et al. have taken this issue further [48]. They found lymphatic spread correlated with the presence of point mutation (the most common *p53* mutation in colorectal cancer) in a study of 187 patients. This mutation occurred in 70% of those with lymph node metastases and in only 40% of those without lymphatic spread.

The same authors have studied *p53* point mutation status and survival along with responses to postoperative adjuvant radiation or chemotherapy [49]. This study demonstrated that the site of point mutation was important in the effectiveness of this treatment. Mutations in the highly conserved regions of the *p53* gene were strongly correlated with lymph node involvement (Table 5). Eighty percent of those with conserved domain point mutations had lymph node metastases. The authors state that in follow-up none of the patients with mutations outside the highly conserved domains have developed distant metastases. Fifty-two percent of those with mutations inside the conserved domains have developed distant metastases. Codon 175 mutations are reported to produce particularly aggressive tumors in regard to dissemination and poor survival.

Might the patients with *p53* mutation–negative tumors or those with a *p53* mutation outside a conserved domain represent the group of T3, N0, M0 rectal cancer patients who can be cured with surgery and total mesorectal excision

Table 5. p53 conserved domain mutations and lymph node spread of colorectal cancer

Site of mutation — domain	Lymph node negative	Lymph node positive
Conserved	9	35
Nonconserved	7	2

Adapted from Goh, Yas, Smith. [48]

alone, as described by Enker and Heald? Also, given the compelling nature of these data, could patients be selected or rejected for local excision procedures based on the likelihood of clinically occult lymph node metastases predicted by their *p53* status? The same authors imply that the success of postoperative adjuvant therapy in improving survival among curatively treated patients was significantly influenced by the presence or absence of a *p53* point mutation. There is already evidence in experimental models, and in other tumor types, that *p53*-dependent apoptosis can correlate with tumor responsiveness to radiation and chemotherapy [50–52].

Gene therapy is being pursued in patients with cancer. Substantial data demonstrate the safe and effective transfer of wild-type *p53* to human cancer cell lines both in vitro and in animal models [53–55]. This gene transfer has resulted in an increased response to anticancer therapy [56].

In summary, three concepts that bear on translational research applicable to rectal cancer management are presented. They are spawned by basic science advances in the understanding of cancer biology. The concepts are (1) the molecular biology of tumor proliferation measurements, (2) the role of angiogenesis in tumor behavior, and (3) the role of *p53* function. All these issues have important roles in predicting outcomes and responses to treatment in our patients. They have the potential to aid us in optimizing cancer treatment. Validation of these advances will come through translational research studies. Translation of these basic science advances into treatment advances for our patients is the next important goal for clinical investigators.

References

1. Nivatvongs S, Wolff BG. Technique of per anal excision for carcinoma of the low rectum. World J Surg 16:447–450, 1992.
2. Morson BC. Factors influencing the prognosis of early cancer of the rectum. Proc Ed 59:607–608, 1966.
3. Minsky BD, Rich TA, Recht A, Harvey W, Mies C. Selection criteria for local excision with or without adjuvant radiation therapy for rectal cancer. Cancer 63:1421–1429, 1989.
4. Nelson JC, Numr AN, Thomford N. Criteria for the selection of early carcinomas of the rectum. Arch Surg 122:533–536, 1987.

5. Graham RA, Gainsey L, Jessup JM. Local excision of rectal carcinoma. Am J Surg 160:306–312, 1990.
6. McDermott FT, Hughes ESR, Phil E, Johnson WR, Price AB. Local recurrence after potentially curative resection for rectal cancer in a series of 1008 patients. Br J Surg 72:34–37, 1985.
7. Ota DM, Skibber JM, Rich TA. M.D. Anderson Cancer Center experience with local excision and multimodality therapy for rectal cancer. Surg Clin North Am 1:147–152, 1992.
8. Quirke P, Durdy P, Dixon MF, et al. Local recurrence of rectal adenocarcinoma due to inadequate surgical resection: Histopathological study of lateral tumor spread and surgical excision. Lancet 2:996–999, 1986.
9. Quirke P, Scott N. The pathologist's role in the assessment of local recurrence in rectal carcinoma. Surg Oncol Clin North Am 1:1–17, 1992.
10. Adam IJ, Mohamdee MO, Martin IG, Scott N, Firan PJ, Johnston D, Dixon MF, Quirke P. Role of circumferential involvement in the local recurrence of rectal cancer. Lancet 344:707–711, 1994.
11. McAnena OJ, Heald RJ, Lockhart-Mummery HE. Operative and functional results of total mesorectal excision with ultra-low anterior resection in the management of carcinoma of the lower one-third of the rectum. Surg Gynecol Obstet 170:517–521, 1990.
12. MacFarlan JK, Ryall RDH, Heald RJ. Mesorectal excision for rectal cancer. Lancet 341:457–460, 1993.
13. Enker WE. Potency, cure, and local control in the operative treatment of rectal cancer. Arch Surg 127:1396–1402, 1992.
14. Fielding LP. Optimizing surgical treatment of rectal cancer. Lancet 340:113, 1995.
15. Krook JE, Moertel CG, Gunderson LL, et al. Effective surgical adjuvant therapy in high risk rectal carcinoma. N Engl J Med 324:709–715, 1991.
16. Byfield JE, Calabro-Jones P, Klisak I, Kulhanian G. Pharmacologic requirements for obtaining sensitization of human tumor cells in vitro to combined 5-fluorouracil for ftorafur and x-rays. Radiat Oncol Biol Phys 8:1923–1933, 1982.
17. Rich TA, Lokich JJ, Chaffey JT. A pilot study of protracted venous infusion of 5-fluorouracil and concomitant radiation therapy. J Clin Oncol 3:402–406, 1985.
18. O'Connell MJ, Martenson JA, Wieand HS, et al. Improving adjuvant therapy for rectal cancer by combining protracted infusion fluorouracil with radiation therapy after curative surgery. N Engl J Med 331:502–507, 1994.
19. Cavaliere F, Pemberton JH, Cosimelli M, Fazio VW, Beast RW. Coloanal anastomosis for rectal cancer: Long-term results at the Mayo and Cleveland Clinics. Dis Colon Rectum 38:807–812, 1995.
20. Lazorthes F, Fages P, Chiotasso P, Lemozy J, Bloom E. Resection of the rectum with construction of a colonic reservoir and coloanal anastomosis for carcinoma of the rectum. Br J Surg 73:136–138, 1986.
21. Drake DB, Pemberton JH, Beast RW, Dozois RR, Wolff BG. Coloanal anastomosis in the management of benign and malignant rectal disease. Ann Surg 205:600–605, 1989.
22. Minsky BD, Cohen AM, Enker WE, Sigurdson E. Phase I/II trial of preoperative radiation therapy and coloanal anastomosis in distal invasive resectable rectal cancer. Int J Radiat Oncol Biol Phys 23:387–392, 1992.
23. Marks G, Mohuiddin M, Eitan A, Masoni L, Rakinic J. High-dose preoperative radiation and radical-sphincter preserving surgery for rectal cancer. Arch Surg 126:1534–1540, 1991.
24. Meterissian S, Skibber JM, Rich TA, Roubein L, Ajani J, Cleary K, Ota DM. Patterns of residual disease after preoperative chemoradiation in ultrasound T3 rectal carcinoma. Ann Surg Oncol 1:111–116, 1994.
25. Minsky BD, Cohen AM, Kemeny N, Enker WE, Kelsen DP, Reichman B, Saltz L, Sigurdson ER, Frankel J. Combined modality therapy of rectal cancer: Decreased acute toxicity with the preoperative approach. J Clin Oncol 10:1218–1224, 1992.
26. Rich TA, Skibber JM, Ajani JA, Bucholz DJ, Cleary KR, DuBrow RA, Levin B, Lynch PM, Meterissian SH, Roubein L, Ota DM. Preoperative infusional chemoradiation therapy for stage T3 rectal cancer. Int J Radiat Oncol Biol Phys 32:1025–1029, 1995.

47

27. Sprangers MAG, Taal BG, Aaronson NK, te Velde A. Quality of life in colorectal cancer: Stoma vs. nonstoma patients. Dis Colon Rectum 38:361–364, 1995.
28. Kollmorgen CF, Meagher AP, Wolff BG, Pemberton JH, Martenson JA, Illstrup, DM. The long-term effects of adjuvant postoperative chemoradiotherapy for rectal carcinoma on bowel function. Ann Surg 220:676–682, 1994.
29. Paty PB, Enker WE, Cohen AM, Minsky BI, Friedlander-Kar H. Long-term functional results of coloanal anastomosis for rectal cancer. Am J Surg 167:90–95, 1994.
30. Weinstein GD, Rich TA, Shumate CR, Skibber JM, Cleary KR, Ajani JA, Ota DM. Preoperative infusional chemoradiation and surgery with or without an electron beam intraoperative boost for advanced primary rectal cancer. Int J Radiat Oncol Biol Phys 32:197–204, 1995.
31. Shumate CR, Rich TA, Skibber JM, Ajani JA, Ota DM. Preoperative chemotherapy and radiation therapy for locally advanced primary and recurrent rectal cancer: A report of surgical morbidity. Cancer 7:3690–3695, 1993.
32. Lowy AM, Rich TA, Skibber JM, Dubrow RA, Curley SA. Preoperative infusional chemoradiation, selective intraoperative radiation and resection for locally advanced pelvic recurrence of colorectal adenocarcinoma. Ann Surg, in press.
33. deHaas WG, Miller MJ, Kroll WJ, Kroll SS, Schusterman MA, Reece GP, Skibber JM. Perineal wound closure with the rectus abdominous flap following tumor ablation. Ann Surg Oncol 1:101–103, 1993.
34. Willet CG, Warland G, Cheek R, Coen J, Efird J, Shellit PC, Compton CC. Proliferating cell nuclear antigen and mitotic activity in rectal cancer: Predictor of response to preoperative irradiation. J Clin Oncol 12:679–682, 1994.
35. Willet CG, Warland G, Hagan MP, Paly WJ, Coen J, Shellito PC, Compton CC. Tumor proliferation in rectal cancer following irradiation. J Clin Oncol 13:1417–1424, 1995.
36. Terry NHA, Peters LJ. The predictive value of tumor-cell kinetic parameters in radiotherapy: Considerations regarding data production and analysis. J Clin Oncol 13:1833–1836, 1995.
37. Folkman J. What is the evidence that tumors are angiogenesis dependent? J Natl Cancer Inst 82:4–6, 1990.
38. Kim KJ, Li B, Winer J, et al. Inhibition of vascular endothelial growth factor induced angiogenesis suppresses tumor growth in vivo. Nature 362:841–844, 1993.
39. Hamada J, Cavanaugh PG, Lotan O, et al. Separable growth and migration factors for large cell lymphoma cells secreted by microvascular endothelial cells derived from target organs for metastatis. Br J Cancer 66:349–354, 1992.
40. Folkman J. Angiogenesis and breast cancer. J Clin Oncol 12:441–443, 1994.
41. Takahashi Y, Kitadai Y, Bucana CD, Cleary KR, Ellis LM. Expressing of vascular endothelial growth factor and its receptor, KDR, correlated with vascularity, metastasis, and proliferation of human colon cancer. Cancer Res 55:3964–3968, 1995.
42. Saclarides TJ, Speziale NJ, Drab E, Szeluga DJ, Dubin DB. Tumor angiogenesis and rectal carcinoma. Dis Colon Rectum 37:921–926, 1994.
43. Zatterstrom UK, Brun E, Willen R, Kjellen E, Wennerberg J. Tumor angiogenesis and prognosis in squamous cell carcinoma of the head and neck. Head Neck 17:312–318, 1995.
44. Greenblatt MS, Bennett WP, Hollstein M, Harris CC. Mutations in the p53 tumor suppressor gene: Clues to cancer etiology and molecular pathogenesis. Cancer Res 54:4855–4878, 1994.
45. Baker SJ, Preisinger AC, Jersup JM, Paraskiva C, Markowitz S, Willson JKV, Hamilton S, Vogelstein B. p53 gene mutations occur in combination with 17P allelic deletions as late events in colorectal tumorigenesis. Cancer Res 50:7717–7722, 1990.
46. Sinicrope FA, Ruan SB, Cleary KR, Stepehens LC, Lee JJ, Levin B. bcl-2 and p53 oncoprotein expression during colorectal tumorigenesis. Cancer Res 50:237–241, 1995.
47. Zeng Z, Sarkis AS, Zhang Z, Klimstra DS, Charaytonowica J, Guillem JG, Cordon-Cardo C, Cohen AM. p53 nuclear overexpression: An independent predictor of survival in lymph node-positive colorectal cancer patients. J Clin Oncol 12:2043–2050, 1904.

48. Goh HS, Chan CS, Khine K, Smith DK. p53 and behavior of colorectal cancer. Lancet 344:233–234, 1994.
49. Goh HS, Yao J, Smith DR. p53 point mutation and survival in colorectal cancer patients. Cancer Res 55:5217–5221, 1995.
50. Lowe SW, Ruley HE, Jacks T, Houseman DC. p53-dependent apoptosis modulates the cytotoxicity of anticancer agents. Cell 74:957–967, 1993.
51. Lowe S, Bodis S, McClatchey A, Remington L, Ruley HE, Fisher DE, Houseman DE, Jacks T. p53 status and the efficacy of cancer therapy *in vivo*. Science 266:807–810, 1994.
52. Rusch V, Klimstra D, Venkatraman E, Oliver J, Martini N, Bralla R, Kris M, Dmitrovsky E. Aberrant p53 expression predicts clinical resistance to Cisplatin-based chemotherapy in locally advanced non-small cell lung cancer. Cancer Res 55:5038–5042, 1995.
53. Zhang WW, Fang X, Mazin W, French BA, Georges RN, Roth JA. High-efficiency transfer and high-level expression of wild-type p53 in human lung cancer cells mediated by recombinant adenovirus. Cancer Gene Ther 1:5–13, 1994.
54. Fujiwara T, Grimm EA, Mukhopudhyay T, Cai DW, Owen-Schaub LB, Roth JA. A retroviral wild-type p53 expression vector penetrates human lung cancer spheroids and inhibits growth by inducing apoptosis. Cancer Res 53:4129–4133, 1993.
55. Zhang NW, Alemany R, Wang J, Koch PG, Ordonez NG, Roth JA. Safety evaluation of Ad5CMV-p53 in vitro and in vivo. Hum Gene Ther 6:155–164, 1994.
56. Fujiwara T, Grimm EA, Mukhopadhyay T, Zhang UW, Owen-Schaub LB, Roth JA. Introduction of chemosensitivity in human lung cancer cells in vivo by adenovirus mediated transfer of wild-type p53 gene. Cancer Res 54:2287–2291, 1994.

3. Molecular and surgical advances in pediatric tumors

Cynthia A. Corpron and Richard J. Andrassy

Introduction

Before the 1950s, less than a third of children with Wilms' tumor, rhabdomyosarcoma (RMS), or neuroblastoma survived. Because of the rarity of these tumors, no single institution could collect enough patients for randomized trials. In the United States, the pediatric cancer study groups joined forces to create the National Wilms' Tumor Study Group (NWTS) in 1969 and the Intergroup Rhabdomyosarcoma Study Committee (IRS) in 1972. Protocols to treat neuroblastoma have been developed by both the Children's Cancer Group (CCG) and the Pediatric Oncology Group (POG). The multinational Société Internationale d'Oncologie Pédiatrique (SIOP) studies form a European counterpart to these groups. The protocols used by these groups that employ multimodality therapy including multiagent chemotherapy, have led to the current long-term survival approaching 40% in neuroblastoma [1], 70% in RMS [2], and 95% in Wilms' tumor [3]. Each group continues to modify risk-adapted therapy based on identified prognostic factors. Recent identifications of molecular level differences may allow for further stratification of risk and adaptation of therapy to maximize survival while minimizing therapy.

Wilms' tumor

Introduction

Wilms' tumor represents approximately 6% of all pediatric cancers [4]. In North America, the annual incidence of Wilms' tumor is approximately seven to either patients per million children. One child in 10,000 will develop a Wilms' tumor, and approximately 350 cases a year are identified in the United States. Ninety-eight percent of children are 7 years of age or younger at the time of diagnosis. Survival approaching 95% can be expected using current multimodality therapy in these children [3].

Raphael E. Pollock (ed.), SURGICAL ONCOLOGY. Copyright © 1997. Kluwer Academic Publishers. ISBN 0-7923-9900-5. All rights reserved.

Staging of Wilms tumor

The staging system used in the National Wilms' Tumor Study (NWTS) is based on extent of disease and is performed after exploration at the time of surgery and histologic examination of resected specimens. Patients are staged by extent of disease, as described in Table 1 [5]. Analysis of the NWTS studies has allowed separation of the histologic/pathologic subtypes of Wilms' tumors by predicted prognosis. The NWTS classifies tumors into favorable or unfavorable histologic subtypes [6]. Anaplastic Wilms' tumors and clear cell sarcomas of the kidney (CCSK) are designated as unfavorable histologic subtypes. CCSK has a particularly poor prognosis unless doxorubicin is included in treatment. Other histologies, including mesoblastic nephromas, are included in favorable histologic subtypes.

Molecular genetics of Wilms' tumors

In 1972, Knudson and Strong proposed a model to explain bilateral presentation and younger ages seen in patients with familial Wilms' tumor [7]. Their model suggested that tumor formation depended on two genetic events, a constitutional lesion, inherited from a parent or resulting from a spontaneous mutation, and a second 'hit' event, which led to tumor development. In sporadic cases, two separate genetic events would have to take place for tumorogenesis. Association between Wilms' tumor, aniridia, genitourinary malformations, and mental retardation (the WAGR syndrome) were first reported in 1964 [8]. Karyotypic analysis of children with this syndrome showed a deletion within the short arm of one copy of chromosome 11 at band p13. Molecular analysis of a series of patients with the WAGR syndrome and a 11p13 deletion allowed identification of several contiguous genes, the PAX 6 gene and the Wilms' tumor suppressor gene WT1 [9]. Loss of one allele of PAX6 causes aniridia [10] and loss or mutation of one allele of WT1 are responsible for genitourinary defects [11] and are the first events in the development of Wilms' tumor. While WT1 mutations are the initial event in Wilms'

Table 1. National Wilms' Tumor Study clinicopathologic staging system

Stage I	Tumor limited to kidney and complete excised. Renal capsule intact. Tumor not ruptured. No residual tumor.
Stage II	Tumor extends beyond kidney but is completely removed. There is penetration of the renal capsule and vessels may be infiltrated or contain tumor thrombus. The tumor may have been biopsied or have had a local tumors spill confined to the flank.
Stage III	Residual tumor confined to the abdomen. Hilar, periaortic, or distant lymph nodes are involved, or there has been diffuse peritoneal rupture of contamination, or tumor has grown through peritoneal surface, or tumor is not completely resectable.
Stage IV	Hematogenous metastases.
Stage V	Bilateral renal involvement at diagnosis.

tumor development in the WAGR syndrome, only 6 of 98 sporadic Wilms' tumors showed WT1 mutations [12]. Denys-Drash syndrome (DDS) involves predisposition to Wilms' tumor, intersex disorders, and mesangial sclerosis. These patients also have WT1 constitutional mutations. However, the severe phenotypic changes suggest that the effect of the WT1 mutation is a dysfunctional rather than a nonfunctional WT1 protein.

The formation of a physical complex by p53 and WT1 proteins was recently described [13]. In the absence of functioning p53, the transcriptional activating activity of WT1 appears to be potentiated. Mutations of the *p53* tumor suppressor gene have been identified in 4 patients with anaplastic histology, while 92 patients with favorable histology lacked *p53* mutations [14].

A second putative Wilms' tumor gene has been suggested by loss of heterozygosity of chromosome 11p15 [15]. This gene has not been isolated but has been named *WT2*. Loss of this allele has been associated with Beckwith-Wiedemann syndrome (BWS), which is characterized by overgrowth, hemihypertrophy, macroglossia, hyperinsulinemic hypoglycemia, and a predisposition to Wilms' tumor development. Insulin-like growth factor II gene encodes a growth factor expressed in fetal kidney and in Wilms' tumors, and is located on chromosome 11p15 [16]. Increased expression of this growth factor resulting from alterations at this site may predispose children to the development of Wilms' tumors. Studies of families with an autosomal dominantly inherited Wilms' tumor in whom 11p13 and 11p15 have been excluded suggest at least one other gene causes predisposition to Wilms' tumors [17].

Loss of heterozygosity studies [18] indicate that deletions of chromosome 16 occur in 20% of Wilms' tumors, and analysis of 232 patients from the National Wilms' tumors study (NWTS) [19] suggests that tumor-specific loss was associated with decreased survival. Deletions at chromosome 1p may also predict a decreased survival [18].

Surgical treatment of Wilms' tumor

Surgical excision is integral to the treatment of Wilms' tumor. The surgeon plays an important role in staging at the time of operation. Incorrect staging can lead to inappropriate therapy. NWTS-4 requires initial nephrectomy for resectable tumors. In NWTS, patients are staged after nephrectomy or identification of distant metastases. Patients with stage I and II, favorable histology tumors, are treated with vincristine and actinomycin D without abdominal irradiation. Stage III patients have abdominal irradiation added, as do those stage IV patients whose abdominal tumors have stage III features. Whole-lung irradiation is added for stage IV patients with lung metastases. Anthracycline (doxorubicin) therapy is included for those patients with favorable histology stage III and IV, anaplastic histology stage II–IV, and CCSK stages I–IV.

Recommendations for surgical treatment include radical nephrectomy through a transperitoneal incision. Of primary importance is the prevention of tumor rupture and spill. Before resection of the primary tumor, the contralateral kidney should be examined by incising Gerota's fascia and palpating the kidney. Data from the NWTS [20] show that contralateral lesions may have unfavorable histology, even if the primary tumor histology was favorable. Isolation of the hilar vessels should be performed, if possible, before mobilization of the kidney. If a large tumor makes identification of vascular anatomy difficult, isolation of the vessels is not necessary and may lead to increased risk of vascular injury. An adequate sample of hilar, periaortic, and any clinically involved nodes should be biopsied. The site of excised nodes, the tumor bed, and any suspicious areas should be marked with clips. If the tumor cannot be removed with adequate margins, resection of contiguous structures may be justified, but only if the tumor can be completely resected.

Intracaval involvement occurs in approximately 4% of Wilms' tumors [21] and should be evaluated prior to operation. Although tumor thrombi can usually be removed by approaches such as thoracoabdominal exposure and infrahepatic caval incision, or by median sternotomy with cardiac bypass, the results of preoperative chemotherapy from NWTS suggest this is a more useful approach.

The approach of the Société Internationale d'Oncologie Pédiatrique (SIOP) is somewhat different from that used in NWTS. The SIOP-1 [22] study randomized 397 patients with nonmetastatic tumors to receive either prenephrectomy radiotherapy or immediate surgery. Survival was similar in both groups. SIOP-2 [23] added a 5-day course of actinomycin D before surgical resection. Tumor rupture occurred in 5% of pretreated patients and in 20% of those who underwent initial resection. SIOP-5 [24] compared preoperative chemotherapy with preoperative radiotherapy and found no difference in the rates of tumor rupture.

SIOP-6 [26] treated all patients with a presumptive diagnosis with preoperative chemotherapy. Fifty-two percent of patients were found to have stage I disease after preoperative treatment and were treated postoperatively with vincristine and actinomycin D. Stage II patients with negative lymph nodes received similar chemotherapy and were randomized to receive or not receive radiotherapy. For stage II node-negative patients, 7 of 50 non-irradiated patients versus 1 of 58 patients who had undergone irradiation had an abdominal relapse. This result led to intensification of therapy, adding epirubicin for stage II node-negative patients. With these preoperative regimens, 84% of stage I–III patients do not receive radiotherapy. Since by the SIOP protocols tumors are not biopsied before chemotherapy, 1% of patients are treated for benign tumors [25]. The current SIOP study uses preoperative chemotherapy for all tumors.

Stage V or bilateral tumors pose a special problem in management [26]. Approximately 5% of patients have bilateral tumors. Since preservation of adequate renal tissue for normal renal function is paramount, current NWTS recommendations involve bilateral biopsy. The largest lesion may not have the least favorable histologic subtype. Complete excision of both tumors may be considered if two thirds of the total renal parenchyma can be preserved, but in most cases biopsy should be followed by chemotherapy. A second-look procedure is performed within 6 months of chemotherapy, and if all tumor can be removed leaving adequate renal parenchyma, resection is performed. If this is not possible, biopsies are repeated and chemotherapy and radiation are continued. A third exploration with a bilateral renal-sparing procedure should be performed within 6 more months. New techniques, such as intraoperative radiation therapy or bench surgery, can be considered in difficult cases. Transplantation has been associated with a high rate of local recurrence and should be avoided if at all possible.

Surgical treatment of metastatic disease

The lung is the most common site of recurrence of Wilms' tumors [27]. Patients with limited, one-lung relapses had over 60% survival in NWTS-1 [28]. Relapse should be confirmed by biopsy. This is usually followed by intensified chemotherapy, with either surgical resection of lung metastases or whole-lung irradiation. Both of these strategies have produced long-term survival. Abdominal, liver, mediastinum, and brain recurrences are associated with a very poor prognosis and should be treated with initial biopsy, intensified chemotherapy, and aggressive local therapy with surgical excision and radiotherapy [28,29].

Surgical complications

Review of NWTS showed a surgical complication incidence of 19.8% [30]. Small bowel obstruction, hemorrhage, wound infection, and vascular injury were the most common. Advanced local tumor may predispose the patient to vascular injuries, especially injuries to the superior mesenteric vessels. Large tumors may displace the mesenteric vessels, and they may be misidentified as renal vessels. Decisions about radical resection in very large tumors should include consideration of biopsy only, followed by postoperative chemotherapy and re-exploration.

Further directions

The SIOP and NWTS studies continue to identify subgroups of patients in whom treatment can be reduced without affecting survival. A subgroup of patients with stage-I, favorable-histology tumors that are less that 550 grams in weight will undergo only resection in NWTS V. Identification of molecular alterations may allow further identification of subgroups of patients with poorer prognosis for more intensive therapy. Biologic tumor markers such as serum renin may allow for better screening and follow-up. Further investigation into the role of oncogenes may allow for molecular level–directed therapy in the treatment of Wilms tumors.

Rhabdomyosarcoma

Introduction

Rhabdomyosarcoma (RMS) is the most common soft tissue sarcoma of childhood and is diagnosed in about 250 children a year in the United States [4]. Prior to the 1960s, children with RMS were treated with local therapy, with or without single-agent chemotherapy, and less than a third survived. The protocols used by the IRS include multiagent chemotherapy, radiotherapy, and surgical treatment, and have led to current long-term overall survival approaching 70% [2]. The IRS continues to modify risk-adapted therapy based on identified prognostic factors. Recent identifications of molecular level differences may allow for further stratification of risk and adapation of therapy to maximize survival while minimizing therapy.

Genetic and molecular features of rhabdomyosarcoma

Evaluation of DNA content in RMS tumors has shown that hyperdiploid tumors are usually embryonal and those with hyperdiploid DNA content may be more sensitive to chemotherapy and irradiation than embryonal tumors without this feature [31]. Tumors with tetraploid DNA content are almost always alveolar and may have a worse prognosis [32]. The value of ploidy as a prognostic factor in RMS is under investigation in a current IRS study.

Embryonal and alveolar tumors can often be distinguished by structural chromosomal abnormalities. Alveolar tumors often have a translocation involving chromosomes 2 and 13, the t(2;13)(q35;q14), which affects the PAX3 and FKHR genes [33,34]. The reciprocal translocation fuses the PAX3 gene to the FKHR gene, and this may result in inappropriate activation of PAX3 transcriptional targets, resulting in dysregulation of cell growth. Several alveolar RMS tumors have had another translocation, t(1;13)(p36;q14) [35], which results in fusion of PAX7 to the FKHR gene, which may result in similar dysregulation of cell growth. Identification of these translocations by reverse-transcriptase polymerase chain reactions of fluorescence in situ hybridization techniques may allow improved identifications of patients with poorer prognoses.

Other genetic abnormalities have been identified in RMS. Mutations of the p53 oncogene have been identified in both RMS tumors and RMS cell lines, and may be present in as many as 50% of tumors [36]. Dias et al. showed amplification of NMYC in 4 of 6 alveolar RMS tumors but no embryonal RMS tumors [37]. No amplification of CMYC was identified in this study. Mutations of the NRAS and KRAS oncogenes have been reported in embryonal tumors [38].

Table 2. IRS Clinical Group classification

Group I	Tumor resected with microscopically negative margins
Group IIa	Tumor grossly resected with microscopic residual tumor
Group IIb	Involvement of regional lymph nodes that have been completely resected
Group IIc	Involvement of nodes but microscopic residual in nodes or margins remains after resection
Group III	Gross residual tumor
Group IV	Distant metastases

Staging of rhabdomyosarcoma

The IRS studies employ a postoperative staging system that classifies patients into clinical groups [39] (Table 2) by completeness of surgical resection and presence of lymphatic and distant metastases. Critics of this system argue that extent of resection is influenced by the surgeon, the surgical approach used, and the adequate evaluation of margin status and nodal status. As responses to preoperative chemotherapy improved, the trend was toward less aggressive resection or amputation. Patients who may have undergone an aggressive resection or amputation in the early IRS studies may undergo initial biopsy and preoperative adjuvant treatment in hopes of avoiding extensive resection. This somewhat subjective shift in classification makes it somewhat difficult to compare results across the IRS studies.

Several authors [40] have suggested staging systems using pretreatment prognostic factors based on the UICC tumor-node-metastasis (TNM) system that include local invasiveness, size, nodal, and distant metastases. Lawrence et al. [41] evaluated this approach using IRS data and showed that this staging system was also predictive of survival. However, in their analysis survival was significantly different in patients with various tumor sites. In 1992 (IRS IV), the IRS began prospectively evaluating a TNM staging system that included tumor site, tumor size, invasion into adjacent structures, and the presence of nodal and distant metastases. As staging improves, therapy can be decreased for those patients in low-risk groups and increased for those at high risk of recurrence. Results from IRS I–III confirmed that survival of similar group patients is different at various sites [2,4,42].

Surgical treatment of rhabdomyosarcoma

The surgical management of RMS is site specific. The goal of surgical treatment is complete resection with preservation of function. The ability to achieve complete resection varies by site and is highest in extremity tumors and lowest in head-and-neck tumors. The efforts of the Intergroup Rhabdomyosarcoma Studies have led to several changes in the surgical treatment of these tumors. Hays et al. [43] analyzed 154 patients with microscopic residual disease after initial surgical resection who were enrolled in the IRS study. Survival was significantly improved for those patients who underwent re-excision before adjunctive therapy when compared with either the group with microscopic residual tumor who did not undergo re-resection or those who had initial complete resection with negative margins. This study suggests that the evaluation of margin status may be difficult, especially if the diagnosis of cancer was unsuspected at the time of initial surgery, and the IRS recommends re-resection for negative margins in any patients in whom completeness of resection is in question.

Because of an emphasis on decreasing extent of surgical resection, IRS III protocols suggested re-exploration after initial preoperative chemotherapy. Of 257 patients with gross residual tumor after initial surgery, 109 underwent a second-look operation [44]. Although re-operation confirmed a complete response in 88%, 12% of patients with a clinically complete response had residual tumor. Seventy-four percent of patients with a clinical partial or nonresponse were categorized as a complete response after operation. Surgical re-resection was responsible for the improvement to a complete response in 28% of patients with a clinical partial response and in 43% of patients with no clinical response. The survival of children who were recategorized from nonresponse to complete response after a second-look operation was not significantly different from those who achieved a complete response after chemotherapy and radiation. As the extent of surgical excision is decreased, many continue to advocate repeated surgical re-evaluation. In contrast, Godzinski et al. [45] from the International Society of Pediatric Oncology reported on 92 patients who had initial biopsy and then only chemotherapy for local control. The rates of local recurrence was not significantly different for biopsied and nonbiopsied patients (51% and 48%, respectively) and suggest that a negative biopsy may not predict risk of relapse, especially when chemotherapy only is used for local therapy. The recommended surgical treatment by site is detailed later.

Extremity rhabdomyosarcoma

Extremity tumors represent approximately 20% of pediatric rhabdomyosarcomas. While many of these patients could be placed in group I by complete resection and/or amputation, there has been an increasing trend towards preoperative chemotherapy and radiation and limb-sparing surgery. Today, less than 5% of patients are treated by amputation. Analysis of the experience with extremity sarcomas in IRS-III [46] confirmed that complete excision with gross and microscopically negative margins is optimal in the treatment of children with extremity rhabdomyosarcomas. When 51 patients with incomplete resection (groups IIa and III) of a distal tumor were compared with those who had complete resection (group I) of distal tumors (many by amputation), the survival difference approached significance. While limb-sparing surgery is very desirable, the effect of less aggressive resection on survival remains unclear. This study also reported that when patients who had histologically proven negative nodes were compared with those who had only clinically negative nodes, survival was significantly better for the first group. This result suggests that histologic evaluation of lymph node status is important in the staging of extremity sarcomas.

Vaginal, vulvar, and uterine rhabdomyosarcomas

Before 1975 children with vaginal or uterine rhabdomyosarcomas were treated with initial radical surgery followed by chemotherapy and irradiation. Starting in 1976 (IRS II) [47], primary hysterectomy and vaginectomy was abandoned for primary chemotherapy with or without radiotherapy, followed by surgical re-exploration. Persistent microscopic tumor required delayed hysterectomy/vaginectomy or partial vaginectomy in most patients. Five patients with a local recurrence had clinical group III tumors and had undergone biopsy only or incomplete gross resection before adjuvant therapy. None of these patients had received doxorubicin as part of their chemotherapy.

In IRS III, all patients with vaginal primaries were treated on a protocol that included vincristine, dactinomycin, cyclophosphamide, and Adriamycin (doxorubicin). This approach included second-look surgery at 20 weeks. The results of IRS III [48] showed 20 patients enrolled with clinical group III tumors. Of these, two patients died of therapy-related complications and one died after achieving a complete response. All of the remaining 17 patients were alive without evidence of disease at the time of the report. Ten of 17 had biopsy as their only surgical resection. Four of these patients underwent irradiation. Six of the seven patients who underwent a secondary resection had no viable tumor found in the resected specimen. The specimen in the seventh patient showed only maturing rhabdomyoblasts. Three clinical group IIa patients (with microscopic residual disease) underwent chemotherapy without further resection. Two of three had irradiation and all survived. All three vulvar tumors could be resected, one received radiotherapy, and all survived. Similar results were suggested by survival of five group III patients with uterine RMS treated with preoperative chemotherapy and/or radiotherapy [49]. Only two of the five required hysterectomy and/or vaginectomy, and all survive.

Bladder rhabdomyosarcoma

The advances of the IRS committee have also led to decreased surgery for children with bladder RMS. Historically, many of these patients were treated with anterior pelvic exenterations. With improvements in chemotherapy, many children underwent only total cystectomy. Hays et al. [50] reported on the results of partial and total cystectomy for bladder RMS. The survival of 40 patients treated with partial cystectomy was 78.5%, while 79.5% of 131 patients with total cystectomy survived. Similar results have been reported by other authors [51]. This suggests that partial cystectomy is a viable alternative to total cystectomy for bladder RMS when the tumor site makes it anatomically feasible.

Paratesticular rhabdomyosarcoma

Surgical treatment of paratesticular RMS requires radical inguinal orchiectomy. Scrotal resection is only used in patients with tumor fixation or if biopsy was done through the scrotum. Traditionally, surgical evaluation of retroperitoneal nodal status has been included [52]. Because of the complications associated with retroperitoneal node dissection (vascular injuries and ejaculatory impotence) [53], the effectiveness of systemic therapy in irradicating nodal micrometastases, and the improved imaging to evaluate retroperitoneal nodes, several authors [54,55] have suggested that routine retroperitoneal nodal dissection is not needed in paratesticular RMS. Paratesticular RMS from IRS III were reviewed by Wiener et al. [56]. Their results describe 127 patients with paratesticular RMS. Retroperitoneal nodal dissection was performed in 93% of patients. The results suggest that radiologic evaluation is not totally reliable (only 57% of imaging studies predicted histologically proven nodal metastases. Since patients were treated on the basis of histologic nodal status, results of treatment by radiologic staging are not clear. Olive et al. [55] have suggested that systemic chemotherapy may adequately treat micrometastatic retroperitoneal disease, but this concept cannot be evaluated by their study or by the IRS results.

Head-and-neck rhabdomyosarcoma

Head-and-neck sites are the most frequent site of involvement with RMS. The development of skull base surgery has allowed resection of a larger percentage of tumors. Patients with orbital tumors have over 90% survival with only biopsy, chemotherapy, and irradiation [2]. The survival of patients with parameningeal sites is lower but has been improved with the addition of cranial irradiation and intrathecal chemotherapy. Superficial head-and-neck sites are more likely to be primarily resectable, and survival in these patients approaches 85%.

Chest wall, trunk, and paraspinal rhabdomyosarcomas

Survival is significantly lower for patients with trunk, thoracic, or paraspinal tumors [2]. The operative procedure of choice for chest wall tumors and abdominal wall tumors is wide local resection with chest wall resection as needed. Because of the high rate of local recurrence, irradiation should be included in all but the smallest tumors. Patients with paraspinal tumors have less than 50% survivals despite very aggressive therapy [57]. Very high rates of recurrence indicate that aggressive local therapy as well as systemic therapy is needed in these patients.

Surgery for lung metastases in rhabdomyosarcoma

The role of surgery in treatment of lung metastases from rhadomyosarcoma is not clear. Several series [58,59] have described resection of lung metastases, but none have evaluated this question in a prospective manner. Results suggest that surgical therapy must be combined with chemotherapy and/or irradiation for successful treatment of lung metastases in rhabdomyosarcoma.

Future directions in therapy of rhabdomyosarcoma

Many questions remain in surgical treatment of RMS. The newly adapted TMN staging system may allow for more objective comparisons between treatments. The comparison of chemotherapy, radiotherapy, and surgery for local control has yet to be performed. The role of lymph node dissection for paratesticular and extremity tumors needs clarification. Surgical therapy may be combined with radiotherapy in new ways using intraoperative radiation therapy [60] and intraoperative placement of catheters for brachytherapy [61]. New treatment strategies, such as high-does chemotherapy with stem cell salvage, may require surgical debulking of the tumor. Each advance in adjunctive therapy requires its evaluation in comparison and combination with surgical therapy. The continued advances in identification of molecular level alterations may allow for better staging of risk and of therapies directed at a molecular level.

Neuroblastoma

Introduction

Neuroblastoma is the most common extracranial malignant solid tumor seen in children [4]. Approximately 500 new cases are diagnosed yearly in the United States. Sixty percent of all cases present in children younger than 2 years, and 97% occur in children younger than 10 years. The higher incidence in young children may be affected by the spontaneous regression seen in some infants, even those with disseminated disease.

Diagnosis

Patients with neuroblastoma may present in many ways. The most common presentation is pain secondary to primary tumor or involvement of bone by metastatic disease. Tumor may cause proptosis and ecchymosis of the orbit. Patients with mediastinal tumors may present with Horner's syndrome. Paraneoplastic syndromes with secretion of a vasoactive intestinal peptide may cause watery diarrhea [62], and children may present with opsoclonus, myoclonus, and ataxia from an acute cerebellar encephalopathy. Suprisingly, this opsoclonus-myoclonus syndrome is most common in low-stage disease [63]. Diagnosis is made by biopsy or by tumor cells in bone marrow combined with elevations of urinary cathecholamine (dopamine, vanillylmandelic acid, or homovanillic acid) excretion.

Screening

Because the diagnosis of neuroblastoma is suggested by elevations of urinary catecholamine excretion, several studies are underway using this technique to screen children for neuroblastoma. Preliminary results [64,65] suggest that most cases are detected in infants who are asymptomatic and that these tumors may be biologically favorable and undergo a high rate of spontaneous regression. Since it seems that many of the tumors identified may have undergone spontaneous regression without treatment, it is unclear if the screening programs have impacted on actual survival. Screening at older ages may identify more children who would benefit from intervention.

Molecular genetics

The majority of neuroblastomas have dipoid karyotypes [68]. The hyperdipoid and near-tripolid tumors in infants frequently have whole chromosome gains with few structural rearrangements. These patients have favorable outcomes. Structural rearrangements are seen in near-diploid tumors in all ages and in hyperdiploid tumors in older patients. These patients have less favorable outcomes.

Deletion of the short arm of chromosome 1(1p) is the most frequently identified cytogenetic alteration in human neuroblastomas and cell lines [66]. This deletion has been identified in 70% of cases. The region of deletion has been identified at the distal end of the short arm of chromosome 1 for 1p36.1 to 1p36.2. Loss of heterozygosity has also been identified for the long arm of chromosome 14 (in up to 50% of cases), which may represent loss of another suppressor gene [67].

Oncogene amplification and expression

The NMYC oncogene has been mapped to the short arm of chromosome 2 [68]. Amplification of NMYC has been identified in 20–30% of children with neuroblastoma and is strongly associated with advanced stage and poor prognosis [69,70]. Studies [71] show that MYCN copy number does not change during the course of the disease, and no patients with a single NMYC copy have developed amplification later in their disease course. Studies [72] have examined HRAS expression in neuroblastoma and have suggested that higher expression may predict a favorable outcome. Overexpression of *p53* has been identified in neuroblastoma cell lines and in tumor specimens from undifferentiated tumors [73]. The role of *p53* in neuroblastoma remains unclear.

Neuronal differentiation markers

Studies [74,75] have shown that increase expression of high-affinity nerve growth factor receptor (gp140^{TRK-A}) correlates significantly with tumors that have a single copy of NMYC and a favorable outcome, while lack of expression of this nerve growth factor correlates significantly with NMYC amplification and poor prognosis. Of special interest is a study [76] showing that transfection of an exogenous TRK-A gene into a neuroblastoma cell line restored the ability of the tumor cells to differentiate in response to nerve growth factors.

Staging

A histologic grading system developed by Chatten et al. [77] has been verified prospectively to predict outcome. Several staging systems have been used to classify patients with neuroblastoma, including those of the Childrens Cancer Study Group, the St. Jude Children's Research Hospital, and the American Joint Committee on Cancer. A combination of these systems is under prospective evaluation. This system focuses of extent of surgical excision and the presence of nodal and distant metastases. Stage 4s is identified as those patients under 1 year of age with tumor dissemination limited to liver skin and/ or bone marrow.

Treatment

Treatment of low-risk patients (those with localized tumor, no or unilateral nodal involvement, and a single copy of MYCN) have an excellent prognosis when primarily treated with surgical resection. Neither radiation nor chemotherapy has been shown to affect survival in this group [78]. Older children with localized tumors and amplification of NMYC are at higher risk and may benefit from more aggressive therapy. Several groups of patients are at intermediate risk. Children under 1 year of age at diagnosis with single copies of NMYC, with disseminated disease (stage IV), or children at any age with favorable Shimada histology, single-copy NMYC, and tumor extending across the midline or with bilateral nodal metastases (stage III) have been treated with surgical resection, local radiation therapy for unresectable disease, and moderately intensive chemotherapy, with survivals of 80–90% [79]. Children with disseminated disease limited to the liver, bone marrow, and skin (stage IVs) may be treated with supportive care without chemotherapy, with survivals of 75–90% [80]. Therapy should be directed at control of symptoms of the tumor by single-agent chemotherapy or limited hepatic irradiation.

High-risk patients include all patients older than 1 year with stage IV disease, stage III patients with unfavorable Shimada histology, and infants with stage IV disease and NMYC amplification. Long-term survival in these patients is only 30% [81] despite multimodality therapy. Current studies are evaluating the use of high-dose ablative therapy and bone marrow transplantation in these patients.

Surgical resection can be curative in localized neuroblastoma. The role of resection in more extensive tumors must be carefully evaluated. While studies [82–84] have suggested that delayed resection of advanced-stage tumors favorably affects survival, surgical exploration also allows determination of response to therapy. Large tumors may require techniques such as hemodilution, hypothermia, and circulatory arrest with cardiopulmonary bypass. The use of lasers, the argon coagulator, and the cavitron ultrasonic dissector [85] has been helpful in the resection of extensive tumors. The goal of these resections is complete resection, with or without microscopic residual tumor. Intraoperative radiation therapy [86] has been suggested in situations where gross resections cannot be accomplished. Intraoperative radiation therapy added to surgical debulking is currently being evaluated in a randomized trial.

Urologic injuries and hemorrhage are the most common complications after extensive resections for neuroblastoma [87]. Nephrectomy was required in 24 of 175 patients reported by a recent CCG study. Resection of debulking of primary or distant disease resulted in fewer local recurrences after high-dose chemotherapy and bone marrow transplantation [88].

New therapies

Several interesting therapies have been developed to treat neuroblastoma. Treatment with radiolabeled ^{131}I-MIBG has been used in over 300 patients with neuroblastoma refractory to other treatment, with a 30% response rate [89]. Myelosuppression at higher doses may theoretically require bone marrow transplantation. Phase I and II trials of monoclonal antibodies to GD_2 ganglinoside have been tested in patients with recurrent disease after bone marrow transplant [90]. While promising responses were seen, addition of IL-2 may further stimulate host responses [91].

Differentiating agents such as retinoic acid have induced maturation in neuroblastoma cell lines in vitro [92]. Trials have shown responses in phase I and II trials, and a randomized phase III trial is now underway [93].

New approaches for treatment of neuroblastoma continue to be developed. Molecular-directed therapy, such as upregulation of TRK-A expression, have be done in the laboratory and may lead to clinical applications. Investigation continues to attempt to identify factors responsible for the spontaneous regression seen in stage IVs neuroblastoma, and once identified may allow for even more successful treatment of neuroblastoma.

References

1. Brodeur GM, Castleberry RP. Neuroblastoma. In Pizzo PA, Poplack DG (eds). Principles and Practice of Pediatric Oncology, 2nd ed. Philadelphia: JB Lippincott, 1993, pp 739–767.

2. Crist W, Gehan EA, Ragab AH, et al. The Intergroup Rhabdomyosarcoma Study-III. J Clin Oncol 13:610–630, 1995.
3. D'Angio GJ, Breslow N, Beckwith JB, et al. Treatment of Wilms' tumors. Results of the Third National Wilms' Tumor Study. Cancer 64:349–360, 1989.
4. Blair V, Birch HM. Patterns and temporal trends in the incidence of malignant disease in children: II. Eur J Cancer 30A:1498–1511, 1994.
5. Breslow NE, Palmer NF, Hill LR, et al. Wilms' tumors: Prognostic factors for patients without metastases at diagnosis. Cancer 41:1577–1589, 1978.
6. Beckwith JB, Palmer NF. Histopathology and prognosis of Wilms' tumor. Results from the first National Wilms' Tumors Study. Cancer 41:1937–1948, 1978.
7. Knudson AG, Strong LC. Mutation and cancer: A model for Wilms' tumors of the kidney. J Natl Cancer Inst 48:313–324, 1972.
8. Miller RW, Fraumeni JF, Manning MD. Association of Wilms' tumor with aniridia, hemihypertrophy and other congenital anomalies. N Engl J Med 270:922–928, 1964.
9. Riccardi VM, Sujansky E, Smith AC, et al. Chromosomal imbalance in the aniridia-Wilms' tumor association: 11p interstitial deletion. Pediatrics 61:604–610, 1978.
10. Ton CC, Hirvonen H, Miwa H, et al. Positional cloning and characterization of a paired box- and homeobox-containing gene from the aniridia region. Cell 67:1059–1074, 1991.
11. Huang A, Campbell CE, Bontetta I, et al. Tissue, developmental and tumor-specific expression of divergent transcripts in Wilms tumors. Science 250:991–994, 1990.
12. Varanasi R, Bardeesy N, Ghahremani M, et al. Fine structure analysis of the WT1 gene in sporadic Wilms' tumor. Proc Natl Acad Sci USA 91:3554–3558, 1994.
13. Maheswaran S, Park S, Bernard A, et al. Physical and functional interaction between WT1 and p53 proteins. Proc Natl Acad Sci USA 89:5100–5104, 1992.
14. Bardeesy N, Falkoff D, Petruzzi M-J, et al. Anaplastic Wilms' tumour, a subtype displaying poor prognosis, harbours p53 gene mutations. Nature Genet 7:91–98, 1994.
15. Koufos A, Grundy P, Morgan K, et al. Familial Weidemann-Beckwith syndrome and a second Wilms' tumor locus both map to 11p15,5. Am J Hum Genet 44:711–719, 1989.
16. Ogawa O, Eccles MR, Szeto J, et al. Relaxation of insulin-like growth factor II gene imprinting implicated in Wilms' tumor. Nature 362:749–751, 1993.
17. Huff V, Compton DA, Chao L, et al. Lack of linkage of familial Wilms' tumor to chromosomal band 11p13. Nature 336:377–378, 1988.
18. Coppes MJ, Bonetta L, Huang A, et al. Loss of heterozygosity mapping in Wilms tumor indicates the involvement of three distinct regions and a limited role for nondisjunction or mitotic recombination. Genes Chromosome Cancer 5:326–324, 1992.
19. Grundy PE, Telzerow PE, Breslow N, et al. Loss of heterozygosity for chromosomes 16q and 1p in Wilms' tumors predicts an adverse outcome. Cancer Res 54:2331–2333, 1994.
20. Blute ML, Kelalis PP, Offord KP, et al. Bilateral Wilms' tumor. J Urol 138:968–973, 1987.
21. Ritchey ML, Kelalis PP, Haase GM, et al. Preoperative therapy for intracaval and atrial extension of Wilms tumor. Cancer 71:4104–4110, 1993.
22. Lemerle J, Voute PA, Tournade MF, et al. Preoperative versus postoperative radiotherapy, single versus multiple courses of actinomycin D in the treatment of Wilms tumors. Preliminary results of a controlled clinical trial conducted by the International Society of Paediatric Oncology (SIOP). Cancer 38:647–654, 1976.
23. Lemerle J, Voute PA, Tournade MF, et al. Effectiveness of preoperative chmoetherapy in Wilms' tumor: Results of an International Society of Paediatric Oncolcogy (SIOP) clinical trial. J Clin Oncol 10:604–609, 1983.
24. Jereb B, Burgers MV, Tournade M-F, et al. Radiotherapy in the SIOP (International Society of Paediatric Oncology) nephroblastoma studies: A review. Med Pediatr Oncol 22:221–227, 1994.
25. deKraker J, Weitzman S, Voute PA, et al. Preoperative strategies in the management of Wilms tumor. Hematol Oncol Clinic North Am 9:1275–1285, 1995.
26. Bishop HC, Teft M, Evans A, et al. Survival in bilateral Wilms' tumor — Review of 30

National Wilms' Tumor Study cases. J Pediatr Surg 12:631–638, 1977.

27. Breslow N, Churchill G, Beckwith JB, et al. Prognosis for Wilms' tumor patients with non-metastatic disease at diagnosis. Results of the Second National Wilms' Tumor Study. J Clin Oncol 3:521–531, 1985.

28. Butow WW, Breslow NE, Palmer NF, et al. Prognosis in children with Wilms' tumor prior to or following primary treatment. Results from the first National Wilms' Tumor Study. Am J Clin Oncol 5:339–347, 1982.

29. Burgers JMV, Tournade MR, Bey P, et al. Abdominal recurrences in Wilms tumours: A report of the SIOP Wilms tumour trial and studies. Radiother Oncol 5:175–182, 1986.

30. Ritchey ML, Kelalis PP, Breslow N, et al. Surgical complications following nephrectomy for Wilms' tumor: A report of National Wilms' Study — 3. Surg Gynecol Obstet 175:507–514, 1992.

31. Pappo AS, Crist WM, Kuttesch J, et al. Tumor cell DNA content predicts outcome in children and adolescents with clinical group III embryonal rhabdomyosarcoma. J Clin Oncol 1:1901–1905, 1993.

32. Shapiro DN, Parham, Douglass, et al. Relationship of tumor cell ploidy to histologic subtype and treatment outcome in children and adolescents with unresectable rhabdomyosarcoma. J Clin Oncol 9:159–166, 1991.

33. Shapiro DN, Sublett JE, Li B, et al. Fusion of PAX3 to a member of the forkhead family of transcription factors in human alveolar rhabdomyosarcoma. Cancer Res 53:5108–5112, 1993.

34. Galili N, Davis RJ, Fredericks WJ, et al. PAX3 in the solid tumor alveolar rhabdomyosarcoma. Nature Genet 5:230–235, 1993.

35. Biegel JA, Meek RS, Parmiter AH, et al. Chromosomal translocation t(1;13)(p36;q14) in a case of rhabdomyosarcoma. Genes Chromosome Cancer 3:480–482, 1991.

36. Felix CA, Kappel CC, Mitsudomi T, et al. Frequency and diversity of p53 mutations in childhood rhabdomyosarcoma. Cancer Res 52:2243–2247, 1992.

37. Dias P, Kumar P, Marsden HB, et al. N-myc gene is amplified in alveolar rhabdoyosarcomas (RMS) but not in embryonel RMS. Int J Cancer 45:593–596, 1990.

38. Stratton MR, Fisher C, Gusterson BA, et al. Detection of point mutations in N-ras and K-ras genes of human embryonal rhabdomyosarcomas using oligonucleotide probes and the polymerase chain reaction. Cancer Res 49:6324–6327, 1989.

39. Maurer HM, Beltangady M, Gehan EA, et al. The Intergroup Rhabdomyosarcoma Study—I: A final report. Cancer 61:209–220, 1988.

40. Lawrence W Jr., Hays DM, Heyn R, et al. Surgical lessons from the Intergroup Rhabdomyosarcoma Study (IRS) pertaining to extremity tumors. World J Surg 12:676–684, 1988.

41. Lawrence WJ, Gehan EA, Hays DM, Beltangady M, Maurer HM. Prognostic significance of staging factors of the UICC staging system in childhood rhabdomyosarcoma: A report from the Intergroup Rhabdomyosarcoma Study (IRS-II). J Clin Oncol 5:46–54, 1987.

42. Maurer HM, Gehan EA, Beltangady M, et al. The Intergroup Rhabdomyosarcoma Study — II. Cancer 71:1904–1922, 1993.

43. Hays DM, Lawrence WJ, Wharam M, et al. Primary re-excision for patients with 'microscopic residual' tumor following initial excision of sarcomas of trunk and extremity sites. J Pediatr Surg 24:5–10, 1989.

44. Hays DM, Raney RB, Crist WM, et al. Secondary surgical procedures to evaluate primary tumor status in patients with chemotherapy-responsive stage II and IV sarcomas. A report from the Intergroup Rhabdomyosarcoma Study (IRS). J Pediatr Surg 25:1100–1105, 1990.

45. Godzinski J, Lamant F, Rey A, et al. Value of postchemotherapy bioptical verification of complete clinical remission in previously incompletely resected (stage I and II pT3) malignant mesenchymal tumors in children: International Society of Pediatric Oncology 1984 Malignant Mesenchymal Tumors Study. Med Pediatr Oncol 22:22–26, 1994.

46. Andrassy RJ, Corpron CA, Hays DM, et al. Extremity sarcomas: An analysis of prognostic factors from the Intergroup Rhabdomyosarcoma Study III. J Pediatr Surg 31:191–196, 1996.

47. Hays DM, Shimada H, Raney RB, Jr., et al. Sarcomas of the vagina and uterus: The Intergroup Rhabdomyosarcoma Study. J Pediatr Surg 20:718–724, 1985.
48. Andrassy RJ, Hays DM, Raney RB, et al. Conservative management of vaginal and vulvar pediatric rhabdomyosarcoma: A report from the Intergroup Rhabdomyosarcoma Study III. J Pediatr Surg 30:1034–1037, 1995.
49. Corpron CA, Andrassy RJ, Hays DM, et al. Conservative management of uterine pediatric rhabomyosarcomas: A report from the Intergroup Rhabdomyosarcoma Study III and IV Pilot. J Pediatr Surg 30:942–944, 1995.
50. Hays DM, Raney RB, Wharam MD, et al. Children with vesical rhabdomyosarcoma (RMS) treated by partial cystectomy with neoadjuvant or adjuvant chemotherapy, with or without radiotherapy. A report from the Intergroup Rhabdomyosarcoma Study (IRS) Committee. J Pediatr Hematol Oncol 17:46–52, 1995.
51. Atra A, Ward HC, Aitken, et al. Conservative surgery in multimodal therapy for pelvic rhabdomyosarcoma in children. Br J Cancer 70:1004–1008, 1994.
52. Raney RB Jr., Tefft M, Lawrence W Jr., et al. Paratesticular sarcoma in childhood and adolescence: A report from the Intergroup Rhabdomyosarcoma Studies I and II 1973–1983. Cancer 60:2342–2343, 1987.
53. Heyn R, Raney RB, Hays DM, et al. Late effects of therapy in patients with paratesticualr rhabdomyosarcoma. For the Intergroup Rhabdomyosarcoma Study Committee. J Clin Oncol 10:614–623, 1992.
54. Fossa SD, Qvist H, Stenwig AE, et al. Is postchemotherapy retroperitoneal surgery necessary in patients with nonseminomatous testicular cancer and minimal residual tumors masses? J Clin Oncol 10:569–573, 1992.
55. Olive D, Lamant F, Zucker JM, et al. Paraaortic lymphadenectomy is not necessary in the treatment of localized paratesticular rhabdomysarcoma. Cancer 54:1283–1287, 1984.
56. Wiener ES, Lawrence W, Hays D, et al. Retroperitoneal node biopsy in paratesticular rhabdomyosarcoma. J Pediatr Surg 29:171–178, 1994.
57. Ortega JA, Wharam M, Gehan EA, et al. Clinical features and end results of therapy for children with paraspinal rhabdomyosarcoma: A report of the Intergroup Rhabdomyosarcoma Study. J Clin Oncol 9:796–801, 1991.
58. Temeck BK, Wexler LH, Steinberg SM, McClure LL, Horowitz M, Pass HI. Metastasectomy for sarcomatous pediatric histologies: Results and prognostic factors. Ann Thorac Surg 59:1385–1390, 1995.
59. Jablons DM, Steinberg SM, Roth J, Johnston MR, Rosenberg SA. Metastasectomy for soft tissue sarcoma: Further evidence for efficacy and pronostic indications. J Thor Cardiovasc Surg 97:695–705, 1989.
60. Haase GM, Meagher DP, Jr., McNeeley LK, et al. Electron beam intraoperative radiation therapy for pediatric neoplasms. Cancer 74:740–747, 1994.
61. Nag S, Grecula J, Ruymann FB. Aggressive chemotherapy, organ-preserving surgery, and high-dose-rate remote brachytherapy in the treatment of rhabdomyosarcoma in infants and young children. Cancer 72:2769–2776, 1993.
62. Mitchell CH, Sinatra FR, Crast, et al. Intractable watery diarrhea, ganglionneuroblastoma, and vasoactive intestinal peptide. J Pediatr 89:593–595, 1976.
63. Fisher PG, Wechsler DR, Singer HS. Anti-Hu antibody in a neuroblastoma-associated paraneoplastic syndrome. Pediatr Neurol 10:309–312, 1994.
64. Naito H, Sasaki M, Yamashiro K, et al. Improvement in prognosis of neuroblastoma through mass population screening. J Pediatr Surg 25:245–248, 1990.
65. Murphy SB, Cohn SL, Craft AW, et al. Do children benefit from mass screening for neuroblastoma? Consensus statement from the American Cancer Society Workshop on neuroblastoma screening. Lancet 337:344–346, 1991.
66. Kanedo Y, Kanda N, Maseki N, et al. Different karyotypic patterns in early and advanced stage neuroblastomas. Cancer Res 47:311–318, 1987.
67. Maris JM, White PS, Beltinger CP, et al. Significance of chromosome 1p loss of heterozygosity

in neuroblastoma. Cancer Res 555:4664–4669, 1995.

68. Schwab M, Varmus HE, Bishop JM, et al. Chromosome localization in normal human cells and neuroblastomas of a gene related to c-myc. Nature 308:288–291, 1984.

69. Seeger RC, Brodeur GM, Sather H, et al. Association of multiple copies of the N-myc oncogene with rapid progression of neuroblastomas. N Engl J Med 313:1111–1116, 1983.

70. Brodeur GM, Seeger RC, Schwab M, et al. Amplification of N-myc in untreated human neuroblastomas correlates with advanced disease stage. Science 224:1121–1124, 1984.

71. Brodeur GM, Hayes FA, Green AA, et al. Consistent N-myc copy number in simultaneous or consecutive neuroblastoma samples from sixty individual patients. Cancer Res 47:4248–4253, 1987.

72. Tanaka T, Slaman DJ, Shimada H, et al. A significant association of Ha-ras p21 in neuroblastoma cells with patients prognosis. Cancer 68:1296–1302, 1991.

73. Moll UM, LaQuaglia M, Benards, et al. Wild-type p53 protein undergoes cytoplasmic sequestion in undifferentiated neuroblastomas but not is differentiated tumors. Proc Natl Acad Sci USA 92:4407–4411, 1995.

74. Nakagawara A, Arima-Nakagawara M, Scavarda NJ, et al. Association between high levels of expression of the TRK gene and favorable outcome in human neuroblastoma. N Engl J Med 328:847–854, 1993.

75. Nakagawara A, Arima M, Azar CG, et al. Inverse relationship between TRK expression and N-myc amplification in human neuroblastomas. Cancer Res 52:1364–1368, 1992.

76. Lavenius E, Gestblom C, Johansson I, et al. Transfection of TRK-A into human neuroblastoma cells restores their ability to differentiate in response to nerve growth factor. Cell Growth Differ Vol 6:727–736, 1995.

77. Chatten J, Shimada H, Sather HN, et al. Prognostic value of histopathology in advanced neuroblastoma: A report from the Children's Cancer Study Group. Hum Pathol 19:1187–1198, 1988.

78. Matthay KK, Sather HN, Seeger RC, et al. Excellent outcome of stage II neuroblastoma is independent of residual disease and radiation therapy. J Clin Oncol 7:234–244, 1989.

79. Haase GM, Atkinson JB, Stram DO, et al. Surgical management and outcome of locoregional neuroblastoma: Comparison of the Childrens Cancer Group and the International Staging Systems. J Pediatr Surg 30:289–295, 1995.

80. Evans AE, Chatten J, D'Angio GJ, et al. A review of 17 IV-S neuroblastoma patients at the Children's Hospital of Philadelphia. Cancer 45:833–839, 1980.

81. Cheung NK, Helelr G. Chemotherapy does intensity correlates strongly with response, median survival and median progression-free survival in metastatic neuroblastoma. J Clin Oncol 9:1050–1058, 1991.

82. Sitarz A, Finklestein J, Grosfeld J, et al. An evaluation of the role of surgery in disseminated neuroblastoma: A report from the Childrens Cancer Study Group. J Pediatr Surg 18:147–151, 1983.

83. Haase GM, Wong KY, deLorimier AA, et al. Improvement in survival after excision of primary tumor in stage III neuroblastoma. J Pediatr Surg 24:194–200, 1989.

84. Martinez DA, King DR, Ginn-Pease ME, et al. Resection of the primary tumor is appropriate for children with stage IV-S neuroblastoma: An analysis of 37 patients. J Pediatr Surg 27:1016–1021, 1992.

85. Loo, R, Applebaum H, Takasugi J, et al. Resection of advanced stage neuroblastoma with the cavitron ultrasonic surgical aspirator. J Pediatr Surg 23:1135–1138, 1988.

86. Aitken DR, Hopkins GA, Archambeau JO, et al. Intraoperative radiotherapy in the treatment of neuroblastoma: Report of a pilot study. J Surg Oncol 2:343–350, 1995.

87. Azizkhan RG, Shaw A, Chandler JG. Surgical complications of neuroblastoma resection. Surgery 97:514–517, 1985.

88. Seeger RC, Villablanca JG, Matthay KK, et al. Intensive chemotherapy and autologous bone marrow tranplantation for poor prognosis neuroblastoma. Prog Clin Biol 366:527–543, 1991.

89. Gaze MN, Wheldon TE, O'Donoghue JA, et al. Multi-modality megatherapy with [^{131}I]

metaiodobenzylguanidine, high dose helphalan and total body irradiation with bone marrow rescue: Feasibility study of a new strategy for advanced neuroblastoma. Eur J Cancer 31A:252–256, 1995.

90. Handgretinger R, Baader P, Dopfer R, et al. A Phase I study of neuroblastoma with the anti-ganglioside GD2 antibody 14 G2a. Cancer Immunol Immunother 24:199–204, 1992.

91. Hank JA, Surfus J, Gan J, et al. Treatment of neuroblastoma patients with antiganglionside GD2 antibody plus interleukin-2 induces antibody-dependent cellular cytotoxicity against neurobastoma detected in vitro. J Immunother 15:29–37, 1994.

92. Sidell N, Altman A, Haussler MR, et al. Effects of retinoic acid (RA) on the growth and phenotypic expression of several human neuroblastoma cell lines. Exp Cell Res 148:21–30, 1983.

93. Villablanca JG, Khan AA, Avramis VI, et al. Phase I trial of 13-cis-retinoic acid in children with neuroblastoma following bone marrow transplantation. J Clin Oncol 13:894–901, 1995.

4. Advances in reconstruction for cancer patients

Mark A. Schusterman, Geoffrey L. Robb, and Helen E. Tadjalli

Introduction

Plastic surgical involvement in surgical oncology was previously limited due to the unreliability of the techniques available. The development of microsurgery in the 1970s revolutionized reconstructive surgery and led to reliable, one-stage, immediate reconstructive techniques [1,2]. This creates the paradox that in many situations the most complicated technique is actually the most reliable and efficacious. Because of these advances, the plastic surgeon, and in particular the reconstructive microsurgeon, has become a full member of the cancer care team.

Reconstructive microsurgery consists of transferring simple or composite units of tissue from distant sites and reattaching them with microscopic aids to restore body structures of contour. These units of tissue, called *free flaps*, have a defined circulatory anatomy that is preserved within the unit to increase the chance of tissue survival. A recipient artery and vein in the ablated area are required for re-establishment of blood flow. The advantages of using free flaps are many. A lesser incidence of wound complications and a greater chance of satisfactory healing have been uniformly observed when even the most challenging defects are repaired using free flaps. When free flaps are used for reconstruction, chronic nonhealing wounds can be avoided following surgical ablations in previously irradiated beds or in tissues treated with preoperative intra-arterial chemotherapy. Such wounds pose unique challenges and are firm indications for microsurgical reconstruction. Versatility in filling dead spaces, padding of vulnerable organs, protection of critical structures, and provision of soft tissue volume in reconstituting form are some other important features of free flaps.

Head and neck reconstruction

Patients with cancers of the oromandibular and pharyngeal regions frequently have poor nutritional status and diminished immune and healing capabilities. In spite of these unfavorable circumstances, a free flap success rate of 95% can

Raphael E. Pollock (ed.), SURGICAL ONCOLOGY. Copyright © 1997. Kluwer Academic Publishers. ISBN 0-7923-9900-5. All rights reserved.

be achieved with immediate reconstruction in this group [3]. Whether the goal of ablation is cure or palliation, a satisfactory reconstruction is necessary to preserve the quality of life; an unrepaired head-and-neck defect is no longer considered acceptable (Fig. 1).

Composite tissue defects, such as those involving the oral lining, mandible, and external skin, can be addressed in single-stage procedures. The vascular anastomoses are commonly done with the external carotid artery and internal jugular vein using an end-to-side technique or with branches of these vessels using an end-to-end technique. Compared with rates for pedicled flaps and nonvascularized grafts, the complication rate using free tissue transfer is favorable [4].

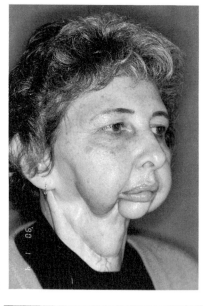

A

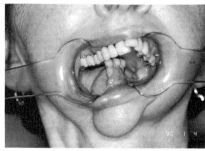

B

Figure 1. **A:** A patient after resection of a portion of the tongue and lateral mandible without reconstruction. Note the external deformity. **B:** Intraoral view demonstrating tethering of the tongue and lateral drift of the remaining mandible, resulting in severe functional impairment.

Soft tissue reconstruction

Soft tissue defects requiring reconstruction are those resulting from wide excisions of the buccal mucosa or retromolar trigone, floor-of-mouth resections, and partial or total glossectomies. Primary closure using the remaining tongue limits tongue mobility and can interfere greatly with speech and swallowing functions. Preserving mobility of the remaining tongue is essential to the promotion or maintenance of oral function. Microvascular surgery has provided a reliable, more effective means of repairing soft-tissue defects of the oral cavity.

The two soft-tissue free flaps used most commonly in the head and neck are the radial forearm flap and the rectus abdominis myocutaneous flap. The radial forearm flap is a fasciocutaneous flap based on the radial artery and the cephalic vein. It is thin, pliable, and ideally suited for wide, shallow defects, such as those of the inner cheek, floor of mouth, partial tongue, and retromolar trigone. The flap is easily and quickly harvested, and has a resulting donor site defect with little to no functional morbidity. The flap's long vascular pedicle and vessel size make it a very reliable flap (Fig. 2).

The other commonly used soft-tissue free flap in the head-and-neck area is the rectus abdominis myocutaneous (RAM) flap. The blood supply to the skin of this flap is derived from blood vessels 'perforating' the muscle. The skin paddle can be oriented either vertically (VRAM flap) or horizontally (TRAM flap). Both versions are based on the deep inferior epigastric artery and vein, which are harvested with the flap. Pedicle length and vessel size are adequate. The main advantage of this flap is that a very large surface area or volume deficit can be restored, making the flap suitable for total glossectomy defects (Fig. 3). The bulk provided with this flap varies depending on the patient's total body fat, but even in the leanest patients there is sufficient subcutaneous fat to fill radical oropharyngeal defects. Donor site morbidity is minimal.

Mandibular reconstruction

Mandibular reconstruction has clearly been revolutionized by the use of free vascularized bone flaps. Several donor sites are now routinely used to repair large segmental losses of the mandible at the time of the resection, even in a radiated bed. A composite defect, including not only the mandible, but intraoral soft tissue as well, can be repaired with a single composite free flap consisting of multiple tissue types.

The free fibula flap is currently the workhorse for mandibular reconstruction. Its advantages are due to specific anatomical characteristics, which include a generous available length and a segmental periosteal blood supply based on the peroneal artery and vein [5,6]. Flap elevation is done through a longitudinal incision in the lateral leg, except for the osteocutaneous version, in which an ellipse of skin is also taken. When a skin paddle is included, a

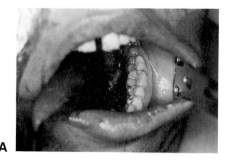 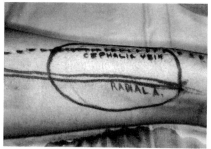

A   **B**

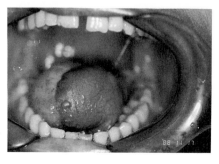

C

Figure 2. **A:** A 30-year-old female with squamous cell carcinoma of the tongue. She has had a hemiglossectomy and a modified neck dissection. She was left with approximately half her tongue remaining. **B:** A free radial forearm flap was planned for transfer. Note that the flap is centered over the radial artery and cephalic vein, which are to be used as the donor vessels. **C:** A photograph of the long-term result demonstrates how this flap nicely approximates the normal tongue.

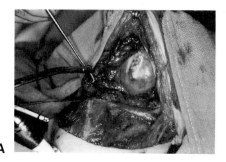 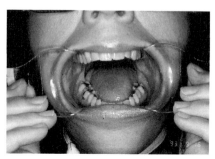

A   **B**

Figure 3. **A:** A 42-year-old female with an advanced carcinoma of the tongue requiring subtotal glossectomy and bilateral neck dissections. Note that the defect is being viewed from below and the maxillary teeth can be seen. The remaining lateral tongue musculature is being retracted laterally. A free transverse rectus myocutaneous flap was used for the reconstruction. (See Figs. 7 and 8.) **B:** The postoperative intraoral photograph demonstrates good restoration of tongue bulk. The patient has retained her larynx and is able to speak and swallow.

correct design is ensured by Doppler localization of the perforating vessels serving the skin. Patients remain fully ambulatory postoperatively, and donor-site morbidity is limited to the cosmetic deficits of the skin graft used to resurface the skin paddle donor area (Fig. 4).

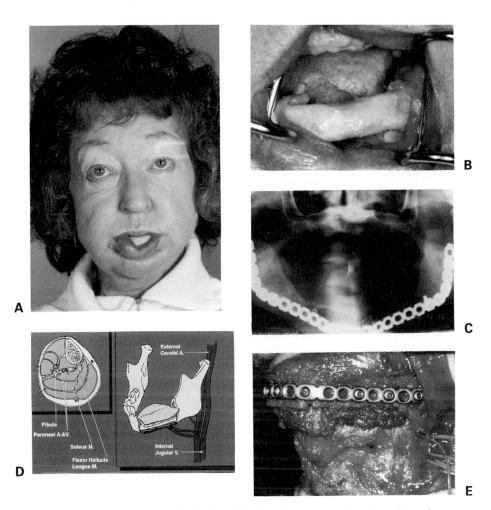

Figure 4. **A,B:** A 60-year-old white female who had undergone a previous floor-of-mouth resection and marginal mandibulectomy for a squamous cell carcinoma. She had received postoperative radiation therapy. Her wound broke down and her anterior mandible became exposed, requiring anterior mandibular resection. **C:** Radiographic image demonstrating the unsuccessful attempt to reconstruct this defect using a reconstruction plate and cadaver, and a nonvascularized autogenous bone graft. **D:** Schematic drawing illustrating the free fibula osteocutaneous flap that was used to reconstruct the patient. **E:** Intraoperative photograph showing the bone flap fixed into the recipient site using a reconstruction plate. **F:** Postoperative result, frontal view. **G:** Postoperative result, lateral view. **H:** Intraoral view showing dental restoration. **I:** Radiograph demonstrating osseointegrated implants in the vascularized bone flap and used to facilitate dental restoration.

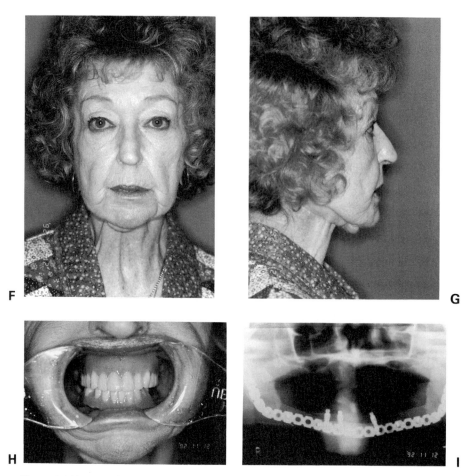

F   G

H   I

Figure 4.4 (Continued).

Reconstruction of the pharynx and cervical esophagus

Microvascular surgery has greatly improved our ability to reconstruct the upper aerodigestive tract. For circumferential defects of the pharynx and cervical esophagus, the free jejunal transfer is the repair method of choice [7,8] (Fig. 5). An abdominal laparotomy is required for tissue harvest. The flap is selected from an area within 20–30 cm of the ligament of Treitz and includes the adjacent vascular arcade leading up to a branch of the superior mesenteric artery; this branch is used as the pedicle. Continuity of the small bowel is re-established with the assistance of a general surgeon.

The patient is not allowed to take anything by mouth for 7–14 days postoperatively, depending on prior history of radiation therapy. A barium swallow study is obtained after 7–14 days, and if no leaks or fistulae are observed, oral intake is begun. If an anastomotic leak is demonstrated, it is most commonly located at the proximal anastomosis. This problem has a tendency to heal spontaneously with proper wound care and continued avoidance of oral intake. Gastrostomy feeding is continued during this interval.

Facial reanimation

One of the most challenging tasks facing a reconstructive microsurgeon is the multistaged process of restoring spontaneous facial animation in cancer patients with complete facial paralysis. Patients undergoing maxillectomy, parotidectomy, or full-thickness cheek excisions for advanced malignant disease may require excision of the facial nerve when it is involved in the malignancy. When both the proximal and distal ends of the facial nerve are available, immediate nerve reconstruction is done with nerve grafting. However, in more extensive resections, the proximal or distal stumps of the facial nerve may not be available for grafting, so the patient will require a staged course of microneurovascular reconstruction for the lower face to achieve spontaneous expressiveness. The paralyzed eye, on the other hand, is a reconstruction priority and is accomplished separately with local procedures to avoid the disconcerting problem of synkinesis.

In certain circumstances, such as when no immediate facial nerve reconstruction was done for oncologic reasons, primary nerve grafting was not successful in providing any spontaneous muscle activity, or the facial paralysis is chronic (beyond several years' duration) so that facial muscle reinnervation is likely beyond probable recovery, a different approach, consisting of free muscle and nerve transfer, must be used to restore delayed spontaneous movement of the lower face with increased perioral and buccal resting tone. Of course, a direct regional muscle transposition can be used for the static support and some dynamic movement of the lower face, but no spontaneous movement can result.

The most popular method currently used to restore spontaneous motion to the oral commissure and upper lip/alar base complex and to attain a reasonably symmetric smile is free muscle transfer following cross-facial nerve grafts from the normal side of the face. The opposite, healthy facial nerve is used as a donor, and facial nerve axons are grafted into the affected side of the face. This two-stage microneurovascular muscle transfer procedure, when successful, can accomplish several important aspects of facial reanimation simultaneously. Besides providing the oblique smile movement for the commissure complex in the lower face, the muscle transfer is also perfectly located to add desirable subcutaneous bulk in the anterolateral cheek, which is otherwise atrophic following the facial nerve denervation. The aesthetic challenge is to avoid excessive volume in the cheek while providing enough muscle power for adequate facial motion.

A number of individual muscles have been described for this facial reani-

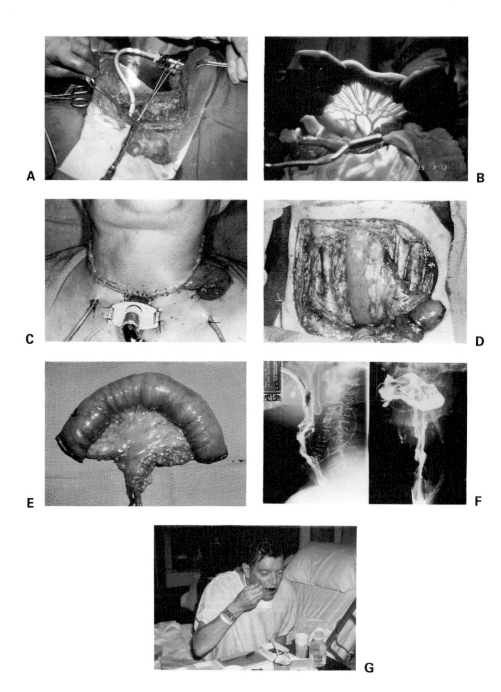

78

mation technique, but the gracilis muscle is probably the preferred muscle because of the ease of harvest, minimal donor site morbidity, and appropriate amount of muscle contraction attained with reinnervation by the nerve grafts from the normal side of the face [9].

The perioral tone is improved immediately following surgery from the muscle's static sling effect on the interior buccal area as well as the commissure complex itself. After approximately 6 months, some motion may be apparent at the commissure; movement increases with time. As the transplanted muscle begins to function, the patient can aid in the recovery of facial movement by practicing facial motions in front of a mirror. These exercises strengthen the new muscle's contractions and help to achieve the final symmetric appearance of the patient's facial expressions (Fig. 6).

Breast reconstruction

Autogenous tissue is the preferred method of breast reconstruction after mastectomy, and microvascular surgery is the preferred method of utilizing autogenous tissue. At our institution, we reserve silicone breast implants for women who are opposed to the use of their own tissue for breast reconstruction and for women in whom there are contraindications to the use of autogenous tissue. With implants, it is harder to obtain symmetry with the contralateral breast than it is with autogenous tissue. In addition, the controversy of whether implants cause connective tissue disease continues to brew. Although there is no hard evidence of a link between silicone gel and rheumatologic or autoimmune diseases, nor any proof that silicone gel induces de novo or recurrent breast cancer [10,11], still the controversy has not been totally resolved. Additionally, there are the standard concerns of implanting foreign material into the human body; implant rupture, capsular contracture, infection, and extrusion are some of the complications associated with breast implant use. The shortcomings of breast implants have made autogenous tissue breast reconstruction much more popular. Furthermore, the cosmetic appearance of reconstructions with autogenous tissue is far superior and more natural looking.

The most common flap used for breast reconstruction is the transverse

◄━━━

Figure 5. **A:** A 52-year-old male underwent laryngopharyngectomy for advanced cancer of the larynx. Note that the clamp is on the esophageal stump. **B:** A laparotomy is performed and the proximal jejunum identified. A loop of jejunum is selected and the mesentery transilluminated in order to select an appropriate vascular arcade. **C:** A jejunal segment of appropriate length is isolated on this vascular arcade. **D,E:** This segment is then transferred to the neck, where it is inset, revascularized, and a small distal portion is retained on a separate portion of mesentery for monitoring purposes, and the neck closed. **F,G:** A contrast study is used to verify the integrity of the anastomoses, and if intact, the patient is restarted on oral intake between postoperative days 7 and 10.

rectus abdominis myocutaneous (TRAM) flap [12]. This flap encompasses a large transverse ellipse of skin with its underlying fat and a representative portion of the rectus abdominis muscle. The skin derives its blood supply from the underlying rectus abdominis muscle, and therefore can be transferred based on either the superior vessel, as a pedicled flap, or based on the inferior vessel, and thus transferred as a free flap. The latter is physiologically more desirable because the inferior system is the dominant blood supply to the lower abdominal skin, thus making the skin paddle more reliable. The microvascular anastomoses are usually carried out with the thoracodorsal artery and vein, just proximal to the takeoff of the branches to the serratus anterior

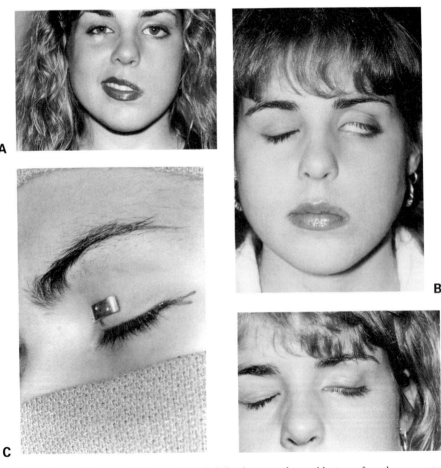

Figure 6. **A:** A 19-year-old Hispanic female following a total parotidectomy for schwannoma of the VIIth nerve with complete facial nerve paralysis. **B:** Incomplete eye closure due to paralysis of lid muscles. **C:** Position of the gold weight in the upper lid. **D:** Complete lid closure following placement of the gold weight. **E:** Significantly improved facial symmetry around the mouth with commissure elevation following cross facial nerve grafts and free muscle transfer to the left cheek.

80

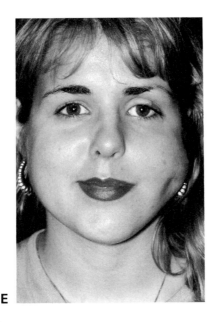

E

Figure 4.6 (Continued).

muscle. It is therefore important to protect these vessels during the axillary node dissection.

The advantages of the free TRAM flap over the pedicled version are multiple: (1) the free flap allows use of the entire skin paddle more reliably; (2) it sacrifices a much smaller amount of muscle and anterior rectus sheath, reducing the potential for hernia or weakness; (3) it is safer in smokers and obese individuals; (4) there is less fat necrosis; (5) it withstands radiation treatments without significant texture or consistency changes; (6) it can be molded into the desired shape more easily; and (7) it achieves a more appealing cosmetic result [13,14] (Fig. 7).

The TRAM flap offers a convenient donor site, allowing flap harvest simultaneously with the mastectomy. Each team uses separate instrument sets, preventing cross-contamination. The donor area is closed by repairing the anterior rectus sheath, with or without plastic mesh, and repositioning the umbilicus. When bilateral free TRAM flaps are being used, one for each breast, symmetry is maximized (Fig. 8). The nipples are reconstructed 3 months postoperatively, and areolar restoration is then done about 3 weeks later using micropigmentation.

Limb salvage

In the past, malignancies of the upper and lower extremities were treated with amputation. However, limb-salvage procedures have been shown to produce

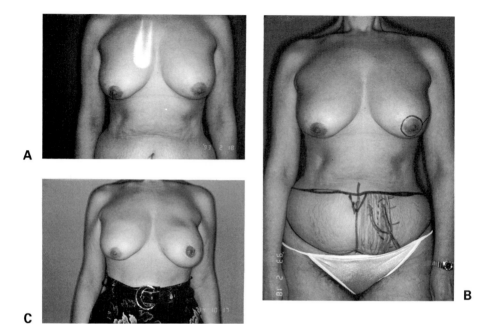

Figure 7. **A:** Preoperative photograph of a 45-year-old female with a T1, stage I breast cancer of the left breast. She is to undergo a modified radical mastectomy. She has elected to have immediate reconstruction using the free TRAM flap. **B:** Patient marking and preoperative plan. Note the plan to harvest the lateral perforators on the free TRAM flap and the use of the skin-sparing mastectomy. **C:** The postoperative result after nipple reconstruction and areolar restoration using micropigmentation techniques.

equivalent survival rates, and today many patients presenting with sarcomas or other malignancies are successfully treated with wide local excision, in conjunction with adjuvant therapy in most cases [15]. Limb-salvage eligibility relates directly to the surgical oncologist's ability to achieve clear surgical margins with a defect for which the reconstructive surgeon can then provide 'form and function' to usefully rehabilitate the extremity. Ablative wounds

Figure 8. **A:** The preoperative view of a 55-year-old white female with cancer of the right breast and a family history of breast cancer. She has elected to undergo bilateral mastectomies with immediate free TRAM reconstruction. **B:** The patient is marked the night before surgery with the surgical plan. Again, note the use of the skin-sparing mastectomy on the right side. The radially oriented biopsy scar on the right lateral breast will also be excised. Note that the plan drawn on the abdomen schematically shows harvest of the lateral myocutaneous perforators, a maneuver that will limit the fascial sacrifice. **C:** Abdominal wall after flap harvest. Note the minimal fascial defect. **D:** The free TRAM flap after harvest, showing the small amount of fascia and muscle harvested and the long pedicle length. **E:** The postoperative result after nipple reconstruction and areolar restoration using micropigmentation techniques.

range from small and simple to extensive and composite in terms of quantitative and qualitative tissue loss. Patients with aggressive extremity tumors usually require considerable soft tissue resection that may include bone or exposed vital structures. For the limb salvage to be successful, reconstructive

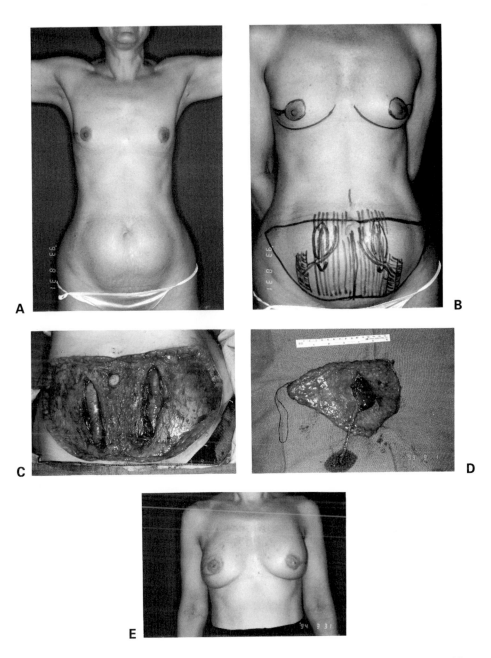

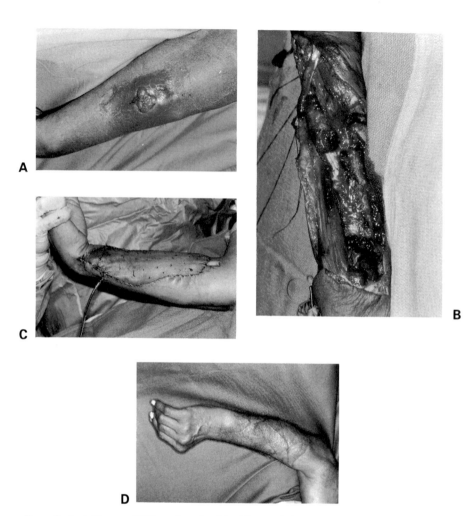

Figure 9. **A:** A 71-year-old Hispanic male with a history of ulcerative sarcoma, right mid forearm, with 5.0 cm recurrence. **B:** Radical resection of the extensor compartment, including the radial nerve and partial ulna. Tendon transfers are completed for wrist and finger extension. **C:** Placement of rectus abdominis free flap and overlying skin graft in the forearm defect. **D:** Healed forearm reconstruction with excellent functional results and good wrist extension.

microsurgeons must then provide adequate, well-vascularized 'like' tissue to cover the vital structures in the extremity and healthy, non-irradiated tissue to obliterate dead space, provide a natural contour, and replace functional units where necessary [16].

Smaller extremity defects following may certainly be repaired using local tissues, such as muscle or skin and fascia flaps. However, many patients will have had preoperative radiotherapy or previous surgery that will significantly limit the local tissues readily available or predictably reliable under these

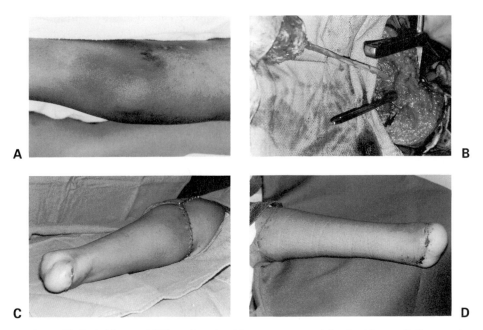

Figure 10. **A:** A 10-year-old Hispanic male with osteosarcoma of the distal femur. **B:** Segmental amputation of the knee with intact sciatic nerve. **C:** Free tissue transfer of the lower leg and heel pad on to the upper leg. **D:** Healed lower leg transfer to the upper leg to provide well-padded stump for AK prosthesis.

circumstances [17]. Furthermore, if the patient requires postoperative radiotherapy after a local tissue reconstruction, the local tissue donor site may need to be included in the radiation field. The quality of the limb-salvage effort must also be considered in terms of the limb function recovery likely after using local tissues, where the patient's potential may be diminished. In contrast, the quality of life achievable with a free tissue transfer for extremity reconstruction can be superior in many ways, reliably increasing the utility or function of the extremity by providing healthy tissue supplemented with an improved blood supply (Figs. 9 and 10).

Chest wall reconstruction

The type of repair needed for chest-wall defects following tumor ablation is directly related to the extent of the missing tissues and the likely resulting functional deficit. In planning the reconstruction, the reconstructive surgeon should consider primarily the postablative condition of the pleural cavity, the integrity of the skeletal support system, the necessity for chest wall reinforcement, and, lastly, the soft-tissue deficit. It is important to achieve skeletal stability and to ensure an airtight closure for optimal postoperative pulmonary function. For full-thickness chest-wall defects limited to a two-rib segment, soft-tissue coverage alone may be sufficient for functional stability. However, for larger defects bony stabilization will usually require additional alloplastic elements, such as mesh or methyl methacrylate, or if infection is present, autogenous fascia or split ribs in conjunction with muscle flap coverage. When the chest wall has been irradiated preoperatively, an even more extensive skeletal defect may remain stable due to the stiff radiation fibrosis in the surrounding tissues.

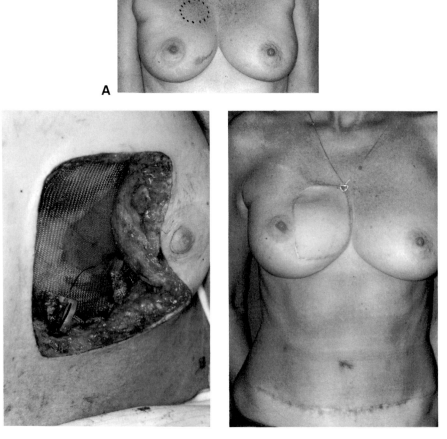

Figure 11. **A:** A 43-year-old white female with chondrosarcoma of right third and fourth ribs of the chest wall. **B:** Medial mastectomy, partial sternectomy, and wide excision of the involved ribs. Plastic mesh is used to stabilize the chest-wall defect. **C:** Free TRAM flap from the lower abdomen is used to reconstruct the chest-wall defect, as well as the form and contour of the breast.

The soft-tissue reconstruction usually requires flaps of muscle, muscle and skin, or skin and fascia to cover exposed bone or pleural cavity. A flap consisting of elongated omentum is also an option, especially when muscle flaps are unavailable. Regional pedicled muscle or myocutaneous flaps are the tissue sources most commonly used to provide well-vascularized coverage for chest-wall defects, especially if the thorax has been irradiated [18]. For larger soft-tissue defects requiring reliable for coverage of vital structures, transfer of free muscle or myocutaneous flap may be necessary. A free flap may also be necessary when pedicled muscle flaps are unavailable or the blood supply of potential regional flaps has been sacrificed in the tumor ablation (Fig. 11).

Groin reconstruction

Difficult acute or chronic defects resulting from the excision of tumors of the groin region can be effectively and reliably repaired with regional muscle, myocutaneous flaps, or fasciocutaneous flaps [19]. Characteristically, these

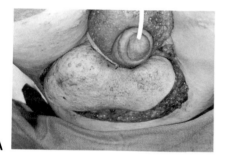
A

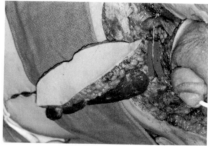
B

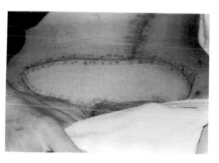
C

Figure 12. **A:** A 23-year-old Caucasian male with extensive lymphangiectatic elephantiasis involving the right leg, hip, anterior abdominal wall, groin, penis, scrotum, and retroperitoneal space. Concern for lymphedema-associated angiosarcoma of the suprapubic area. **B:** Subtotal excision of the groin lymphangioma with lympho-lymphatic shunt and rectus abdominis myocutaneous flap for soft tissue coverage. **C:** Healed groin reconstruction with the rectus abdominis myocutaneous flap and significant improvement in the lymphedema present through the groin and right leg.

wounds are extensive, deep, and, because of the proximity of the urethra and anus, susceptible to urinary and fecal contamination. Previous irradiation of the area adds further difficulty to the reconstruction because of potential wound healing problems and can necessitate a larger soft-tissue excision to achieve healthy wound margins, beyond the excision needed for tumor-free margins. As with most reconstructive efforts, the best results are achieved with immediate repair of defects, while the area hygiene is optimal, and using well-vascularized flap tissue to obliterate dead space and cover any exposed bone or major neurovascular structures in the anterior pelvic or groin region. The rectus abdominis muscle or myocutaneous flap based on the deep inferior epigastric vessels is the workhorse for reconstruction of the lower abdomen or groin. The flap offers a significant volume of muscle and skin, with a wide arc of rotation that allows it to be rotated downward and inset into the anterior pelvic or groin defect. The donor site morbidity is modest, although the possibility of postoperative abdominal bulge is a known risk. Other local and regional muscle flaps, such as the sartorius, tensor fascia lata, rectus femoris, and gracilis flaps, act as back up options to the rectus abdominis muscle flap for most groin reconstructive applications. Each of these muscle or myocutaneous flaps has certain advantages or specific uses in lower abdominal or groin reconstruction, such as abdominal fascial repair with the rectus femoris or the tensor fascia lata flap, large vessel coverage with the sartorius flap, or deep perineal coverage with the gracilis muscle flap (Fig. 12). These muscle or myofascial flaps are associated with relatively modest donor site mortality. However, the rectus femoris muscle flap is often a secondary choice in ambulatory patients because of possible knee-extension deficiencies following sacrifice of the muscle. The muscle flaps with split-thickness skin graft coverage have excellent utility in repairing superficial soft-tissue defects of the groin or pelvis, with a distinct advantage over the thicker myocutaneous flaps, especially in obese patients.

References

1. Daniel RK, Taylor GI. Distant transfer of an island flap by microvascular anastomoses. Plast Reconstr Surg 52:111, 1973.
2. Harashina T, Fujino T, Aoyagi F. Reconstruction of the oral cavity with a free flap. Plast Reconstr Surg 58:412, 1976.
3. Schusterman MA, Miller MJ, Reece GP, Kroll SS, Marchi M, Goepfert H. A single center's experience with 308 free flaps for repair of head and neck cancer defects. Plast Reconstr Surg 93:472, 1994.
4. Schusterman MA, Kroll SS, Weber RS, Byers RM, Guillamondegui OM, Goepfert H. Intraoral soft tissue reconstruction after cancer ablation: A comparison of the pectoralis major flap and the free radial forearm flap. Am J Surg 162:397, 1991.
5. Schusterman MA, Reece GP, Miller MJ, Harris S. The osteocutaneous free fibula flap: Is the skin paddle reliable? Plast Reconstr Surg 90:787, 1992.
6. Hidalgo DA. Fibula free flap: A new method of mandible reconstruction. Plast Reconstr Surg 84:71, 1989.

7. Reece GP, Bengtson BP, Schusterman MA. Reconstruction of the pharynx and cervical esophagus using free jejunal transfer. Clin Plast Surg 21:125, 1994.
8. Schusterman MA, Shestak KC, deVries EJ, Swartz WM, Jones NF, Johnson JT, Myers EN, Reilly J. Reconstruction of the cervical esophagus: Free jejunal transfer versus gastric pull-up. Plast Reconstr Surg 85:16, 1990.
9. Sassoon EM, Polle MD, Rushworth G. Reanimation for facial palsy using gracilis muscle grafts. Br J Plast Surg 44:195–200, 1991.
10. Berkel H, Birdsell DC, Jenkins H. Breast augmentation: A risk factor for breast cancer? [Comments]. N Engl J Med 326:1649, 1992.
11. Sanchez-Guerrero J, Colditz GA, Karlson EW, Hunter DJ, Speizer FE, Liang MH. Silicone breast implants and the risk of connective-tissue diseases and symptoms. N Engl J Med 332:1666, 1995.
12. Hartrampf CR, Jr., Scheflan M, Black PW. Breast reconstruction with a transverse abdominal island flap. Plast Reconstr Surg 69:216, 1982.
13. Schusterman MA, Kroll SS, Weldon ME. Immediate breast reconstruction: Why the free TRAM over the conventional TRAM flap? Plast Reconstr Surg 90:255, 1992.
14. Schusterman MA, Kroll SS, Miller MJ, Reece GP, Baldwin BJ, Robb GL, Altmyer CS, Ames FC, Singletary SE, Ross MI, Balch CM. The free transverse rectus abdominis musculocutaneous flap for breast reconstruction: One center's experience with 211 consecutive cases. Ann Plast Surg 32:234, 1994.
15. Sim FH, Bowman WE, Wilkins RN, Chao EY. Limb salvage in primary malignant bone tumor. Orthopaedics 8:574, 1985.
16. Serafin D, Sabatier R, Morris R. Reconstruction of the lower extremity with vascularized composite tissue: Improved tissue survival and specific indication. Plast Reconstr Surg 66:230, 1980.
17. Manktelow RT. *Microvascular Reconstruction*. Heidelberg: Springer-Verlag, 1986, chapters 6 and 19.
18. Boyd AD, Shaw WW, McCarthy JG, Baker D, Trehan NK, et al. Immediate reconstruction of full thickness chest wall defects. Ann Thorac Surg 32:337, 1981.
19. Bostwick JB, Hill HL, Nahai F. Repairs in the lower abdomen and groin or perineum with myocutaneous or omental flaps. Plast Reconstr Surg 63:186, 1979.

5. New developments in soft tissue sarcoma

Peter W.T. Pisters, Barry W. Feig, Denis H.Y. Leung,
and Murray F. Brennan

Introduction

This chapter focuses on recent developments in soft tissue sarcoma of the
extremities. Rather than provide a broad overview of the disease, which has
been thoroughly reviewed in several recent book chapter [1,2], we wanted to
provide a more in-depth perspective on developments in the field. We have
selected four specific issues in extremity soft tissue sarcoma: prognostic factors, surgery without adjuvant irradiation, adjuvant chemotherapy, and isolated limb perfusion. In this manner, we hope to provide greater insight into
current controversies in the evaluation and management of patients with soft
tissue sarcoma.

Refinement of clinicopathologic prognostic factors

In many areas of clinical oncology, recent attention has been focused on
prognostic factors. In part, such studies have emanated from the substantial
amounts of clinical data gained during efforts to validate and further expand
the present staging systems for individual diseases. In other instances, studies
have been carried out in an effort to define additional clinical criteria for the
application of specific primary and adjuvant therapies.

Purpose and requirements for prognostic factor analysis

Prognostic factor analyses are undertaken for a number of reasons: to provide
outcome expectations for individual patients, to develop and refine staging
systems, to identify stratification criteria for clinical trials, to define clinical
criteria for the application of adjuvant therapies, and to support treatment
planning in individual cases. The underlying goal of these types of analyses is
to provide accurate assessment of risk for relapse and death. In the case of soft
tissue sarcoma, it is particularly important to define and distinguish the specific
forms of relapse (local failure, distant failure, or disease-related mortality)

Raphael E. Pollock (ed.), SURGICAL ONCOLOGY. Copyright © 1997. Kluwer Academic Publishers.
ISBN 0-7923-9900-5. All rights reserved.

because it has become apparent that the clinicopathologic factors that predict these various endpoints are different.

A number of potential problems are inherent in any effort to analyze prognostic factors. These are outlined in Table 1. It is important to note that the statistical power of a prognostic factor study is not strictly governed by the number of patients analyzed. This is because the analysis is performed to determine specific clinicopathologic factors that significantly impact event-free survival (local-recurrence–free survival, distant-recurrence–free survival, disease-free survival, or overall survival). As such, the critical factor impacting the statistical power of such an analysis is the number of *events* observed. For example, the statistical power of a multivariate analysis designed to identify prognostic factors for disease-specific survival in a cohort of 1000 patients among whom there are 50 disease-related deaths is the same as that of a study of 75 patients among whom there are 50 disease-related deaths. Thus, a large number of patients is required only to the extent that it is needed to obtain a large number of observed events. Follow-up of the cohort of patients must be long term and complete. This is essential to ensure that all possible events are indeed detected.

Prognostic factor analyses require accurate and complete documentation of a range of clinical, pathologic, and treatment-related factors. These factors are then examined for their prognostic significance. Since the statistical methodology employed, multivariate regression analysis, is designed to evaluate the independent prognostic significance of separate clinicopathologic parameters, it is critical that the documentation of clinicopathologic factors be complete.

Table 1. Multivariate analyses of prognostic factors in extremity soft tissue sarcoma

Institution/site	Ref.	Year	Accrual period (yr)	Data collection	No. patients
Multicenter (n = 13)	Heise [19]	1977	5	Retrospective	594
Fox Chase	Sears [4]	1980	10	Retrospective	70
Uppsala, Sweden	Markhede [5]	1982	21	Retrospective	97
Bordeaux, France	Trojani [6]	1984	11	Retrospective	155
Lund, Sweden	Rydholm [7]	1984	15	Retrospective	237
MSKCC	Collin [8]	1987	10	Retrospective	423
Osaka, Japan	Tsujimoto [9]	1988	24	Retrospective	163
Osaka, Japan	Ueda [10]	1988	24	Retrospective	163
Lund, Sweden	Rooser [11]	1988	15	Retrospective	82
Caen, France (CFB)	Mandard [12]	1989	12	Retrospective	109
Princess Margaret	Bell [13]	1989	7	Retrospective	100
Lund, Sweden	Alvegard [14]	1990	5	Retrospective	148
St. Mary's, London	Stotter [15]	1990	6	Retrospective	175
MSKCC	Gaynor [16]	1992	10	Retrospective	423
Harvard	Singer [17]	1994	23	Retrospective	182
MSKCC	Pisters [18]	1996	10	Prospective	1041

MSKCC = Memorial Sloan-Kettering Cancer Center; CFB = Centre Francois Baclesse, Caen, France.

92

Although statistical methods can adjust for missing data in a multivariate analysis, the discriminant statistical power of the analysis will be diluted to the extent that there are missing specific data elements.

Clinicopathologic prognostic factors in soft tissue sarcoma

Table 1 outlines the published multivariate analyses of prognostic factors in extremity soft tissue sarcoma. Until recently, the largest such analysis was the multicenter study evaluating retrospectively collected data on 594 patients from 13 institutions [19]. With two exceptions [16,18], the remaining single-institution studies all contain fewer than 300 patients. The initial study of prognostic factors in extremity sarcoma from the Memorial Sloan-Kettering Cancer Center (MSKCC) evaluated clinicopathologic prognostic factors in a series of 423 patients with extremity soft tissue sarcoma seen from 1968 to 1978 at MSKCC [16]. The analysis was among the first to discriminate between specific clinical endpoints, and it clearly established the clinical profile of what is now accepted as the high-risk patient with extremity soft tissue sarcoma — the patient with a large (>5 cm), high-grade, deep lesion.

In 1982, a prospective soft tissue sarcoma database was established at MSKCC. It enabled prospective collection of data on an array of clinico-pathologic factors. The importance of *prospective* data collection cannot be overemphasized. It is exceedingly difficult, if not impossible, to retro-spectively examine patient charts for these variables. Using this database, a comprehensive analysis of 1041 consecutively treated patients with extremity soft tissue sarcoma was conducted and recently reported [18]. The endpoints for the multivariate analyses were local recurrence, distant recurrence (metastasis), and disease-specific survival. The results of the regression analy-ses for each of these endpoints are outlined in Table 2. These results, using prospectively acquired data, confirm the observations made initially by Gaynor et al. [16]. In addition, the previously unappreciated prognostic signifi-cance of specific histopathologic subtypes and the increased risk for adverse outcome associated with presentation with locally recurrent disease were noted.

Until recently, with few exceptions, the specific histopathologic subtype of extremity soft tissue sarcoma was considered to be of comparatively little prognostic significance because of the general impression that for extremity lesions, individual histologic subtypes of comparable histologic grade behaved similarly [1,2]. However, the recent multivariate analyses of prospectively collected data demonstrate that patients with fibrosarcomas and malignant peripheral nerve tumors are at increased risk for local recurrence. In addition, the histologic subtype leiomyosarcoma is an independent adverse prognostic factor for distant recurrence and tumor-related mortality. Conversely, the subtype liposarcoma is a *favorable* prognostic factor compared with the other histologic subtypes. These findings lend support to clinical treatment algo-rithms for extremity soft tissue sarcoma that include assessment of histologic

Table 2. Multivariate analysis of prognostic factors in 1041 patients with extremity soft tisue sarcoma

Endpoint	Adverse prognostic factors	Relative risk	95% confidence interval
Local recurrence	Age >50 yr	1.6	1.1–2.1
	Local recurrence at presentation	2.0	1.4–2.7
	Microscopically positive margin	1.8	1.3–2.5
	Fibrosarcoma	2.5	1.4–4.4
	Malignant peripheral nerve tumor	1.8	1.2–2.7
Distant recurrence	Size 5–9.9 cm	1.9	1.3–2.8
	Size ≥10 cm	1.5	1.0–2.0
	High grade	4.3	2.6–6.9
	Deep location	2.5	1.5–4.1
	Local recurrence at presentation	1.5	1.0–2.1
	Leiomyosarcoma	1.7	1.0–2.6
	Non-liposarcoma histology	1.6	1.1–2.2
Disease-specific survival	Size ≥10 cm	2.1	1.5–3.0
	Deep location	2.8	1.6–4.8
	Local recurrence at presentation	1.5	1.0–2.2
	Leiomyosarcoma	1.9	1.1–3.0
	Malignant peripheral nerve tumor	1.9	1.2–3.2
	Microscopically positive margin	1.7	1.2–3.2
	Lower extremity site	1.6	1.3–2.0

Adverse prognostic factors identified are independent by Cox regression analysis.
Adapted from Pisters et al. [18], with permission.

subtype in addition to histologic grade, tumor size, and tumor depth. It is also interesting to note that presentation with locally recurrent disease has emerged as an independent adverse prognostic factor for not only subsequent local recurrence but also distant recurrence and disease-related mortality. Clearly, local recurrence is a reflection of the inherent biologic aggressiveness of the lesion and portends increased risk for adverse outcome. This factor should clearly be used as a stratification criterion for clinical trials.

The results of the multivariate analyses from MSKCC also have important clinical implications vis-à-vis the staging system for extremity soft tissue sarcoma. The analyses demonstrate that the adverse prognostic factors for local recurrence in extremity soft tissue sarcoma are different from those that predict distant metastasis and disease-specific mortality. Thus, staging systems that are designed to stratify patients for risk of distant metastasis and tumor-related mortality using these prognostic factors will not stratify patients for risk of local recurrence. Conversely, patients with a constellation of adverse prognostic factors for local recurrence are not necessarily at increased risk for distant metastasis or tumor-related mortality. This suggests that for this specific solid tumor, perhaps there should be two separate staging systems — one that stratifies patients for risk of local recurrence and a second staging system that stratifies patients for risk of distant metastasis and tumor-related mortality. Clearly, the discordant nature of these prognostic factors by clinical endpoint and the implications for staging of patients further diminish the utility of the present American Joint Committee on Cancer (AJCC) staging system. The data from these analyses should be incorporated into the design of new staging systems for soft tissue sarcoma, the design of clinical trials, and the identification of individual patients at high risk for distant recurrence and death.

Role of surgery alone

Advances in the treatment of patients with soft tissue sarcoma have paralleled progress made against other cancers. The parallels between soft tissue sarcoma and breast cancer are instructive. For patients with localized or locoregional breast cancer, mastectomy has been largely replaced by conservative surgery combined with adjuvant irradiation [20], and recent attention has been focused on defining the population of patients with localized breast cancer who can be treated by surgery alone [21]. Parallel advances have been made in soft tissue sarcoma: limb-sparing therapy has become the mainstay of treatment for patients with extremity soft tissue sarcoma. At the outset, this therapeutic approach incorporated adjuvant irradiation together with surgical resection. However, several recent reports suggest that adjuvant irradiation is not required for many patients with completely resected, small soft tissue sarcomas. As a consequence, many centers now employ surgery alone for specific groups of patients treated for localized, small soft tissue sarcomas.

The initial observation that patients with small primary sarcomas of the extremities have an excellent overall prognosis was made by Geer et al. in a report of 174 patients with small (<5 cm) primary soft tissue sarcomas treated at MSKCC [22]. The majority of these patients (114, 66%) had high-grade sarcomas. Seventeen (10%) experienced a local recurrence. Distant metastases were observed in only 8 (7%) of 114 patients with high-grade tumors. The overall survival rate for the entire group was 94% at 5 years, with a median follow-up for all patients of 48 months. These data demonstrate the uniformly favorable prognosis of patients with small (<5 cm) primary extremity sarcomas irrespective of histologic grade.

Additional evidence substantiating the excellent prognosis of patients with small extremity sarcomas treated by surgery alone comes from Sweden. Rydholm et al. have reported their experience with 70 patients with subcutaneous or intramuscular extremity sarcomas [23]. The patients were treated with wide surgical resection and microscopic assessment of margins. Negative histologic margins were obtained for 32 of 40 subcutaneous and 24 of 30 intramuscular tumors. The 56 patients with microscopically negative margins received no postoperative radiotherapy, yet only 4 (7%) developed a local recurrence. These favorable local recurrence rates are comparable with the local recurrence rates observed with conventional multimodality therapy incorporating adjuvant irradiation [24–26].

Similarly, a recent report from the Brigham & Women's Hospital outlined the treatment results of 54 patients with small (<5 cm) soft tissue sarcomas (AJCC stage IA, IIA, or IIIA) treated by surgical resection without adjuvant irradiation [27]. Resection margins were microscopically clear for all but one patient. Only 4 (7%) of 54 patients developed subsequent local recurrence, and distant metastases were observed in 4 patients (7%) with intermediate- or high-grade lesions. Taken together, the reports from the MSKCC, Brigham & Women's Hospital, and Sweden strongly support the hypothesis that patients with small primary soft tissue sarcomas treated by surgical resection alone require no form of adjuvant therapy.

With the presently available data, it is difficult to define precise criteria identifying the subset of patients who can be treated by surgery alone. The most conservative recommendation that can be made based on current data would be that patients with a small primary extremity sarcoma who undergo complete surgical resection with unequivocally microscopically negative surgical margins can be safely observed without adjuvant irradiation. It is even more difficult to provide a precise estimation of what, if any, size restriction should be placed on this recommendation. In the Swedish study, the median tumor size of the deep lesions treated with wide surgical resection was 7 cm. The other studies, however, used a smaller tumor size as a criterion for application of surgical therapy without adjuvant radiotherapy. The most conservative recommendation that can be made at this time would be to use 5 cm as an approximate cutoff size. Treatment of patients with large (>5 cm) primary lesions by surgery alone should not be done outside the confines of a clinical trial or prospective current practice program.

Status of adjuvant chemotherapy

The role of adjuvant chemotherapy in the management of soft tissue sarcoma remains highly controversial. Table 3 outlines the 10 published randomized trials evaluating adjuvant chemotherapy in patients with extremity sarcoma. Each of these trials had a control arm who received no adjuvant therapy and a treatment group who received doxuorubicin-based postoperative systemic therapy. The combination chemotherapy regimens incorporated cyclophosphamide, methotrexate, vincristine, or dactinomycin with doxorubicin. Four of the trials reported significantly improved relapse-free survival, but only 1 of 10 trials has found an improvement in overall survival [35,36].

The single positive trial, from the Istituto Ortopedico Rizzoli [35,36], used a rather unusual pair-matched randomization schema to randomize 76 patients to receive either doxorubicin (total dose 450 mg/m^2) or no adjuvant chemotherapy. With a median follow-up of 120 months (95–156 months), 18 (56%) of 32 patients in the treatment group were relapse-free as compared with 12 (27%) of 44 patients in the control group. Actuarial disease-free survival rates have not been reported yet, although univariate comparison of

Table 3. Randomized trials of adjuvant doxorubicin-based chemotherapy versus observation in extremity soft tissue sarcoma

Group	Regimen	Total no. patients	Median follow-up (mo)	Disease-free survival (%)			Overall survival (%)		
				CTx	Obs	p value	CTx	Obs	p value
EORTC [28]	ACVD	317	80	56	43	0.007	63	56	NS
MDACC [29]	ACVAd	43	120	60	35	0.05	75	61	NS
NCI [30]	ACM	67	85	75	54	0.037	83	60	NS
Mayo [31,32]	AVDAd	48	64	88	67	NS	83	63	NS
UCLA [33]	A	119	28	58	54	NS	84	80	NS
Scand [34]	A	154	40	62	56	NS	75	70	NS
Rizzoli [35,36]	A	76	120	56	27	<0.02	NR	NR	0.04
MGH/DFCI [37–39]	A	26	46	90	71	NS	89	81	NS
ISTSS [40]	A	41	20	77	50	NS	72	62	NS
ECOG [37,38]	A	18	59	70	63	NS	61	63	NS

Studies of extremity lesions only and subset analyses of studies that included extremity lesion.
CTx = chemotherapy; Obs = observation; NS = not significant; NR = not reported; EORTC = European Organization for Research and Treatment of Cancer; MDACC = M.D. Anderson Cancer Center; NCI = National Cancer Institute; Mayo = Mayo Clinic; UCLA = University of California at Los Angeles; Scand = Scandinavian Sarcoma Group; Rizzoli = Istituto Ortopedico Rizzoli; MGH/DFCI = Massachusetts General Hospital/Dana Farber Cancer Institute; ISTSS = Intergroup Sarcoma Study Group; ECOG = Eastern Cooperative Oncology Group; A = doxorubicin (Adriamycin); C = cyclophosphamide; V = vincristine, D = dacarbazine; Ad = dactinomycin; M = methotrexate.

these survivals suggests a statistically significant difference in favor of the treatment group. Details of the subgroup analyses also have not been reported yet. However, in the preliminary report from this group there was a marked imbalance of high-risk pelvic and thigh tumors in the control group (57% vs. 37.5% in the doxorubicin group) [35]. In addition, for unexplained reasons a survival benefit from adjuvant chemotherapy has been apparent only in the subgroups who underwent amputation or scar re-excision. No survival benefit has been demonstrated in patients who underwent limb-sparing surgery [35].

Results of the largest randomized prospective trial of adjuvant chemotherapy in soft tissue sarcoma were recently reported by the European Organization for Research and Treatment of Cancer (EORTC) [28]. A total of 145 randomized, eligible, and evaluable patients received CYVADIC chemotherapy (cyclophosphamide, 500 mg/m^2 intravenously on day 1; vincristine, 1.4 mg/m^2 by intravenous bolus on day 1; doxorubicin, 50 mg/m^2 intravenously on day 1; and dacarbazine, 400 mg/m^2 by 1-hour intravenous infusion on days 1–3). CYVADIC was repeated every 28 days for a total of 8 courses. The results of the treatment group were compared with those in the control group, which consisted of 172 patients who received no adjuvant chemotherapy. With a median follow-up of 80 months (39–165 months), overall survival rates were not significantly different between the treatment and control groups (63% vs. 56%, p = 0.64). Similarly, no difference in the frequency of distant metastasis was observed between the groups (32% for CYVADIC vs. 36% for control, p = 0.42). However, relapse-free survival rates were higher for CYVADIC-treated patients than for control patients (56% vs. 43%, p = 0.007). Subset analysis of patients with non-extremity lesions also demonstrated an improvement in local control: 17% of those who received adjuvant chemotherapy versus 31% of those in the control group had local failures (p = 0.004).

The EORTC trial illustrates many of the difficulties in performing multi-institutional randomized studies. The trial required 11 years to complete, and despite careful control of eligibility criteria and histopathologic review, fully 32% of the original 468 randomized patients were considered ineligible for a variety of reasons. Notwithstanding these difficulties, this randomized trial lends additional support to the body of randomized data (see Table 3), suggesting that there is no impact of adjuvant chemotherapy on the development of distant metastasis or on overall survival in patients with soft tissue sarcoma. While the impact of CYVADIC therapy on local control is noteworthy, this improvement in local control was manifest only in the patients with non-extremity lesions, and the local control rates achieved with CYVADIC (83%) in this group were at best equivalent, if not inferior, to those reported with surgery and adjuvant irradiation.

There are a number of recognized deficiencies in the design and conduct of all the randomized clinical trials of adjuvant chemotherapy for soft tissue sarcoma. The most commonly cited deficiency of these trials as a group relates to the relatively small sample size and to the fact that small differences in survival require relatively large numbers of patients to detect with sufficient statistical power. The statistical tool of meta-analysis is designed to address this systematic deficiency of a group of similarly designed clinical trials. The performance and limitations of meta-analysis are beyond the scope of this review but have been addressed in detail elsewhere [44].

A from of meta-analysis has been applied to the randomized prospective trials of adjuvant doxorubicin chemotherapy in soft tissue sarcoma [45]. The endpoints for this analysis were overall survival and disease-free survival. In 10 of the 11 evaluable trials, data were abstracted from the narrative text and tables. In the remaining trial, from Scandinavia, proportions of patients were determined from interpolation of survival and disease-free survival curves at the median follow-up time. With this form of meta-analysis, the relative risk of relapse in the control group compared with the adjuvant chemotherapy group was 1.89 ± 0.42. The relative risk of death in the control group compared with the adjuvant therapy group was 1.72 ± 0.49. Both of these relative risks are significantly different from 1.0 at the p = 0.05 level of statistical significance. On this basis, the authors concluded that meta-analysis of the randomized prospective trials demonstrates improvement in relapse-free and overall survival with adjuvant chemotherapy. However, it is important to note that this statistical technique generally requires pooling of the individual trials' raw data to facilitate analysis of the combined data. As such, the form of meta-analysis employed in this study deviates from the standard statistical approach employed for meta-analysis. Consequently, clinicians should be appropriately cautious in applying conclusions generated based on statistical manipulation of the abstracted data to broad groups of patients.

The paradox that has arisen from the meta-analysis of these clinical trials in soft tissue sarcoma centers on the fact that 10 of the 11 published randomized trials showed no benefit from adjuvant chemotherapy and that the only study that showed a benefit has been highly criticized, yet a form of meta-analysis demonstrated an increased relative risk (significantly different from unity) for the patients who did not receive adjuvant doxorubicin-based chemotherapy. It is important to remember, however, that meta-analysis is a statistical technique: it is not a definitive clinical trial.

Proponents of the meta-analysis results have concluded that it will be difficult, if not impossible, to conduct a definitive randomized trial of adjuvant chemotherapy in this disease that has sufficient statistical power to detect clinically significant improvements in overall or disease-free survival within a reasonable time frame. Furthermore, there was a uniform but not statistically significant improval in disease-free and overall survival for patients who received adjuvant chemotherapy in each of the randomized trials. Some investigators have therefore concluded that the results generated from the meta-analysis should be extrapolated to the entire population of patients with high-risk soft tissue sarcomas. This population is generally believed to include patients with adverse prognostic factors, such as large tumor size and high histologic grade. However, while it is accepted that this group has a high risk of distant recurrence and disease-related mortality, it is difficult to advocate a treatment algorithm employing routine use of adjuvant chemotherapy in this setting based on the available published data.

The most cautious interpretation of the available published data, including the meta-analysis of Zalupski and colleagues [45], would be that adjuvant doxorubicin-based chemotherapy should be employed in selected patients with high-grade soft tissue sarcomas, ideally within the confines of a clinical trial or focused current practice program. A conventional form of meta-analysis employing the original data from published randomized trials may ultimately help to address some of the criticisms that have been raised about the present meta-analysis. Until such an analysis is performed or until more definitive data are available for review, the routine use of adjuvant chemotherapy cannot to advocated for patients with soft tissue sarcoma. In the absence of such data, potentially toxic adjuvant chemotherapy should be reserved for selected patients who present with adverse prognostic factors for overall survival. These factors include tumor size greater than 5 cm, deep tumor location, and high histologic grade [16,18]. Patients should be offered adjuvant chemotherapy only with the express understanding that it is empiric therapy to treat micrometastatic disease and not based on a body of conclusive data documenting a survival benefit. Future research on this disease should be directed toward identifying additional prognostic factors and/or molecular determinants that may more precisely identify the patients who are most likely to have relapses.

Table 4. Randomized phase III trials with ifosfamide-containing treatment arms in advanced soft tissue sarcoma

Group	Treatment Arm drug regimen	Dose (mg/m²)	No. patients	Response rate (%)	Median survival (mo)
SWOG/CALGB [41]	1. AD	A (60), D (1000)	170	17	12
	2. ADI	A (60), D (1000), I (7.5)	170	32[a]	13[a]
ECOG [42]	1. A	A (80)	90	20	9
	2. AI	A (60), I (7.5)	88	34[a]	12
	3. MAP	M (8), A (40), P (60)	84	32	10
EORTC [43]	1. A	A (75)	263	23	13
	2. AI	A (50), I (5)	258	28	12.8
	3. CyVAD	Cy (500), V (1.5), A (50), D (750)	142	28	13.8

SWOG = Southwest Oncology Group; CALGB = Cancer and Leukemia Study Group B; ECOG = Eastern Cooperative Oncology Group; EORTC = European Organization for Research and Treatment of Cancer, A = doxorubicin (Adriamycin); I = ifosfamide; D = dacarbazine; M = mitomycin C; P = cisplatin; V = vincristine; Cy = cyclophosphamide; response rate = complete respone + partial response.
[a] $p < 0.05$.

Ifosfamide, an analogue of cyclophosphamide, has been reported to produce significant response rates in the range of 30–40% in adults with advanced soft tissue sarcoma. Higher response rates have been reported with small cell sarcomas, such as rhabdomyosarcoma and synovial sarcoma. The evaluable phase III trials with ifosfamide-containing treatment arms are summarized in Table 4. The most comprehensive comparative study performed to date was reported by the EORTC [43]. In that study, 663 eligible patients were randomly assigned to receive doxorubicin, 75 mg/m² (arm A); cyclophosphamide, vincristine, doxorubicin, and dacarbazine (CYVADIC; arm B); or ifosfamide, 5 mg/m², plus doxorubicin, 50 mg/m² (arm C). There was no statistically significant difference detected among the three study arms in terms of response rate (arm A, 23.3%; arm B, 28.4%; and arm C, 28.1%), remission duration, or overall survival (median 52 weeks on arm A, 51 weeks on arm B, and 55 weeks on arm C). The degree of myelosuppression was significantly greater for the combination of ifosfamide and doxorubicin than for the other two regimens. Cardiotoxicity was also more frequent in arm C. This study and others suggest that single-agent doxorubicin is still the standard chemotherapy against which more intensive or new drug treatments should be compared. Although it is clear that a dose-response relationship exists for both doxorubicin and ifosfamide, further studies will be required to define the response rates and toxicity with high-dose ifosfamide-based combination regimens. At this time there is no evidence to substantiate the use of adjuvant ifosfamide-based chemotherapy in soft tissue sarcoma outside the confines of a clinical trial.

Isolated limb perfusion of extremity soft tissue sarcoma

Traditionally, limb-salvage therapy for extremity sarcomas has consisted of a combination of surgery and radiotherapy. In most recent series, this has resulted in a limb-salvage rate of approximately 90% [25]. There remains a group of patients, however, with tumors that are in proximity to bones or major neurovascular structures for whom limb salvage is not an option owing to technical considerations. In addition, an important quality of life issue exists in those patients who are not candidates for a traditional limb-salvage procedure and who already have distant metastatic disease. In an effort to achieve limb salvage in an even larger group of patients, several investigators have used hyperthermic isolated limb perfusion (HILP) as a means of achieving tumor cytoreduction and limb salvage.

Isolated limb perfusion (ILP) was first introduced in 1958 by Creech et al. at Tulane University [46]. The majority of studies involving ILP were initially designed for patients with melanoma confined to an extremity. As almost an afterthought, sarcoma patients with large, advanced lesions who were otherwise ineligible for limb-salvage protocols were included in ILP protocols on an ad-hoc basis. The first report of the results of ILP in sarcoma patients alone was published by McBride from M. D. Anderson Cancer Center in 1974 [47]. Over the ensuing 22 years, eight retrospective reviews of individual institutional experience with ILP for sarcoma have been published in the scientific literature [48–54]. In addition, multiple studies of hyperthermic isolated limb perfusion (HILP) for melanoma have included scattered sarcoma patients [55,56]. In all, there have been over 500 reported cases of ILP or HILP for extremity sarcomas during this period. There has been a wide range of response rates (18–60%) and 5-year survival rates (50–69%) in these studies. The heterogeneous response of soft tissue sarcomas to ILP in these studies is most likely multifactorial in nature. As mentioned earlier, these studies have all been retrospective, single-institution reviews. There has not been, to date, a prospective randomized study comparing HILP with any other treatment modality using either response rate or survival as an endpoint. All of the studies have treated a variety of histologic subtypes, stages, and grades of tumor without any stratification for these variables. Additionally, a variety of different drugs have been used, not only among different studies but also within the same study. The most commonly used drugs in these series were melphalan, dactinomycin, mechlorethamine (nitrogen mustard), doxorubicin, and cisplatin, perfused singly and in various combinations. For all of these reasons, it is difficult to evaluate the actual tumor response to and the clinical efficacy of ILP for sarcoma. However, the consensus of those performing ILP/HILP is that it has significant antitumor activity.

Despite this initial antitumor activity seen in patients with melanoma and sarcoma, ILP fell out of favor, in part because of the significant morbidity associated with the procedure. No significant new advances were made in the technical or pharmacologic aspects of ILP until the late 1980s, when Lienard et al. added tumor necrosis factor (TNF) to the chemotherapeutic agents given during HILP [57]. TNF was first cloned by Pennica and associates in 1985 [58], and subsequently was shown to cause hemorrhagic necrosis of subcutaneously implanted tumors in mice [59]. Based on promising preclinical studies, multiple phase I and II clinical trials of systemic TNF were initiated with relatively disappointing results. Unfortunately, the maximally tolerated dose of TNF in the clinical trials was significantly lower than what was observed to be tumoricidal animal models, and it was hypothesized that the lack of efficacy of TNF in the clinical trials was secondary to inadequate blood and tissue levels. In this regard, isolated perfusion of an extremity would provide an ideal clinical model to test this hypothesis. Lienard et al. [57] were the first to realized the potential suitability of TNF for administration via an HILP circuit. In the animal models, pathologic responses occurred after a single intravenous bolus of TNF, with a response time on the order of hours. In addition, by confining TNF to the circulation of only the involved extremity, the dose-limiting toxic effect, hypotension, could potentially be avoided, and increased blood and tissue levels could thereby be achieved. However, despite these attributes of TNF, which would appear to make it an ideal agent for HILP, efforts using TNF as the single agent in the perfusion circuit have been rather unsuccessful. Unfortunately, a prospective randomized trial comparing TNF alone with TNF in combination with other chemotherapeutic agents has not been performed. Although only a few patients have been treated with HILP using TNF alone and most of them had melanoma, the uniform lack of tumor responsiveness has led more investigators to conclude that there is no role for TNF as a single agent in HILP [60].

In contrast, the results using TNF in combination with melphalan have been remarkable. The initial report by Lienard et al. [57] included five perfusions in four patients with recurrent sarcomas of the extremity. There were four complete responses (CR) and one partial response (PR). Three of these responses were documented pathologically, while the remaining two responses were documented only clinically. The single patients with the PR had a multifocal synovial sarcoma invading bone and was reperfused, resulting in a pathologic CR. (No information was given about the time interval between the two perfusions.) The duration of responses at the time of this report ranged from 5 to 23 months. Similar results were seen in the melanoma patients in this study (100% overall response rate, with 89% being CRs). The authors note that the CRs were in patients with 'bulky' tumors; however, no actual measurements were given. The number of tumor nodules per extremity perfused ranged from 1 to 10.

Two other reports have been published documenting the results of this TNF/ melphalan/interferon-gamma therapy HILP for extremity sarcomas. Both reports are from the Rotterdam Cancer Center. The initial report of 16 patients showed a limb-salvage rate of 92%. Systemic toxicity was confined to those patients in whom more than 10% of the drugs leaked out of the perfusion circuit and into the systemic circulation [61]. In a follow-up report, a similar limb-salvage rate (93%) was obtained in a series of 23 patients. In that series, the follow-up ranged from 6 to 38 months, and the median tumor size was 21×18 cm. Systemic toxicity was similar to that seen in the previous study [62].

The use of melphalan as the chemotherapeutic agent in HILP for soft tissue sarcomas has been somewhat controversial. When melphalan is used systemically, it has minimal activity against soft tissue sarcomas. Therefore, there has been some question as to whether melphalan is the drug of choice for sarcoma HILP therapy. Melphalan began being used a in HILP for sarcomas as a result of its activity in patients with melanoma being treated by HILP. As most systemic chemotherapy regimens for soft tissue sarcomas are doxorubicin based, it is natural to ask whether doxorubicin would be more effective against soft tissue sarcomas in an HILP circuit. Because of the significant tissue toxicity seen with systemic doxorubicin, most investigators have been reticent to use this agent in HILP for fear of significant local tissue toxicity. However, recently Rossi et al. reported phase I and II trials using doxorubicin in HILP for soft tissue sarcomas [63,64]. These studies showed a limb-salvage rate of 91%, comparable with that seen with the triple-drug regimen of Lejeune et al. In addition, the locoregional toxicity was comparable with that in previous HILP studies.

Many questions remain to be answered concerning the role of HILP in treating soft tissue sarcomas of the extremities. As mentioned previously, no randomized trial has been performed comparing HILP with standard treatment (either limb salvage or amputation) to validate the efficacy of HILP. Currently, the National Cancer Institute is sponsoring a phase II trial to evaluate the role of TNF and melphalan administered by HILP for otherwise unresectable sarcomas of the extremities. Questions regarding the role of interferon-gamma in the triple-drug regimen are awaiting the results of a European randomized trial. Eventually, randomized trials comparing different chemotherapeutic agents (e.g., doxorubicin and melphalan) as well as combinations of drugs and biologic agents (e.g., TNF and interferon) will need to be performed to adequately address all of the remaining questions regarding HILP for extremity sarcomas.

Acknowledgments

The authors gratefully acknowledge the tremendous assistance of Vivian Z. Garcia in the preparation of this manuscript.

References

1. Pisters PWT, Brennan MF. Sarcomas of soft tissue. In Abeloff M, Armitage J, Lichter A, Niederhuber J (eds). Clinical Oncology. New York: Churchill Livingstone, 1995, pp 1799–1832.
2. Yang JC, Glatstein EJ, Rosenberg SA, Antman KH. Sarcomas of soft tissues. In DeVita VT Jr., Hellman S, Rosenberg SA (eds). Cancer: Principles and Practice of Oncology, 4th ed. Philadelphia: J.B. Lippincott, 1993, pp 1436–1488.
3. Russell WO, Cohen J, Enzinger F, et al. A clinical and pathological staging system for soft tissue sarcomas. Cancer 4:1562–1570, 1977.
4. Sears HF, Hopson R, Inouye W, Rizzo T, Grotzinger PJ. Analysis of staging and management of patients with sarcoma: A ten year experience. Ann Surg 191:488–493, 1980.
5. Markhede G, Angervall L, Stener B. A multivariate analysis of the prognosis after surgical treatment of malignant soft-tissue tumors. Cancer 49:1721–1733, 1982.
6. Trojani M, Contesso G, Coindre JM, et al. Soft-tissue sarcomas of adults: Study of pathological prognostic variables and definition of a histopathological grading system. Int J Cancer 33:37–42, 1984.
7. Rydholm A, Berg NO, Gullberg B, Persson BM, Thorngren KG. Prognosis for soft-tissue sarcoma in the locomotor system. A retrospective population-based follow-up study of 237 patients. Acta Pathol Microbiol Immunol Scand [A] 92:375–386, 1984.
8. Collin C, Godbold J, Hajdu S, Brennan M. Localized extremity soft tissue sarcoma: An analysis of factors affecting survival. J Clin Oncol 5:601–612, 1987.
9. Tsujimoto M, Aozasa K, Ueda T, Morimura Y, Komtsubara Y, Doi T. Multivariate analysis for histologic prognostic factors in soft tissue sarcomas. Cancer 62:994–998, 1988.
10. Ueda T, Aozasa K, Tsujimoto M, et al. Multivariate analysis for clinical prognostic factors in 163 patients. Cancer 62:1444–1450, 1988.
11. Rooser B, Attewell R, Berg NO, Rydholm A. Prognostication in soft tissue sarcoma. A model with four risk factors. Cancer 61:817–823, 1988.
12. Mandard AM, Petiot JF, Marnay J, et al. Prognostic factors is soft tissue sarcomas. A multivariate analysis of 109 cases. Cancer 63:1437–1451, 1989.
13. Bell RS, O'Sullivan B, Liu FF, et al. The surgical margin in soft-tissue sarcoma. J Bone Joint Surg Am 71:370–375, 1989.
14. Alvegard TA, Berg NO, Baldetorp B, et al. Cellular DNA content and prognosis of high-grade soft tissue sarcoma: The Scandinavian Sarcoma Group experience. J Clin Oncol 8:538–547, 1990.
15. Stotter AT, Ahern RP, Fisher C, Mott AF, Fallowfield ME, Westbury G. The influence of local recurrence of extremity soft tissue sarcoma on metastasis and survival. Cancer 65:1119–1129, 1990.
16. Gaynor JJ, Tan CC, Casper ES, et al. Refinement of clinicopathologic staging for localized soft tissue sarcoma of the extremity: A study of 423 adults. J Clin Oncol 10:1317–1329, 1992.
17. Singer S, Corson JM, Gonin R, Labow B, Eberlein TJ. Prognostic factors predictive of survival and local recurrence for extremity soft tissue sarcoma. Ann Surg 219:165–173, 1994.
18. Pisters PWT, Leung DHY, Woodruff J, Shi W, Brennan MF. Analysis of prognostic factors in 1041 patients with localized soft tissue sarcomas of the extremities. J Clin Oncol 14:1679–1689, 1996.
19. Heise HW, Myers MH, Russell WO, et al. Recurrence-free survival time for surgically treated soft tissue sarcoma patients. Cancer 57:172–177, 1986.
20. Fisher B, Anderson S, Redmond CK, Wolmark N, Wickerham DL, Cronin WM. Reanalysis and results after 12 years of follow-up in a randomized trial comparing total mastectomy with

lumpectomy with or without irradiation in the treatment of breast cancer. N Engl J Med 333:1456–1461, 1995.

21. Recht A, Houlihan MJ. Conservative surgery without radiotherapy in the treatment of patients with early-stage invasive breast cancer. Ann Surg 222:9–18, 1995.

22. Geer RJ, Woodruff J, Casper ES, Brennan MF. Management of small soft-tissue sarcoma of the extremity in adults. Arch Surg 127:1285–1289, 1992.

23. Rydholm A, Gustafson P, Rooser B, et al. Limb-sparing surgery without radiotherapy based on anatomic location of soft tissue sarcoma. J Clin Oncol 9:1757–1765, 1991.

24. Pisters PWT, Harrison LB, Leung DHY, Woodruff JM, Casper ES. Long-term results of a prospective randomized trial of adjuvant brachytherapy in soft tissue sarcoma. J Clin Oncol 14:859–868, 1996.

25. Brennan MF, Casper ES, Harrison LB, Shiu MH, Gaynor J, Hajdu SI. The role of multimodality therapy in soft-tissue sarcoma. Ann Surg 214:328–337, 1991.

26. Suit HD, Mankin HJ, Wood WC, et al. Treatment of the patient with stage M0 soft tissue sarcoma. J Clin Oncol 6:854–862, 1988.

27. Healey B, Corson J, Demetri G, Singer S. Surgery alone may be adequate treatment for select stage IA–IIIA soft tissue sarcomas (abstr). Proc Am Soc Clin Oncol 14:517, 1995.

28. Bramwell V, Rouesse J, Steward W, et al. Adjuvant CYVADIC chemotherapy for adult soft tissue sarcoma — reduced local recurrence but no improvement in survival: A study of the European Organization for Research and Treatment of Cancer Soft Tissue and Bone Sarcoma Group. J Clin Oncol 12:1137–1149, 1994.

29. Benjamin RS, Terjanian TO, Fenoglio CJ, et al. The importance of combination chemotherapy for adjuvant treatment of high risk patients with soft-tissue sarcomas of the extremities. In Salmon S (ed). Adjuvant Therapy of Cancer, 5th ed. Orlando: Grune & Stratton, 1987, pp 735–744.

30. Chang AE, Kinsella T, Glatstein E, et al. Adjuvant chemotherapy for patients with high-grade soft-tissue sarcomas of the extremity. J Clin Oncol 6:1491–1500, 1988.

31. Edmonson JH, Fleming TR, Ivins JC, Burgert EO Jr, Soule EH. Randomized study of systemic chemotherapy following complete excision of nonosseous sarcomas. J Clin Oncol 2:1390–1396, 1984.

32. Edmonson JH. Role of ajduvant chemotherapy in the management of patients with soft tissue sarcomas. Cancer Treat Rep 68:1063–1066, 1984.

33. Eilber FR, Giuliano AE, Huth JF, Morton DL. A randomized prospective trial using postoperative adjuvant chemotherapy (Adriamycin) in high-grade extremity soft-tissue sarcoma. Am J Clin Oncol 11:39–45, 1988.

34. Alvegard TA, Sigurdsson H, Mouridsen H, et al. Adjuvant chemotherapy with doxorubicin in high-grade soft tissue sarcoma: A randomized trial of the Scandinavian Sarcoma Group. J Clin Oncol 7:1504–1513, 1989.

35. Gherlinzoni F, Pignatti G, Fontana M. Soft tissue sarcomas: The experience at the Istituto Ortopedico Rizzoli. Chir Organi Mov 75:150–154, 1990.

36. Gherlinzoni F, Picci P, Sangiorgi A, Cazzola A, Zherly H. Late results of a randomized clinical trial for soft tissue sarcomas of the extremities (abstr). Proc Connect Tissue Oncol Soc 1:A6, 1995.

37. Antman K, Amato D, Lerner H. Eastern Cooperative Oncology Group and Dana-Farber Cancer Institute/Massachusetts General Hospital study. In Jones S, Salmon S (eds). Adjuvant Therapy of Cancer, 4th ed. Orlando: Grune & Stratton, 1984, pp 611–620.

38. Antman K, Amato D, Lerner H, et al. Adjuvant doxorubicin for sarcoma: Data from the Eastern Coooperative Oncology Group and Dana-Farber Cancer Institute/Massachusetts General Hospital studies. Cancer Treat Symp 3:109–115, 1985.

39. Antman K, Suit H, Amato D, et al. Preliminary results of a randomized trial of adjuvant doxorubicin for sarcomas: Lack of apparent difference between treatment groups. J Clin Oncol 2:601–608, 1984.

40. Antman K, Amato D, Pilepich M, et al. A preliminary analysis of a randomized intergroup (SWOG, ECOG, CALBG, NCOG) trial of adjuvant doxorubicin for soft tissue sarcomas. In Salmon S (ed). Adjuvant Therapy of Cancer, 5th ed. Orlando: Grune & Stratton, 1987, pp 725–734.

41. Antman K, Crowley J, Balacerzak SP, et al. An intergroup phase III randomized study of doxorubicin and dacarbazine with or without ifosfamide and mesna in advanced soft tissue and bone sarcomas. J Clin Oncol 11:1276–1285, 1993.

42. Edmonson JH, Ryan LM, Blum RH, et al. Randomized comparison of doxorubicin alone versus ifosfamide plus doxorubicin or mitomycin, doxorubicin, and cisplatin against advanced soft tissue sarcomas. J Clin Oncol 11:1269–1275, 1993.

43. Santoro A, Tursz T, Mouridsen H, et al. Doxorubicin versus CYVADIC versus doxorubicin plus ifosfamide in first-line treatment of advanced soft tissue sarcomas: A randomized study of the European Organization for Research and Treatment of Cancer Soft Tissue and Bone Sarcoma Group. J Clin Oncol 13:1537–1545, 1995.

44. Simon R. Meta-analysis and cancer clinical trials. In DeVita VT, Jr., Hellman S, Rosenberg SA (eds). Cancer: Principles and Practice of Oncology, Vol. 5, No. 6, Updates. 1991.

45. Zalupski M, Ryan J, Hussein M, Baker L. Defining the role of adjuvant chemotherapy for patients with soft tissue sarcomas of the extremities. In Salmon S (ed). Adjuvant Therapy of Cancer, 7th ed. Philadelphia: W.B. Saunders, 1993, pp 385–392.

46. Creech O, Krementz ET, Ryan RF, Winblad JN. Chemotherapy of cancer: Regional perfusion utilizing an extracorporeal circuit. Ann Surg 148:616–632, 1958.

47. McBride CM. Sarcomas of the limbs, results of adjuvant chemotherapy using isolation perfusion. Arch Surg 109:304–308, 1974.

48. Krementz ET, Carter RD, Sutherland CM, Hutton I. Chemotherapy of sarcomas of the limbs by regional perfusion. Ann Surg 185:555–564, 1977.

49. Stehlin JS, de Ipolyi PD, Giovanella BC, Gutierrez AE, Anderson RF. Soft tissue sarcomas of the extremity: Multidisciplinary therapy employing hyperthermic perfusion. Am J Surg 130:643–646, 1975.

50. Hoekstra HJ, Schraffordt Koops H, Molenaar WM, Oldhoff J. Results of isolated regional perfusion in the treatment of malignant soft tissue tumors of the extremities. Cancer 60:1703–1707, 1987.

51. Lethi PM, Stephens MH, Janoff K, Stevens K, Fletcher WS. Improved survival for soft tissue sarcoma of the extremities by regional hyperthermic perfusion, local excision, and radiation therapy. Surg Gynecol Obstet 162:149–152, 1986.

52. Klaase JM, Kroon BBR, Benckhuijsen C, van Geel AN, Albus-Lutter E, Wieberdink J. Results of regional isolated perfusion with cytostatics in patients with soft tissue tumors of the extremities. Cancer 64:616–621, 1989.

53. Schraffodt-Koops H, Eibergen R, Oldhoff J, van der Ploeg E, Vermey A. Isolated regional perfusion in the treatment of soft tissue sacomas of the extremities. Clin Oncol 2:245–252, 1976.

54. Ghussen F, Nagel K. Die regionale hypertherme cytostatica-perfusion als alternative bei der behandlung von malignen weichgewebetumoren der extremitaten. Chirurg 55:505–507, 1984.

55. Pommier RF, Moseley HS, Cohen J, Huang CS, Townsend R, Fletcher WS. Pharmacokinetics, toxicity, and short-term results of cisplatin hyperthermic isolated limb perfusion for soft-tissue sarcoma and melanoma of the extremities. Am J Surg 155:667–671, 1988.

56. Roseman JM. Effective management of extremity cancers using cisplatin and etoposide in isolated limb perfusion. J Surg Oncol 35:170–172, 1987.

57. Lienard D, Ewalenko P, Delmotte J-J, Renard N, Lejeune FJ. High-dose recombinant tumor necrosis factor alpha in combination with interferon gamma and melphalan in isolation perfusion of the limbs for melanoma and sarcoma. J Clin Oncol 10:52–60, 1992.

58. Pennica DG, Hayflick JS, Bringman TS, Palladinl MA, Goeddel DV. Cloning and expression in *Escherichia coli* of the cDNA for murine tumor necrosis factor. Proc Natl Acad Sci USA 82:6060–6064, 1985.

59. Asher A, Mule JJ, Reichert CM, Shiloni E, Rosenberg SA. Studies on the anti-tumor efficacy of systemically administered recombinant tumor necrosis factor against several murine tumors in vivo. J Immunol 138:963–974, 1987.

60. Posner MC, Lienard D, Lejeune FJ. Hyperthermic isolated limb perfusion with tumor necrosis factor alone for melanoma. Cancer J Sci Am 1:274–280, 1995.

61. Eggermont AMM, Lienard D, Schraffordt-Koops H, van Geel AN, Hoekstra HJ, Lejeune FJ. Limb salvage by high dose tumor necrosis factor-alpha (TNF), gamma-interferon (IFN) and melphalan isolated limb perfusion (ILP) in patients with irresectable soft tissue sarcomas (abstr). Am Soc Clin Oncol 11:412, 1992.

62. Schraffordt-Koops H, Lienard D, Eggermont AM, Hoekstra HJ, van Geel BN, Lejeune FJ. Isolated limb perfusion with high dose TNF-alpha, gamma-IFN, and melphalan in patients with irresedtable soft tissue sarcomas. A highly effective limb salving procedure (abstr). Soc Surg Oncol 1993; [Abstract].

63. Rossi CR, Vecchiato A, Da Pian PP, et al. Adriamycin in hyperthermic perfusion for advanced limb sarcomas. Ann Oncol 3:511–513, 1992.

64. Rossi CR, Vecchiato A, Foletto M, et al. Phase II study on neoadjuvant hyperthermic-antiblastic perfusion with doxorubicin in patients with intermediate or high grade limb sarcomas. Cancer 73:2140–2146, 1994.

6. Advances in the diagnosis and treatment of adenocarcinoma of the pancreas

Douglas B. Evans, Jeffrey E. Lee, Peter W.T. Pisters,
Chusilp Charnsangavej, Lee M. Ellis, Paul J. Chiao, Renato Lenzi,
and James L. Abbruzzese

Introduction

Pancreatic cancer is the flfth leading cause of adult cancer mortality. The etiology of cancer of the pancreas remains a mystery despite the implication of various agents, such as coffee, alcohol, and cigarettes. The current management of patients with pancreatic cancer at our institution involves: (1) a selective approach to the use of laparotomy based on accurate radiographic imaging techniques, and the availability of reliable minimally invasive techniques for biliary decompression; (2) the use of multimodality therapy in all patients with localized, potentially resectable disease; and (3) a standardized approach to surgery and perioperative patient management. The goals of this approach are to maximize the length and quality of patient survival while minimizing treatment-related toxicity and limiting the social and economic impact of complicated, multimodality therapy. However, less than 5% of patients with adenocarcinoma of the pancreas will be alive 5 years after diagnosis. Therefore, clinical and basic science research is proceeding in parallel: while attempting to optimize the length and quality of life of patients with localized pancreatic tumors, research is also focusing on developing improved strategies for early diagnosis and effective systemic therapy.

Diagnostic imaging

Surgical resection remains the only potentially curative treatment strategy for patients with adenocarcinoma of the pancreatic head. Patients who undergo successful resection of the primary tumor combined with either pre- or postoperative chemoradiation have a 5-year survival rate of up to 20% and a median survival of 18–19 months [1,2]. In contrast, patients with locally advanced, unresectable disease treated with palliative chemoradiation have a median survival of only 10–12 months, with virtually no chance for long-term survivorship [3,4]. Importantly, patients who undergo pancreaticoduodenectomy but are found to have a positive margin of resection also have a median survival of only 10 months (Table 1) [5–10]. Therefore,

Raphael E. Pollock (ed.), SURGICAL ONCOLOGY. Copyright © 1997. Kluwer Academic Publishers.
ISBN 0-7923-9900-5. All rights reserved.

Table 1. Median survival for patients who underwent surgical resection for adenocarcinoma of the pancreas and were found to have a positive margin of resection

Reference (yr)	No.	Margin	Median survival (mo)
Tepper [10] (1976)	17[a]	G/M	8
Trede [6] (1990)	54	G/M	10
Whittington [7] (1991)	19	G	[b]
Willet [8] (1993)	37	G/M	11
Nitecki [5] (1995)	28	G	9
Yeo [9] (1995)	58	G/M	10

[a] All patients also had positive regional lymph nodes.
[b] Two patients alive at 18 months of follow-up.
G = grossly positive margin; M = microscopically positive margin.
From Staley, et al. [1], with permission.

it is essential that surgery be applied only to patients with localized pancreatic cancer amenable to a margin-negative pancreaticoduodenectomy. However, only 16–30% of patients who undergo operations with curative intent have their pancreatic cancers successfully removed; the remaining patients are found to have unsuspected liver or peritoneal metastases or, most commonly, local tumor extension to the superior mesenteric vein (SMV) or superior mesenteric artery (SMA) [11]. Laparotomy in patients who are found to be unresectable at surgery is associated with a mortality rate of 2.5–5.0%, a morbidity rate of approximately 30%, and a mean hospital stay of 2 weeks [12,13]. Further, laparotomy for palliation in this subgroup of patients is often unnecessary because of recent advances in endoscopic, percutaneous, and laparoscopic methods of biliary decompression. In patients with unresectable disease, laparotomy should be avoided, when possible, due to the morbidity (and recovery time) of surgery and the relatively short life expectancy of these patients. Therein lies the importance of how the clinician defines resectability.

Advocates of limited preoperative evaluation followed by surgical exploration in all patients with presumed nonmetastatic pancreatic cancer believe that intraoperative evaluation is the most sensitive method of determining resectability [13,14]. At the time of surgical exploration for pancreatic head cancer, a Kocher maneuver is the first procedure performed to assess the relationship of the tumor to the SMA by palpation (Fig. 1). This maneuver has proved to be an insensitive method of evaluationg this vital tumor–vessel relationship as demonstrated by the high incidence of positive-margin resections recently reported [8,9]. Direct intraoperative assessment of the extent of retroperitoneal tumor growth in relation to the SMA origin is not completed

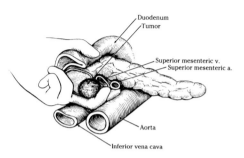

Figure 1. Intraoperative palpation to determine the relationship of the tumor to the mesenteric vessels at the time of the Kocher maneuver. The tumor is palpated with the left hand. The difficulty in accurately assessing the tumor–vessel relationship by palpation emphasizes the importance of preoperative thin-section, contrast-enhanced, helical CT. (From Cusack et al. [37] with permission.)

until the final step in tumor resection, after gastric and pancreatic transection, when the surgeon is committed to resection even if all of the tumor cannot be safely removed. The second intraoperative maneuver performed to assess local tumor resectability is to develop a plane of dissection between the anterior surface of the superior mesenteric-portal vein (SMPV) confluence and the posterior surface of the neck of the pancreas (Fig. 2); tumor encasement of this region, in the opinion of most surgeons, precludes resection. However, the rationale for this maneuver early in the operation is unclear as tumors of the pancreatic head or uncinate process are prone to invade the lateral or posterior wall of the SMPV confluence; the anterior wall is rarely involved in the absence of encasement of the celiac axis or SMA orgin (as seen in locally advanced tumors of the pancreatic neck or body). The relationship of a pancreatic head tumor to the lateral and posterior walls of the SMPV confluence (and the SMA) can be *directly* inspected only after gastric and pancreatic transection and, therefore, needs to be accurately assessed by preoperative imaging studies [15,16].

Data from our institution have demonstrated improved rates of resectability when thin-section contrast-enhanced CT is combined with objective criteria for resectability [11]. Only patients with radiographic evidence of a resectable tumor are candidates for laparotomy. CT criteria for resectability include (1) the absence of extrapancreatic disease, (2) a patent SMPV confluence, and (3) no direct tumor extension to the celiac axis or SMA (Fig. 3). Patients whose tumors are deemed unresectable by these radiographic criteria are not considered candidates for a potentially curative pancreaticoduodenectomy. To assess the accuracy of this CT criteria for resectability, we studied 145 consecutive patients who were referred with a presumed resectable pancreatic neoplasm. Only 42 patients fulfilled the criteria for resectability. However, 37 (88%) of the 42 patients underwent successful pancreaticoduodenectomy. The other five patients (12%) were found to have unresectable tumors at laparotomy. Final pathologic evaluation of the

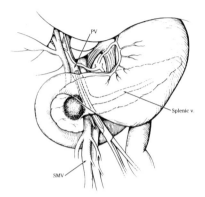

Figure 2. Tumor-free plane between the anterior surface of the superior mesenteric-portal vein confluence and the posterior surface of the pancreas. This plane can often be developed despite fixation of the tumor to the lateral wall of the superior mesenteric vein (SMV). PV = portal vein.

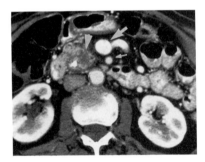

Figure 3. Contrast-enhanced CT scan demonstrating a resectable adenocarcinoma of the pancreatic head. Note the normal fat plane between the low-density tumor (arrowhead) and both the superior mesenteric artery (smally arrow) and the superior mesenteric vein (large arrow). The intrapancreatic portion of the common bile duct contains a stent, which was endoscopically placed for biliary drainage.

retroperitoneal margin (Fig. 4) was used to confirm the accuracy of our CT criteria to predict resectability. No patient had a grossly positive margin of resection, and only 5 of 25 patients with adenocarcinoma of pancreatic head origin were found to have a microscopic focus of adenocarcinoma at the retroperitoneal margin. This was despite the fact that many patients had undergone a previous nontherapeutic laparotomy prior to referral to our institution, and nine patients required resection of the SMV or SMPV confluence.

The development of helical or spiral CT scanning has improved scan speed allowing the pancreas to be scanned in approximately 30 seconds compared with 2 minutes with a conventional scanner. The faster scan speed is made

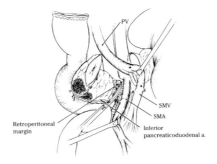

Figure 4. Illustration of the final step in pancreaticoduodenectomy. They retroperitoneal margin is defined as the tissue directly adjacent to the proximal 3–4 cm of the superior mesenteric artery (SMA). PV = portal vein; SMV = superior mesenteric vein. From Fuhrman et al. [11], with permission.

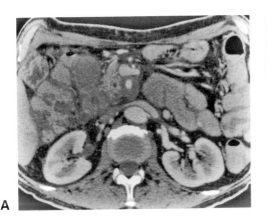

A

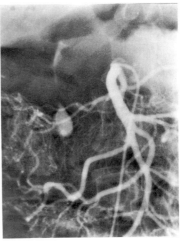

B

Figure 5. **A:** Contrast-enhanced CT scan illustrating an unresectable adenocarcinoma of the uncinate process of the pancreas with tumor encasement of the superior mesenteric artery. **B:** Visceral angiography in the same patient illustrating a normal superior mesenteric artery (despite tumor encasement seen on CT scan).

possible by continuous rotation of the x-ray tube around the gantry, and offers several advantages: (1) imaging of the entire pancreas during the bolus phase of contrast enhancement, (2) improved visualization of vascular anatomy, and (3) improved detection of hepatic metastases as the liver is scanned during the proper phase of contrast enhancement. Helical CT performed with contrast enhancement and a thin-section technique can accurately assess the relationship of the low-density tumor to the celiac axis, SMA, and SMPV confluence.

However, design of the scanning protocol and interpretation of scans must be done by experienced physicians who understand the clinical importance of accurate staging and assessment of resectability in patients with pancreatic cancer.

Contrast-enhanced helical CT has also reduced the role of preoperative angiography. Angiography does not provide the detail that is needed to determine the anatomic relationship between the tumor and the SMA that is provided by high-quality contrast-enhanced CT. Angiography allows contrast enhancement of only the vessel lumen; the surrounding tumor and soft tissue cannot be evaluated (Fig. 5A,B). We limit the use of angiography to reoperative cases in which identification of aberrant hepatic arterial anatomy may prevent iatrogenic injury during portal dissection when there is extensive scarring from a previous biliary procedure. Tyler and Evans reported a replaced or accessory right hepatic artery arising from the SMA in 26% of patients who underwent reoperative pancreaticoduodenectomy [17]. Preoperative knowledge of this common anatomic variant may help prevent operative misadventure in the reoperative setting.

Combined modality therapy

External-beam radiation therapy (EBRT) and concomitant 5-fluorouracil (FU) chemotherapy (chemoradiation) were shown to prolong survival in patients with locally advanced adenocarcinoma of the pancreas [3,18,19]. Those data were the foundation for a prospective randomized study of adjuvant chemoradiation ($500 \, mg/m^2/day$ of 5-FU for 6 days and 40 Gy of radiation) following pancreaticoduodenectomy conducted by the Gastrointestinal Tumor Study Group; that trial also demonstrated a survival advantage from multimodality therapy compared with resection alone [20,21]. However, owing to a prolonged recovery, 5 (24%) of the 21 patients in the adjuvant chemoradiation arm could not begin chemoradiation until more than 10 weeks after pancreaticoduodenectomy. Further, published studies advocating postoperative adjuvant chemoradiation are prone to selection bias; the patients likely to be considered for protocol entry are those who recover rapidly from surgery and have a good performance status. The slow patient accrual of postoperative adjuvant therapy studies [20,22] and the positive correlation of survival with performance status in the Gastrointestinal Tumor Study Group trial validate this concern [20]. Additional data regarding the potential benefit of postoperative adjuvant therapy will come from the European Organization for Research and Treatment of Cancer (EORTC) and the European Study Group for Pancreatic Cancer (ESPCA). The EORTC initiated a study in 1987 comparing adjuvant 5-FU–based chemoradiation following pancreatectomy versus surgery alone [23]. Over 150 patients have been entered, but the results are not yet available. In 1994 a study was initiated by the ESPCA randomizing patients following pancreatectomy to one of four treatment groups: (1) no adjuvant therapy, (2) 5-FU–based chemoradiation, (3) 5-FU–based chemoradiation followed by systemic 5-FU and leucovorin, and (4) 5-FU and leucovorin without EBRT [23].

The risk of delaying adjuvant therapy, combined with small published experiences of successful pancreatic resection following EBRT [24–26] prompted many institutions to initiate studies in which chemoradiation was given before pancreaticoduodenectomy for patients with potentially resectable (or locally advanced) adenocarcinoma of the pancreas [27–30]. The preoperative use of chemoradiation is supported by the following considerations [31]: (1) Radiation therapy is more effective on well-oxygenated cells that have not been devascularized by surgery. (2) Peritoneal tumor cell implantation caused by the manipulation of surgery may be prevented by preoperative chemoradiation. (3) The high frequency of positive-margin resections recently reported supports the concern that the retroperitoneal margin of excision, even when negative, may be only a few millimeters; surgery alone may therefore be an inadequate strategy for local tumor control. (4) Patients with disseminated disease evident on restaging studies after chemoradiation will not be subjected to laparotomy. (5) Because radiation therapy and chemotherapy are given first, delayed postoperative recovery will have no effect on the delivery of multimodality therapy, a frequent problem in adjuvant therapy studies.

In patients who receive chemoradiation prior to surgery, a repeat staging CT scan after chemoradiation reveals liver metastases in 25% [32]. If these patients had undergone pancreaticoduodenectomy at the time of diagnosis, it is possible that the liver metastases would have been subclinical; these patients would therefore have undergone a major surgical procedure only to have liver metastases found soon after surgery. In the MDACC trial, patients who were found to have disease progression at the time of restaging had a median survival of only 6.7 months [32]. The avoidance of a lengthy recovery period and the potential morbidity of pancreaticoduodenectomy in patients with such a short expected survival duration represents a distinct advantage of preoperative over postoperative chemoradiation. When delivering multimodality therapy for any disease, it is beneficial, when possible, to deliver the most toxic therapy last, thereby avoiding morbidity in patients who experience rapid disease progression not amenable to currently available therapies.

The most recent report from our institution involved 39 patients who received preoperative 5-FU–based chemoradiation, pancreaticoduodenectomy, and electron-beam intraoperative radiation therapy for adenocarcinoma of the pancreatic head [1]. The median survival of all 39 patients was 19 months, with a median follow-up of 19 months (range 4–56 months). Thirty-eight patients were evaluable for patterns of treatment failure; there was one perioperative death. Overall, there were 38 recurrences in 29 patients: 8 (21%)

were locoregional (pancreatic bed and/or peritoneal cavity), and 30 (79%) were distant (lung, liver, and/or bone). The liver was the most frequent site of tumor recurrence, and liver metastases were a component of treatment failure in 53% of patients (69% of all patients who had recurrences). Fourteen patients (37% of all patients; 48% of patients who had recurrences) had liver metastases as their only site of recurrence. Isolated local or peritoneal recurrences were documented in only four patients (11%). This improvement in locoregional control was seen despite the fact that 14 of 38 evaluable patients had undergone laparotomy with tumor manipulation and biopsy prior to referral for chemoradiation and reoperation. If these 14 patients were excluded, only 2 patients (8%) would have experienced local or peritoneal recurrence as any component of treatment failure. Improved locoregional tumor control translated into only a small improvement in median survival compared with that in other recently published studies because of the large percentage of patients who developed distant metastatic disease, predominantly in the liver. Therefore, in the absence of effective systemic therapy, the goal of chemoradiation (preoperative or postoperative) and pancreatectomy should be to maximize locoregional tumor control while minimizing treatment-related toxicity and cost.

The first report of standard-fractionation preoperative chemoradiation (50.4 Gy over 5.5 weeks with concomitant 5-FU) from MDACC documented gastrointestinal toxic effects (nausea, vomiting, and dehydration) that required hospital admission in one third of patients [27]. A similar experience was recently reported from the multicenter Eastern Cooperative Oncology Group trial [33]. Placement of a jejunostomy tube (laparoscopically) prior to the initiation of chemoradiation has prevented subsequent hospital admission due to gastrointestinal toxicity in the experience at MDACC [31], a finding previously also observed with the delivery of postoperative chemoradiation [34]. However, adhesions from prior operations prevent the successful laparoscopic placement of a jejunostomy tube in many patients, and the need for general anesthesia makes it an expensive procedure. The gastrointestinal toxicity of standard-fractionation (5.5 week) preoperative chemoradiation caused us to study the use of rapid-fractionation chemoradiation (30 Gy over 2 weeks with concomitant 5-FU) in an effort to decrease the length of treatment and thereby reduce cost, toxicity, and patient inconvenience while attempting to maintain therapeutic efficacy [35]. Initial data on the use of 5-FU–based rapid-fractionation chemoradiation, pancreaticoduodenectomy, and electron-beam intraoperative radiation therapy have demonstrated the safety of this treatment program. Rapid-fractionation chemoradiation is currently being combined with new radiation sensitizing agents (paclitaxel, gemcitabine); treatment effect is assessed by histologic evaluation of the resected specimen. Future treatment programs will combine locoregional chemoradiation with the systemic or regional delivery of novel agents that inhibit essential steps in tumor cell growth (inhibitors of angiogenesis, *Ras*).

Vascular resection at the time of pancreaticoduodenectomy

The first resection and anastomosis of the SMV as part of pancreaticoduodenectomy was reported by Moore et al. from the University of Minnesota in 1951 [36]. The resection was prompted by their finding of tumor involvement of the SMV after gastric and pancreatic transection:

> An exploratory laparotomy May 25, 1950, was done . . . the superior mesenteric vessels and the portal veins were not thought to be involved . . . the pancreas was cut across . . . further dissection revealed the tumor to be firmly attached to the *lateral* wall of the superior mesenteric vein for a distance of 2 cm. At this point it was decided to remove the vein wall involved with tumor . . .

As illustrated in this case, tumor involvement of the SMV or SMPV confluence may not be apparent to the surgeon until after gastric and pancreatic transection, a point in the operation when nonresectional procedures are no longer an option. Tumor invasion of the lateral wall of the SMV is the most frequent unexpected finding at the time of pancreaticoduodenectomy [37]. In contrast to tumor involvement of the SMA, tumor invasion of the SMV can occur in the absence of extensive retroperitoneal invasion and therefore may represent the only barrier to the performance of a negative-margin pancreaticoduodenectomy. In addition, the relationship between a pancreatic head tumor and the SMV is not as accurately defined (as is the SMA) on preoperative imaging studies [38].

The published experience with regional pancreatectomy convinced most surgeons that vascular resection, when combined with regional lymphadenectomy for adenocarcinoma of the pancreatic head, was associated with increased patient death and morbidity with little improvement in the length of patient survival [39,40]. Therefore, most surgeons consider tumor invasion of the SMV or SMPV confluence a contraindication to pancreaticoduodenectomy. However, our recent results suggest that tumor invasion of the SMV or SMPV confluence can be successfully managed by surgical resection and is not associated with a higher incidence of margin or lymph node positivity [38]. During a 3-year period, 59 consecutive patients with adenocarcinoma of the pancreatic head or periampullary region underwent either pancreaticoduodenectomy (36 patients) or pancreaticoduodenctomy with en-bloc resection of the SMV or SMPV confluence (23 patients). The only perioperative death occurred in a patient who, prior to referral, had received two previous operations, radiation therapy (including external-beam and intraoperative radiation therapy), and chemotherapy for a localized adenocarcinoma of duodenal origin. Perioperative complications occurred in 7 (30%) of the 23 patients who required venous resection, and in 10 (28%) of the 36 patients who underwent standard pancreaticoduodenectomy. Pathologic findings for the 59 patients who underwent

Table 2. Pathologic findings for 59 consecutive patients who underwent pancreaticoduo-denectomy or pancreaticoduodenectomy with en-bloc segmental venous resection

Surgery	No. patients	Median tumor size (cm)	No. with positive retroperitoneal margin	No. with positive nodes
P	36	3.0	5 (14%)[a]	22 (61%)
VR	23	3.7	4 (17%)[b]	9 (39%)
p value		NS	NS[c]	NS[d]

[a] One specimen classified as margin negative had acelluar mucin within the perineural tissue.
[b] In one specimen (classified as margin positive), tumor cells were seen in perineural tissue at the retroperitoneal margin in the absence of direct extension from the primarly tumor.
Differences assessed by unpaired Student's t-test, [c] Fisher's exact test, or [d] chi-squared analysis.
NS = not significant; VR = venous resection; P = pancreaticoduodenectomy.
Adapted from Fuhrman, et al. [38].

pancreaticoduodenectomy are listed in Table 2. No significant differences in median tumor size, retroperitoneal margin positivity, or nodal positivity were observed between patients who required venous resection and those who did not. The apparent trend toward larger tumor size and node negativity in patients who underwent venous resection awaits further study.

It is important to emphasize the distinction between regional pancreatectomy and pancreaticoduodenectomy with segmental resection of the SMV or SMPV confluence as performed at our instutution. We do not perform venous resection in an attempt to improve lymphatic and soft tissue clearance as is performed in regional pancreatectomy. It is unlikely that larger locoregional resections in poorly selected patients with advanced disease will impact survival. We perform venous resection in carefully selected patients who have no evidence of tumor extension to the SMA or celiac axis. In such patients, the only apparent barrier to resection with a negative retroperitoneal margin is tumor adherence to the SMV or SMPV confluence.

Systemic therapy

The most recent systemic agent demonstrating activity in patients with pancreatic cancer is gemcitabine. Gemcitabine (2',2'-difluorodeoxycytidine; Gemzar) is a deoxycytidine analogue with structural and metabolic similarities to cytosine arabinoside [41]. As a prodrug, gemcitabine must be phosphorylated to its active metabolites gemcitabine diphosphate and gemcitabine triphosphate. In both preclinical and clinical testing, gemcitabine has demonstrated activity greater than that of ara-C [42]. These observations can be explained by the following properties of gemcitabine: (1) It is three to four times more

118

lipophilic than ara-C, resulting in greater membrane permeability and celular uptake; (2) it has higher affinity to deoxycytidine kinase; and (3) gemcitabine triphosphate has a long intracellular retention. Following phase I study [43], gemcitabine was evaluated in a multicenter trial involving 44 patients with advanced pancreatic cancer [44]. While only five objective responses were documented, the investigators noted frequent subjective symptomatic beneflt, often in the absence of an objective tumor response. Based on these observations, two subsequent trials of gemcitabine in patients with advanced pancreatic cancer have been completed. In one trial, gemcitabine was randomized against 5-FU in previously untreated patients [45]. Patients treated with gemcitabine achieved modest but statistically significant improvements in response rate and median survival compared with those treated with 5-FU. More clinically meaningful effects on disease-related symptoms (pain control, performance status, weight gain) were seen with gemcitabine compared with 5-FU–treated patients. Similar effects were documented in patients treated with gemcitabine after progression on 5-FU [46]. These results suggest that gemcitabine will become the accepted first-line therapy for patients with advanced pancreatic adenocarcinoma.

Despite the recent encouraging results with gemcitabine, median survival for patients with metastatic pancreatic cancer continues to be less than 6 months, with few patients achieving long-term stabilization of their disease process. Some of the effects attributed to chemotherapy may not be substantially different from what can be achieved with aggressive supportive care alone, prompting many physicians to consider less toxic alternatives for systemic therapy.

Johnson and Corbishley first noted that pancreatic tumors contained sex steroid hormone receptors [47]. In addition, serum testosterone concentrations were lower in both men and women with pancreatic cancer as compared to patients with other cancers or healthy controls [48–50]. Laboratory evidence that exocrine pancreatic cancers are sensitive to gastrointestinal hormones, sex steroids, and growth factors led to the use of hormonal manipulation in patients with pancreatic cancer. Several uncontrolled clinical studies have suggested improved survival in patients with pancreatic cancer treated with tamoxifen [51–53], yet other studies have failed to confirm this observation [54–56]. A case control study involving 80 patients did suggest a survival advantage for patients treated with tamoxifen [57]. However, in a prospective, randomized, double-blind trial, patients receiving tamoxifen had a median survival of 115 days compared with 122 days for the placebo-treated patients; 8% of patients were alive at 1 year in both groups [55]. Studies with sandostatin [57], steroids, and LHRH agonists [58], as well as combinations of these agents [59,60], have failed to show an increase in survival for patients with pancreatic cancer. A pilot study of MK329, a cholecystokinin (CCK) antagonist, in 18 patients with pancreatic cancer demonstrated no antitumor activity [61]. However, the CCK receptor status of the patients was unknown.

Basic and translational research

Studies using archival human pancreatic tumor tissue and human pancreatic cancer cell lines have identified an increasing number of characteristic genetic abnormalities. Point mutations at codon 12 of the K-*ras* oncongene have been reported in 75–90% of pancreatic adenocarcinoma specimens [62–65]. *Ras* proto-oncogene products are transmembrane proteins that are believed to transduce an external stimulus (i.e., growth factors) through the binding and activation of intracellular GTP-binding proteins. *Ras* bound to GTP is maintained in an active configuration that triggers other enzymatic second messengers, such as the phosphatidylinositol and protein kinase C pathways. This leads to nuclear signals resulting in cellular division and proliferation. The mutated *ras* oncogene is not able to convert GTP to inactive GDP, resulting in a constitutively active *ras* protein product, unregulated cellular proliferation signals, and a transformed cell [66]. The specific cause and role of the K-*ras* mutations in pancreatic carcinogenesis are unknown, but the mutations have been proposed to be an early, somatic event in pancreatic tumor progression [67].

Additional genetic alterations that have been described in human pancreatic cancer include overexpression of oncogenes such as c-*myc* [68,69] and mutations in the adenomatous polyposis coli gene [70]. Mutations in the *p53* gene are found frequently but are heterogeneous [71]. The RB1 gene product was found by immunoprecipitation in 5 of the 7 human pancreatic cancer cell lines analyzed and in the 10 primary pancreatic carcinomas evaluated [71]. Recently, frequent mutations in the *p16* (MTS1) inhibitor of cyclin D/CdK-4 complexes have been described [71]. Based on the frequency with which mutations in K-*ras*, *p53*, and *p16* are found, a model of pancreatic carcinogenesis has been suggested whereby the malignant clone evolves from cells driven by a dominant oncogene (K-*ras*) with subsequent deregulation of cell growth precipitated by abnormal cell-cycle control resulting from mutations in *p53* and/or *p16* [72].

Exactly how the cellular biochemical changes produced by the molecular alterations described thus far in human pancreatic cancer interact during pancreatic carcinogenesis is still unclear. A recent report from Brentnall and colleagues examined *ras* oncogene mutations and microsatellite instability (MIN) in pancreatic juice obtained during endoscopic retrograde cholangiopancreatography (ERCP) from patients with and without pancreatic cancer [73]. MIN was also studied in tumor DNA obtained from paraffin blocks. Their results suggested that MIN was an early event in pancreatic carcinogenesis and was possibly induced by reactive oxygen species generated in the development of acute or chronic pancreatitis. The events leading to MIN may eventually cause mutations in a number of genes (K-*ras*, *p53*, *bcl*-2), resulting in the malignant phenotype.

Our current challenge is to translate the expanding body of basic science knowledge into effective diagnostic techniques and therapy for patients with pancreatic cancer. Patient survival will be improved either by developing strategies for early diagnosis, thereby allowing more patients to undergo potentially curative surgery, or by developing more effective systemic therapy. Detection of cancer-derived gene products from biologic fluids is an important emerging approach to the diagnosis of malignant diseases. Tumor-derived oncogene and suppressor gene DNAs have been isolated from a variety of biologic sources, including urine, stool, and, more recently, blood and pancreatic fluid [74]. We have demonstrated that identification of mutant K-*ras* DNA from FNA specimens may complement the standard cytologic diagnosis of malignancy [75]. Detection of K-*ras* DNA in bile, pancreatic juice, or stool may be used to develop a strategy for the early diagnosis of pancreatic cancer in groups at higher risk than the general population. The use of bile obtained from duodenal aspiration would not require cannulation of the ampulla of Vater and avoids the complexity of processing stool samples for molecular analysis [76].

The majority of patients who undergo a potentially curative pancreaticoduodenectomy develop recurrent disease in the liver. Central to the development of organ-selective processes of metastases are cell adhesion, cell-matrix interactions, growth stimulation, and neovascularization. Angiogenesis is essential for tumors to grow larger than $1\,mm^3$, the maximal distance of oxygen transport and nutrient diffusion. In addition, angiogenesis must occur for metastasis formation and growth. Specific factors must be expressed and the appropriate receptors must be present on the target endothelium in order to initiate basement membrane degradation, endothelial cell proliferation and migration, and capillary tubule formation. Vascular endothelial growth factor (VEGF), also known as vascular permeability factor, was initially found to be a protein that increases vascular permeability [77]. VEGF is 50,000 times more potent than histamine in inducing capillary permeability and plays a role in formation of the extracellular matrix [77]. Overexpression of VEGF has been demonstrated in several tumors when compared with controls [78]. Vessel density and VEGF staining have been associated with tumor metastasis and survival in patients with colon cancer [79]. VEGF mRNA has also been shown to be overexpressed in a Syrian hamster pancreatic cancer cell line [80]. Recent data suggest that upregulation of VEGF may occur due to activating mutations of the *ras* oncogene [81]. Therefore, *ras* mutations may contribute to pancreatic carcinogenesis not only by promoting tumor cell proliferation, but indirectly through the stimulation of tumor angiogenesis.

Recent data also suggest that *ras* and *src* oncogenes mediate their effects on gene expression, partly by activating transcription factors AP-1 and Rel/NF-*k*B. These transcription factors have been shown to upregulate a number of genes whose protein products play important roles in tumor invasion, angiogenesis, and metastasis [82,83]. Agents that inhibit angiogenesis and agents that inhibit post-translational farnesylation of the *ras* protein are currently in phase I testing in the United States.

References

1. Staley CA, Lee JE, Cleary KA, et al. Preoperative chemoradiation, pancreatico-duodenectomy, and intraoperative radiation therapy for adenocarcinoma of the pancreatic head. Am J Surg, 171:118–125, 1996.
2. Geer RJ, Brennan MF. Prognostic indicators for survival after resection of pancreatic adenocarcinoma. Am J Surg 165:68–73, 1993.
3. Gastrointestinal Tumor Study Group. A multi-institutional comparative trial of radiation therapy alone and in combination with 5-fluorouracil for locally unresectable pancreatic carcinoma. Ann Surg 189:205–208, 1979.
4. Whittington R, Neuberg D, Tester WJ, et al. Protracted intravenous fluorouracil infusion with radiation therapy in the management of localized pancreaticobiliary carcinoma: A phase I Eastern Cooperative Oncolongy Group trial. J Clin Oncol 13:227–232, 1995.
5. Nitecki SS, Sarr MG, Colby TV, vanHeerden JA. Long-term survival after resection for ductal adenocarcinoma of the pancreas. Is it really improving? Ann Surg 221:59–66, 1995.
6. Trede M, Chir B, Schwall G, Saeger H. Survival after pancreaticoduodenectomy: 118 consecutive resections without an operative mortality. Ann Surg 211:447–458, 1990.
7. Whittington R, Bryer MP, Haller DG, Solin LJ, Rosato EF. Adjuvant therapy of resected adenocarcinoma of the pancreas. Int J Radiat Oncol Biol Phys 21:1137–1143, 1991.
8. Willet CG, Lewandrowski K, Warshaw AL, et al. Resection margins in carcinoma of the head of the pancreas: Implications for radiation therapy. Ann Surg 217:144–148, 1993.
9. Yeo CJ, Cameron JL, Lillemore KD, et al. Pancreaticoduodenectomy for cancer of the head of the pancreas: 201 patients. Ann Surg 221:721–733, 1995.
10. Tepper J, Nardi G, Suit H. Carcinoma of the pancreas: Review of MGH experience from 1963–1973. Cancer 37:1519–1524, 1976.
11. Fuhrman GM, Charnsangavej C, Abbruzzese JL. Thin-section contrast enhanced computed tomography accurately predicts resectability of malignant pancreatic neoplasms. Am J Surg 167:104–113, 1994.
12. de Rooij PD, Rogatko A, Brennan MF. Evaluation of palliative surgical procedures in unresectable pancreatic cancer. Br J Surg 78:1053–1058, 1991.
13. Lillemoe KD, Sauter PK, Pitt HA, et al. Current status of surgical palliation of periampullary carcinoma. Surg Gynecol Obstet 176:1–10, 1993.
14. Alvarez C, Livingston EH, Ashley SW, et al. Cost-benefit analysis of work-up for pancreatic cancer. Am J Surg 165:53–60, 1993.
15. Evans DB, Lee JE, Leach SD, et al. Vascular resection and intraoperative radiation therapy during pancreaticoduodenectomy: Rationale and technique. Adv Surg 29:235–262, 1995.
16. Evans DB, Lee JE, Pisters PWT. Pancreaticoduodenectomy (Whipple operation) and total pancreatectomy for cancer. In Nyhus LM, Baker RJ, Fishcer JF (eds). Mastery of Surgery, 3rd ed. Boston: Little, Brown 1997, pp 1233–1249.
17. Tyler DS, Evans DB. Reoperative pancreaticoduodenectomy. Ann Surg 2:211–221, 1994.
18. Moertel CG, Childs DS, Reitemeier RJ, et al. Combined 5-fluorouracil and supervoltage radiation therapy of locally unresectable gastrointestinal cancer. Lancet 2:865–867, 1969.
19. Moertel CG, Frystak S, Hahn RG, et al. Therapy of locally unresectable pancreatic carcinoma: A randomized comparison of high dose (6000 rads) radiation alone, moderate dose radiation and 5-fluorouracil. Cancer 48:1705–1710, 1981.
20. Gastrointestinal Tumor Study Group. Furgher evidence of effective adjuvant combined radiation and chemotherapy following curative resection of pancreatic cancer. Cancer 59:2006–2010, 1987.
21. Kalser MH, Ellenberg SS. Pancreatic cancer: Adjuvant combined radiation and chemotherapy following curative resection. Arch Surg 120:899–903, 1985.
22. Bakkevold KE, Arnesjo B, Dahl O, Kambestad B. Adjuvant combination chemotherapy

(AMF) following radical resection of carcinoma of the pancreas and papilla of vater — results of a controlled, prospective, randomized multicentre study. Eur J Cancer 29A:698, 1995.

23. Neoptolemos JP, Kerr DJ. Adjuvant therapy for pancreatic cancer. Br J Surg 82:1012–1014, 1995.
24. Ishikawa O, Ohhigashi H, Teshima T, et al. Clinical and histopathological appraisal of preoperative irradiation for adenocarcinoma of the pancreaticoduodenal region. J Surg Oncol 40:143–151, 1989.
25. Pilepich MV, Miller HH. Preoperative irradiation in carcinoma of the pancreas. Cancer 46:1945–1949, 1980.
26. Kopelson G. Curative surgery for adenocarcinoma of the pancreas/ampulla of Vater: The role of adjuvant pre- or postoperative radiation therapy. Int J Radiat Oncol Biol Phys 9:911–915, 1983.
27. Evans DB, Rich TA, Byrd DR, et al. Preoperative chemoradiation and pancreaticoduodenectomy for adenocarcinoma of the pancreas. Arch Surg 127:1335–1339, 1992.
28. Hoffman JP, Weese JL, Solin LJ, et al. A single institutional experience with preoperative chemoradiation for stage I–III pancreatic adenocarcinoma. Am Surg 59:772–781, 1993.
29. Jessup JM, Steele G, Mayer RJ, et al. Neoadjuvant therapy for unresectable pancreatic adenocarcinoma. Arch Surg 128:559–564, 1993.
30. Wanebo HJ, Posher M, Glicksman M, et al. Integrated modality protocol for carcinoma of the pancreas: Pilot program (abstr). Proc Am Soc Clin Oncol 10:158, 1991.
31. Spitz FR, Abbruzzese JL, Lee JE, et al. Preoperative and Postoperative Chemoradiation Strategies in Patients Treated with Pancreaticoduodenectomy for Adenocarcinoma of the Pancreas. J Clin Oncol. 15:928–937, 1997.
32. Evans DB, Abbruzzese J, Lee J, et al. Preoperative chemoradiation and pancreaticoduodenectomy for adenocarcinoma of the pancreas (abstr). Proc Am Soc Clin Oncol 13:226, 1994.
33. Hoffman JP, Weese JL, Solin LJ, et al. Preoperative chemoradiation for patients with resectable pancreatic adenocarcinoma: An Eastern Cooperative Oncology Group (ECOG) phase II study (abstr). Proc Am Soc Clin Oncol 14:201, 1995.
34. Whittington R, Bryer MP, Haller DG, Solin LJ, Rosato EF. Adjuvant therapy of resected adenocarcinoma of the pancreas. Int J Radiat Oncol Biol Phys 21:1137–1143, 1991.
35. Evans DB, Abbruzzese JL, Rich TA. Cancer of the pancreas. In DeVita VT Jr, Hellmans, Rosenberg SA (eds). Cancer: Principles and Practice of Oncology (eds). Philadelphia, PA, Lippin cott, 1997, pp 1054–1087.
36. Moore GE, Sako Y, Thomas LB. Radical pancreaticoduodenectomy with resection and reanastomosis of the superior mesenteric vein. Surgery 30:550–553, 1951.
37. Cusack JC, Fuhrman GM, Lee JE, et al. Management of unsuspected tumor invasion of the superior mesenteric-portal venous confluence at the time of pancreaticoduodenectomy. Am J Surg 168:352–354, 1994.
38. Fuhrman G, Leach SD, Staley CA, et al. Rationale for en-bloc vein resection in the treatment of pancreatic adenocarcinoma adherent to the superior mesenteric-portal venous confluence. Ann Surg, 223:154–162, 1996.
39. Fortner JG, Kim DK, Cubilla A, et al. Regional pancreatectomy. Ann Surg 186:42–50, 1977.
40. Nagakawa T, Konishi I, Veno K, et al. Surgical treatment of pancreatic cancer. The Japanese experience. Int J Pancreatol 9:135–143, 1992.
41. Hertel LW, Kroin JS, Misner JW, et al. Synthesis of 2-deoxy-2′,2′ difluro-D-ribose and 2-deoxy-2′,2′difluro-D-fibofuranosyl nucleosides. J Organ Chem 53:2406–2409, 1988.
42. Hertel LW, Boder GB, Kroin JS, et al. Evaluation of the antitumor activity of gemcitabine (2′,2′-difluoro-2′-deoxycytidine). Cancer Res 50:4417–4422, 1990.
43. Abbruzzese JL, Grunewald R, Weeks EA, et al. A phase I clinical, plasma and cellular pharmacology study of gemcitabine. J Clin Oncol 9:491–498, 1991.
44. Casper ES, Green MR, Kelsen DP, et al. Phase II trial of gemcitabine (2′,2′-

difluorodeoxycytidine) in patietns with adenocarcinoma of the pancreas. Invest New Drugs 12:29–34, 1994.

45. Moore M, Andersen J, Burris H, et al. A randomized trial of gemcitabine versus 5-FU as first-line therapy in advanced pancreatic cancer (abstr). Proc Am Soc Clin Oncol 14:199, 1995.

46. Rothenberg ML, Burris HA III, Andersen JS, et al. Gemcitabine: Effective palliative therapy for pancreas cancer patients failing 5-FU (abstr). Proc Am Soci Clin Oncol 14:198, 1995.

47. Johnson PJ, Corbishley TP. Sex steroid receptors and antisteroid agents in the treatment of pancreatic adenocarcinoma. Monogr Ser Eur Organ Res Treat Cancer 18:99–104, 1987.

48. Greenway B, Iqbal MJ, Johnson PJ, et al. Oestrogen receptor proteins in malignant and fetal pancreas. Br Med J 283:751–753, 1981.

49. Iqbal MJ, Greenway BA, Wilkinson ML, et al. Sex steroid enzymes, aromatase and 5-alpha-reductase in the pancreas: A comparison of normal adult, foetal and malignant tissue. Clin Sci 65:71, 1983.

50. Greenway B, Iqbal MJ, Johnson PJ, Williams R. Low serum testosterone concentrations in patients with carcinoma of the pancreas. Br Med J 286:93–95, 1983.

51. Theve NO, Pousette A, Carlstrom K. Adenocarcinoma of the pancreas — a hormone sensitive tumor? A preliminary report on Nolvadex treatment. Clin Oncol 9:193–197, 1983.

52. Tonnesen K, Kamp-Jensen M. Antiestrogen therapy in pancreatic carcinoma: A preliminary report. Eur J Surg Oncol 12:69–70, 1984.

53. Wong A, Chan A, Arthur K. Tamoxifen therapy in unresectable adneocarcinoma of the pancreas. Cancer Treat Rep 71:7–14, 1987.

54. Taylor OM, Benson IA, McMahon MJ. Clinical trial of tamoxifen in patients with irresectable pancreatic adenocarcinoma. The Yorkshire Gastrointestinal Tumor Group. Br J Surg 80:384–386, 1993.

55. Bakkevold KE, Pattersen A, Ames JB, et al. Tamoxifen therapy in unresectable adenocarcinoma of the pancreas and the papilla of Vater. Br J Surg 77:725–730, 1990.

56. Keating JJ, Johnson PJ, Cochrane AM, et al. A prospective randomized trial of tamoxifen and cytoproterone acetate in pancreatic carcinoma. Br J Cancer 60:789–792, 1989.

57. Zeitoun G. Hormonal therapy by somatostatin and/or LH-RH has no benefit on survival in adenocarcinoma of the pancreas (meeting abstr). Third International Conference on Neo-adjuvant chemotherapy, Paris, France, Feb. 6–9, 1991; p 51.

58. Allegretti A, Lionetto R, Saccomanno S, et al. LH-RH analogue treatment in adenocarcinoma of the pancreas: A phase II study. Oncology 50:77–80, 1993.

59. Philip PA, Carmichael J, Tonkin K, et al. Hormonal treatment of pancreatic carcinoma; a phase II study of LHRH agonist goserelin plus hydrocortisone. Br J Cancer 67:379–382, 1993.

60. Swarovsky B, Wolf M, Havemann K, et al. Tamoxifen or cytoproterone acetate in combination with buserelin is ineffective in patients with pancreatic adenocarcinoma. Oncology 50:226–229, 1993.

61. Abbruzzese JL, Gholson CF, Daugherty K, et al. A pilot clinical trial of the cholecystokinin receptor antagonist MK 329 in patients with advanced pancreatic cancer. Pancreas 7:165–171, 1992.

62. Almoguera C, Shibata D, Forrester K, et al. Most human carcinomas of the exocrine pancreas contain mutant c-K-ras genes. Cell 53:549–554, 1988.

63. Smit VT, Boot AJ, Smits AM, et al. KRAS codon 12 mutations occur very frequently in pancreatic adenocarcinomas. Nucleic Acids Res 16:7773–7782, 1988.

64. Masson P, Andren-Sandberg A. Crude isolation of DNA from unselected human pancreatic tissue and ampliflcation by the polymerase chain reaction of Ki-ras oncogene to detect point mutations in pancreatic cancer. Acta Oncol 31:421–424, 1992.

65. Pellegata NS, Losekoot M, Foddie R, et al. Detection of K-ras mutations by denaturing gradient gel electrophoresis (DGGE): A study on pancreatic cancer. Anticancer Res 12:1731–1736, 1992.

66. Bos JL. Ras oncogenes in human cancer: A review. Cancer Res 49:4682–4689, 1989.

67. Pellegata NS, Sessa F, Renault B, et al. K-ras and p53 gene mutations in pancreatic cancer:

Ductal and nonductal tumors progress through different genetic lesions. Cancer Res 54:1556–1560, 1994.

68. Yamada H, Sakamoto H, Taira M, et al. Ampliflcation of both c-Ki-ras with a point mutation and c-myc in a primary pancreatic cancer and its metastatic tumors in lymph nodes. Jpn J Cancer Res 77:370–375, 1986.

69. Yamada H, Yoshida T, Sakamoto H, et al. Establishment of a human pancreatic adenocarcinoma cell line (PSW-1) with amplifications of both c-myc and activated c-Ki-ras by a point mutation. Biochem Biophys Res Commun 140:167–170, 1986.

70. Horii A, Nakaturu S, Miyoshi Y, et al. Frequent somatic mutations of the APC gene in human pancreatic cancer. Cancer Res 52:6696–6698, 1992.

71. Ruggeri B, Zhang SY, Caamano J, et al. Human pancreatic carcinomas and cell lines reveal frequent and mulitple alterations in the p53 and Rb-1 tumor-suppressor genes. Oncogene 7:1503–1511, 1992.

72. Caldas C, Hahn SA, da Costa LT, et al. Frequent somatic mutations and homozygous deletions of the p16 (MTSl) gene in pancreatic adenocarcinoma. Nature Genet 8:27–32, 1994.

73. Brentnall TA, Chen R, Lee JG, et al. Microsatellite instability and K-*ras* mutations associated with pancreatic adenocarcinoma and pancreatitis. Cancer Res 55:4264–4267, 1995.

74. Tada M, Omata M, Kawai S, et al. Detection of *ras* gene mutations in pancreatic juice and peripheral blood of patients with pancreatic adenocarcinoma. Cancer Res 53:2472–2474, 1993.

75. Evans DB, Frazier ML, Charnsangavej C, et al. Molecular diagnosis of exocrine pancreatic cancer using a percutaneous technique. Ann Surg Oncol, 3:241–246, 1996.

76. Abbruzzese JL, Evans DB, Larry L, et al. Molecular diagnosis of pancreatic cancer (abstr). Proc Am Soc Clin Oncol 13:119, 1994.

77. Senger DR, Water LVD, Brown LF, et al. Vascular permeability factor (VPF, VEGF) in tumor biology. Cancer Metastasis Rev 12:303–324, 1993.

78. Brown LF, Berse B, Jackman RW, et al. Expression of vascular permeability factor (vascular endothelial growth factor) and its receptors in adenocarcinomas of the gastrointestinal tract. Cancer Res 53:4727–4735, 1993.

79. Takahashi Y, Kitadai Y, Bucana CD, et al. Expression of vascular endothelial growth factor and its receptor, KDR, correlates with vascularity, metastasis, and proliferation of human colon cancer. Cancer Res 55:3964–3968, 1995.

80. Egawa S, Tsutsumi M, Konishi Y, et al. The role of angiogenesis in the tumor growth of syrian hamster pancreatic cancer cell line HPD-NR. Gastroenterology 108:1526–1533, 1995.

81. Rak J, Mitsuhashi Y, Bayko L. Mutant *ras* oncogenes upregulate VEGF/VPF expression: Implications for induction and inhibition of tumor angiogenesis. Cancer Res 55:4575–4580, 1995.

82. Bours V, Dejardin E, Goujon-Letawe F, Merville M, Castronovo V. The NF-kB transcription factor and cancer: High expression of NF-kB- and IkB-related proteins in tumor cell lines. Biochem Pharmacol 47:145–149, 1994.

83. Grilli M, Chiu JJ-S, Lenardo MJ. NF-*k*B and Rel: Participants in a multiform transcriptional regulatory system. Int Rev Cytol 143:1–62, 1993.

7. Recent advances in bone sarcomas

Alan W. Yasko and Mark E. Johnson

Primary bone sarcomas are rare neoplasms that present many challenges for the musculoskeletal oncologist. Current strategies have been shaped by the experience of the last two decades, during which time a transition from ablative to limb-sparing surgery has evolved. The long-term oncologic and functional outcomes of this major advance are just recently being reported in the literature (A.W. Yasko, unpublished) [1–4].

Enthusiasm over the success of local disease control with limb preservation has been tempered by the limitations of current limb-sparing reconstructive approaches to preserve function long term. In response to emerging data, current initiatives have focused on two principal unresolved clinical issues: redefining the nature and scope of diagnostic and surgical interventions, and optimizing current biological and nonbiological skeletal and soft-tissue reconstruction methods. We focus on these clinical issues and discuss the research efforts that currently are being undertaken to advance the understanding and management of bone sarcomas, including recent investigations into molecular aspects, cytogenetics, and novel reconstructive strategies using innovative techniques to engineer new bone, cartilage, and soft tissues through guided tissue regeneration.

Molecular biology of bone tumors

Recent advances in molecular and cytogenetics have provided new insights into the biology of bone tumors, have yielded powerful new diagnostic techniques, and may provide staging and prognostic data that will prove complementary and more powerful than current data generated from light microscopy and radiographic imaging studies. Tumor grading systems incorporating molecular data promise a more precise approach to stratifying patients enrolled in clinical trials and to formulating rational treatment plans based on lesions described at the genomic level. On the more distant horizon is the possibility of gene therapy, using retroviral vectors to introduce active copies of defective nucleoproteins into dedifferentiated cells, in the hopes of

Raphael E. Pollock (ed.), SURGICAL ONCOLOGY. Copyright © 1997. Kluwer Academic Publishers.
ISBN 0-7923-9900-5. All rights reserved.

either downregulating such cells into a more normal phenotype or forcing them into a pathway leading to apoptosis.

The techniques of molecular genetics have provided useful tools for diagnosing Ewing's sarcoma (ES) and primitive neuroectodermal tumor (PNET). Although the characteristic translocations in ES were initially discovered using classical cytogenetic analysis, this technically demanding process is not an ideal method for routine diagnosis because accurate karyotyping requires tissue in amounts that cannot be provided by fine-needle aspiration. With the cloning and sequencing of the chromosomal breakpoints in ES, DNA probes identifying the sequences flanking the breakpoints can be used to perform fluorescent in-situ hybridization analysis (FISH). McManus and coworkers reported the successful application of this technique to fine-needle aspirates [5]. Other investigators have reported the use of reverse transcription of tumor-derived RNA in conjunction with polymerase chain reaction amplification (RT-PCR) to identify expression of the abnormal fusion protein EWS/FLI-1 [6–8]. Recently, a monoclonal antibody (HBA71) has been developed that recognizes a cell-surface glycoprotein (p30/32^{MIC2}) in human Ewing's sarcoma and primitive neuroectodermal tumor (PNET) [9,10]. Strong immunoreactivity of HBA71 in Ewing's sarcoma and PNET distinguishes these tumors from other small round cell tumors of childhood and adolescence [9–11]. In one recent comparison of the immunoperoxidase assay with a cDNA probe for the EWS breakpoint region, the MIC2 assay was expressed in 19 of 20 cases, including 3 cases that did not show EWS rearrangement [12].

Molecular genetic investigations of osteosarcoma have focused on two hereditary syndromes, both of which are characterized by an abnormally high incidence of osteosarcoma. In 1968, Li and Fraumeni [13] reviewed 648 pediatric rhabdomyosarcoma patients and identified four families in which first- or second-degree relatives had childhood sarcomas. This work led to the identification of a distinct genetic syndrome, transmitted as an autosomal dominant, and associated with a remarkably high incidence of breast carcinoma, soft tissue and bone sarcomas, brain tumors, and leukemia.

In 1990, Malkin et al. [14] found germ-line mutations of the tumor suppressor gene p53 in 5 out of 5 Li-Fraumeni families that they analyzed. The p53 gene is located on the short arm of chromosome 17 (17p) and encodes a 53 kDa nuclear phosphoprotein [15]. Mutation of the p53 locus is the most common molecular genetic abnormality found in human cancers [16] and is found in many different tumor types [17]. The presence of p53 mutations in germ-line cells of patients with sporadic osteosarcoma is rather rare (~3%) [18]; however, approximately 30% of osteosarcoma tumor samples exhibit p53 mutations [19,20]. The most common form of p53 mutation found in carcinoma is substitution of a single base pair, leading to a mutant protein that, due to its binding affinity for other intranuclear proteins, exhibits an abnormally long half-life and is thus detectable using monoclonal antibody assays. Wadayama et al. analyzed 113 bone and soft tissue sarcomas using immunohistochemical assays and DNA analysis. They found that 75% of the p53 mutations in

128

osteosarcoma led to absence of expression of the protein [20]. Although the occurrence of the *p53* mutation has not been correlated with overall prognosis in osteosarcoma, point mutations in the *p53* gene were found in 4 out of 4 patients with multifocal osteosarcoma [21], a clinical subtype with a very low survival. In addition to the mechanism of genetic mutation, *p53* tumor suppressor activity may be inactivated by other intracellular events. In particular, the expression of MDM2, a protein that binds and inactivates *p53* in vivo, has been shown to be amplified in locally recurrent and metastatic, but not in primary, osteosarcomas [12].

Retinoblastoma, a childhood eye tumor, is associated with loss of the RB-1 gene, which is located in chromosome band 13q14. Because patients who survive childhood retinoblastoma have an abnormally high probability of developing osteosarcomas later in life [22], the RB-1 gene, and its protein product, a 105 kDa nuclear phosphoprotein that binds DNA, have been the subject of a number of recent investigations. The RB protein is known to be bound by several viral oncogene proteins [23] and has also been shown to suppress the neoplastic phenotype in cultured RB− osteosarcoma cells transfected with cloned wild-type RB genetic material [24]. The incidence of structural alteration of the RB gene in osteosarcoma biopsy specimens has been reported to be between 20% and 40% [25–28]. The molecular pathophysiology of RB− tumors is presumed to involve inactivation of the normal RB allele (the 'two-hit' hypothesis), leading to loss of the tumor-suppressing activity of the normal gene product. Interestingly, one recent study demonstrated that loss of heterozygosity (LOH) at the RB locus was associated with a poor prognosis, but that absence of RB protein expression was found as often in cells without LOH as in cells with LOH [29]. These investigators speculated that the poor prognosis observed in patients with LOH at the RB locus might be due to alteration of other genes mapping to 13q or might be a general index of genomic instability.

Mechanisms for tumor resistance to chemotherapy are the subject of active investigation because response to preoperative chemotherapy is the single most important prognostic indicator of patient outcome. One promising line of research has targeted the *mdr*1 (multiple drug resistance) gene, which is commonly overexpressed in osteosarcoma cell lines [30,31]. The protein product of the *mdr*1 gene is a 170 kDa membrane-bound glycoprotein (p170) that functions as a transmembrane ATP-dependent pump. Overexpression of the p-glycoprotein is associated with resistance to Vinca alkaloids and anthracycline derivatives. Imanishi and coworkers [32], using RT-PCR and Northern blot analysis, found a direct correlation between overexpression of p-glycoprotein and poor tumor response to chemotherapy. In this investigation, RT-PCR revealed MDR1 expression in 9 of 20 osteosarcomas studied. Of those nine, eight tumors failed to respond to chemotherapy. The clinical correlation was highly significant ($p < 0.01$). Gebhardt et al. [33] reported an assay for intranuclear concentration of Adriamycin (doxombicin) in murine osteosarcoma cells. This method, which involves cytofluorometry of cells incubated with Adriamycin, was able to reliably distinguish between Adriamycin-resistant and Adriamycin-sensitive cell lines. The clinical utility of the technique and its relationship to p-glycoprotein expression, have not yet been established.

Potential autocrine mechanisms in the propagation of osteosarcoma have been the subject of much recent investigation. Yoshikawa et al. [34] have described a subtype of osteosarcoma exhibiting production of bone morphogenic protein (BMP) as determined by the ability of tumor cell lysates to induce bone formation in the subcutaneous tissue of mice. Twelve of 30 osteosarcomas assayed exhibited bone induction in this model. The incidence of pulmonary metastasis was 83% in the patients with BMP-producing tumors, compared with 44% in the 18 patients with BMP− tumors. The BMP family of proteins are cytokines that are important in stimulating division of osteoprogenitor cells during fracture healing. Because of the lack of specificity of the bioassay employed in this study, the authors were unable to determine which of the eight BMP proteins were being expressed by the tumors.

The BMP proteins have now been cloned and sequenced, thus opening the possibility of a less cumbersome method of assaying BMP formation in biopsy material and of more precisely delineating which of the proteins are being overproduced. The poor prognosis associated with BMP production by osteosarcoma cells certainly suggests that a self-sustaining autocrine loop may be important in the pathophysiology of pulmonary metastasis. In a more recent study, Ferracini [35] and colleagues found overexpression of the c-MET proto-oncogene and its ligand, HGF (hepatocyte growth factor), in 60% of osteosarcoma samples studied. The Met/HGF receptor is normally expressed in cells of epithelial origin. HGF has been found to promote the motility and invasiveness of carcinoma cells into adjacent collagenous matrices. Because HGF is widely distributed in human tissues, the authors suggested a possible paracrine mechanism of action for osteosarcoma cells overexpressing the HGF receptor alone, or an autocrine mechanism in those cells aberrantly expressing both the receptor and the ligand. It remains to be seen whether osteosarcomas exhibiting expression of the Met/HGF receptor represent a subtype with a poorer clinical outcome. The c-FOS protooncogene has been found in a large proportion of osteosarcomas by Wu et al. [36]. The *ras* family of oncogenes have not been detected in human osteosarcomas [37], and amplification of the MYC protooncogene was found in only 2 of 27 tumors studied by Ladanyi et al. [38]. Again, the possible clinical significance of these findings is yet to be determined.

From the standpoint of molecular biology, chondrosarcoma is the least well understood of the common primary malignant tumors of bone. Because the typical low- or intermediate-grade chondrosarcoma grows slowly when compared with high-grade sarcomas, these lesions are not sensitive to radiotherapy or chemotherapy. Pulmonary metastases do not occur frequently, and generally only appear after a prolonged period of local growth or in the setting of multiple local recurrences. The current system of histological grading is effective in distinguishing between the two extremes of low- and high-grade lesions, but is less useful in predicting the growth characteristics of lesions that fall into the broad middle ground. It is likely that histological grading of chondrosarcoma will someday be supplanted, or at the very least augmented, by immunohistochemical or molecular methods. The search for consistent cytogenetic abnormalities in cartilaginous malignancies has thus far revealed a tendency toward translocation of the q12 band of chromosome 22 with various portions of the long arm of chromosome 9 [39–41] in extraskeletal myxoid chondrosarcomas. This cytogenetic abnormality has not been detected in other types of chondrosarcoma [42]. This finding is intriguing because the identified breakpoint on chromosome 22 is in the region of the EWS gene described in Ewing's sarcoma, suggesting a link between the molecular pathogenesis of these two otherwise disparate tumor types. One recently reported investigation found a direct correlation between expression of *p53* (determined by immunohistochemical assay) and tumor grade, with weakly positive staining of 3 of 4 low-grade chondrosarcomas, and intense staining of all 3 high-grade lesions studied [43]. Future investigations into the molecular genetics of cartilaginous malignancies are certain to be most rewarding.

Surgical advances

The increased understanding of tumor biology, advances in diagnostic imaging modalities, development of effective multiagent chemotherapy regimens, and application of new technologies and techniques for surgical resection and reconstruction have altered the criteria for the selection of patients eligible for limb-sparing surgery. These advances have helped shape current surgical strategies and have prompted more tissue-conserving, yet more technically demanding, surgical procedures. Refinements in diagnostic and operative approaches, bone and joint reconstructive techniques, and soft-tissue coverage methods have resulted in an expanding pool of patients who have been deemed candidates for limb conservation without placing them at a significantly increased risk for local tumor recurrence.

The growing interest and experience with minimally invasive diagnostic techniques have altered our initial diagnostic approach to primary bone sarcomas. Percutaneous needle techniques have enjoyed much success outside the realm of bone sarcomas; however, acceptance of this recognized diagnostic modality has not been widespread.

Since the late 1970s, percutaneous biopsy techniques have been used at the University of Texas M.D. Anderson Cancer Center for the diagnosis of bone lesions. Our experience with over 800 biopsies of sarcomas using a cutting core (Tru-cut®) and/or fine-needle aspiration has demonstrated percutaneous biopsy to be a safe, highly accurate, and economic diagnostic procedure when performed by experts in percutaneous musculoskeletal biopsy techniques [44]. Currently, the accuracy of the biopsy has reached 90% in our center but remains highly variable in other institutions [45]. The primary concern with this technique is the limited amount of tissue obtained to establish the diagnosis and for research investigations. However, tissue obtained by this technique can be processed for standard histologic and cytologic preparations, immunohistochemical studies, electron microscopy, flow cytometry, and molecular studies.

There are several significant advantages of this technique over surgical biopsy for the surgeon. In-continuity excision of a surgically created biopsy tract with the resected tumor specimen has been emphasized to reduce the incidence of local recurrence of tumor in the biopsy tract. As a consequence, potentially contaminated skin, fat, fascia, and muscle, along with the tumor-bearing bone specimen, need to be resected, even when well-executed surgical biopsies are performed. The results of a multiinstitutional study examining the hazards of surgical biopsy revealed that poorly placed or performed surgical biopsies can adversely affect patient outcome, leading to more radical resections, increased morbidity, limb amputation, and increased local tumor recurrences [46].

Our experience does not indicate that a radical alteration of the planned surgical procedure is indicated for a poorly placed, but properly performed, needle biopsy [47]. A retained needle biopsy tract was not a negative prognostic variable for local recurrence in patients with extremity osteosarcoma who underwent limb-salvage surgery and pre- or postoperative chemotherapy. Amputation, complex wound closures with soft tissue reconstructions, and large soft tissue resections were avoided using this technique. Moreover, the incidence of wound-related complications and patient morbidity was negligible.

The extent of the skeletal resection for both long bone and pelvis tumors determines the functional deficient and influences the decision regarding the type of reconstruction to be offered to the patient to optimize function. The ability to more precisely delineate the extent of the primary tumor through the use of magnetic resonance imaging has prompted reexamination of the nature and scope of the surgical approach taken to achieve adequate surgical margins.

New formal and informal classification schemes based on more precise determination of the extent of the primary tumor, as determined by currently available imaging methods, are evolving to more accurately identify the scope of the procedure necessary for any given tumor [48]. Preservation of bone stock, joint surfaces, and ligamentous structures of the joint results in a significant improvement in limb function with the prospects of maintaining near-normal function long term. Tumors associated with soft tissue extension have been treated historically by extraarticular joint resection and sacrifice of the surrounding muscle because of concerns for soft tissue invasion, intraarticular contamination, and tracking of tumor along ligamentous and capsular structures. However, for selected tumors with minimal soft tissue extension, or for patients whose tumor has responded favorably to preoperative chemotherapy, the resection may be performed safely through the joint. Motor function may be optimized without compromising local tumor control [49]. The preservation of these structures provides more favorable soft tissue coverage of the reconstruction, decreases the risk of infection, increases joint stability, improves function, and provides a more cosmetic result.

Current approaches to skeletal reconstruction

Reconstruction alternatives have expanded due to advances in biomechanical engineering, allograft biology, and microvascular techniques. Although the reconstructive method chosen must be individualized, multiple factors influence the type of reconstruction selected and the probability of successfully maintaining long-term function. Current methods of reconstruction of the skeletal defects following tumor excision include prosthetic arthroplasty, osteoarticular allografts, allograft/prosthesis composites, and vascularized and nonvascularized large segment autografts. The advantages and disadvantages of these reconstructive techniques have been the focus of several reports [50–53].

One of the most common methods of reconstruction is prosthetic arthroplasty. Short-term results have been excellent in our experience (A.W. Yasko, unpublished), resulting in early return to function with low perioperative morbidity (<2%). This has tremendous implications for patients who must undergo chemotherapy postoperatively. Although well tolerated, late complications, including infection, polyethylene component wear debris, loosening at the prosthesis–bone interface, and mechanical failures have severely compromised the utility of this method to provide long-term durability. Improvements in metallurgy and prosthetic design have reduced many implant-related complications and have resulted in satisfactory function in the majority of patients [3,4,54]. An alternative to nonbiological reconstructions is allogeneic materials, including large bone segments and bone/cartilage composites. There are several limitations of these biological reconstructions, which include possible disease transmission, graft rejection, resorption, fracture, infection, and nonunion [55,56]. Late consequences have included joint instability and degenerative arthritis.

Method-specific complications impact on both short- and long-term outcome. Regardless of the type of reconstruction, the principal perioperative concern is infection, which may place the patient's life and limb in jeopardy. Reconstruction durability is the primary issue limiting long-term maintenance of meaningful function. Despite the limitations of current reconstructive techniques, meaningful function for a significant percentage of patients with limb sarcomas can be restored. Several unresolved problem areas of clinical concern for which no satisfactory solution has been determined to date include (1) limb reconstruction in the skeletally immature patient, (2) reconstruction of the pelvis, and (3) the salvage of failed limb-sparing reconstructions.

Limb-sparing surgery in skeletally immature patients

Techniques of reconstruction that have proven successful in adults are problematic when applied to growing children. The immature skeleton rapidly expands longitudinally, leading to the problem of limb-length inequality, and circumferentially, causing early loosening of implants fitted to the intramedullary canal. Children and adolescents frequently place great demands on implants, and, as the proportion of osteosarcoma and Ewing's sarcoma survivors increases with effective chemotherapy, the life expectancy of the reconstructed limb is likely to be many times shorter than the life expectancy of the patient. For these reasons, amputation has, until relatively recently, been the treatment of first resort in the surgical management of osseous malignancies in children. The functional and psychological outcome expected with ablative surgery remains the standard against which any form of limb reconstruction must be measured. Techniques to salvage a functional, long-lived extremity in the pediatric patient include: (1) allografts, either osteoarticular or intercalary; (2) rotationplasty; (3) arthrodesis, using allograft or autograft bone to bridge the defect; and (4) expandable endoprostheses.

Allografts may be used either to bridge a defect in the diaphysis of a long bone, with preservation of the adjacent joints (intercalary), or as a primary reconstruction for one half of a diarthrodial joint (osteoarticular). In the former case, a segment of fresh-frozen tubular bone is interposed into the defect, where it is secured using appropriate fixation devices — either plates and screws or intramedullary rods. The reported experience with intercalary allografts has been favorable, with better than 90% good or excellent outcomes in one recent large series [57]. Other authors have experienced a higher complication rate with intercalary allografts and advocate the use of vascularized fibular autografts for the reconstruction of diaphyseal defects [58]. Recently, Manfrini, Capanna, and coworkers reported the use of intercalary allografts in conjunction with vascularized fibular grafts, with encouraging results [59]. Intercalary allografts may not be suitable for use in the lower extremities of very young children with substantial growth potential because the ability to lengthen such grafts, even after successful incorporation, has not been demonstrated.

Osteoarticular allografts offer the chance to reconstitute a functional diarthrodial joint in cases requiring resection of the epiphysis of a long bone. Patients considering such a reconstruction should be informed that there is a high rate of early complications (infection, nonunion, and fracture), and that the initial period of activity restriction is longer than that required for other forms of reconstruction [57,60]. The use of osteoarticular allografts should be reserved for patients with little (≤4 cm) or no remaining growth because these grafts are not able to remodel their transverse dimensions, and size

134

mismatch at the joint surface would eventually result in premature degradation of the joint surface. Bearing these admonitions in mind, osteoarticular allografts offer the only chance at a truly biological reconstruction of a joint surface and should be offered as a reconstruction option to appropriately selected patients.

Rotationplasty was originally described for reconstruction after resection of the distal femur for osteosarcoma by Kotz and Salzer [61]. This technique attempts to substitute the ankle joint for the absent knee joint, thus converting an above-knee amputation into the functional equivalent of a below-knee amputation. Winkelmann has applied variations of the Van Nes principle of transposing joints one level proximally to reconstruction following proximal femoral resection [62]. Gait analysis and oxygen consumption studies of rotationplasty patients have shown that the level of function is closer to below-than above-knee amputation [63,64]. The overall complication rate of this procedure is low, but care must be taken in determining the proper level at which to place the ankle relative to the contralateral knee [65].

The major objection to this procedure is cosmetic; many patients and their parents are initially shocked by the appearance of a shortened extremity with the 'foot on backwards.' In this regard, we have found at M. D. Anderson that meetings with former patients who are now successfully using their prostheses are very helpful to candidates for rotationplasty and their families. Videotapes showing the appearance of the operated limb with and without the prosthesis are also useful in counseling patients considering this procedure. On one occasion, we have performed a proximal transfer of the tibia to the proximal femur, with a Syme amputation of the foot, for a patient who was unwilling to accept the appearance of a classic Van Nes rotationplasty. Rotationplasty is an excellent method for restoring function in children younger than 8 years, and offers a reconstruction with excellent function and a low risk of complications to the older patient who is able to accept the appearance of the extremity.

Arthrodesis using allograft, autograft, or a combination of the two has been used successfully for limb salvage following joint resection in growing patients. A retrospective long-term follow-up of 45 pediatric patients who had been reconstructed by this technique found 26% good, 26% fair, and 48% poor functional results [66]. These researchers related the poor results of knee arthrodesis to the occurrence of limb-length inequality. The technique of limb lengthening by distraction using external fixators has been described in a small group of patients [67] with knee arthrodeses, with good short-term results. The introduction of the Ilizarov limb-lengthening methodology into musculoskeletal oncology raises the likelihood that poor results secondary to limb-length discrepancy may be salvageable.

The implantation of longitudinally extensible prosthetic bone and joint replacements for pediatric patients was begun in Great Britain in 1975 [68]. Several centers have now reported long-term follow-up experience with these devices. Kenan and Lewis [69] found 91% excellent or good functional results in 12 patients with distal femoral expanding prostheses followed for 2–4 years.

One third of these patients required revision surgery for stem loosening. The results of proximal tibial replacement were discouraging, with only 2 of 9 good results, 5 of 9 fair, and 2 of 9 poor [69]. In a study of 6 pediatric patients followed to the point of skeletal maturity, Schiller et al. reported that a total of 53 planned lengthening procedures and 7 revision operations for complications were necessary to achieve an average length gain of 13 cm [70]. Functional results were excellent or good in all cases.

All authors stress the use of the Anderson et al. [71] or Moseley [72] methods for predicting limb growth during the preoperative planning phase. These standard methods of calculating expected growth may be used without modification for children receiving chemotherapy; although skeletal growth is retarded during the administration of chemotherapy, overall growth is only slightly affected [73]. When a malignant tumor located about the knee is resected, only one of the two physeal plates is usually removed with the specimen; the remaining growth plate, however, is transfixed with an intramedullary stem. It has been reported that when a smooth stem is cemented into the proximal tibia, the physeal plate continues to grow, as evidenced by fracture of the cement mantle in this region [74]. This fact is of considerable importance when designing the prosthesis.

The first generation of limb-lengthening prostheses has been plagued by mechanical failures, resulting in prosthesis fracture, inability to lengthen the prosthesis, or cataclysmic shortening [70,75]. Many prosthetic designs are now incorporating disclike spacers to provide a redundant system protecting against sudden mechanical failure with shortening of the device [68,75]. At our institution we have used a mechanically simple device, which incorporates a metal piston fitted within a polyethylene-lined cylinder in the body of the expansion module. Distraction of the device is achieved using a ratchet that fits into slots machined into the prosthesis. Length and rotation are controlled by a clip that fits into machined grooves in a piston. Additional stability is provided by metal shims, which are fastened about the piston. The device is fully modular, permitting the surgeon to exchange the expansion mechanism for a definitive prosthesis after the patient has achieved full growth, or for a longer expansion mechanism, if required. Our experience with this device is still in the earliest stages of clinical investigation.

All of the expandable prostheses described thus far require numerous operative procedures during the period of active skeletal growth. A limb cannot be lengthened more than about 2 cm at one sitting without risking major neurovascular complications [70]. Multiple operative exposures of the implant increase the risk of infection. Newer designs that provide for lengthening without an invasive procedure have been described. One such device incorporates a permanent magnet within the prosthesis, which is driven by an externally applied magnetic field [76]. Another purely mechanical solution allows lengthening of the prosthesis when the knee is repeatedly flexed beyond a certain angle [77]. Both of these implants are still in the investigational stage of development.

Novel approaches are focused on the preservation of the native joint and skeletal growth of the affected bone in selected pediatric patients. Techniques to safely perform transphyseal resections in an attempt to preserve the growth plate, as well as the integrity of the adjacent joint, are currently being reported. This approach, when applicable, has substantial advantages over the afore-mentioned therapies currently available.

Reconstruction of the pelvis

Pelvic resections and reconstructions are the most challenging clinical issues in limb-salvage surgery. The surgical principles for resection of tumors arising within the bones of the pelvis are similar to those of the long bones of the extremity. Two aspects of this surgery remain unresolved. The first is the choice of reconstruction to be used for a given type of resection in order to provide optimal functional results. The second is the high incidence of complications related to the complex nature of the surgical procedure.

The reconstruction method used is dependent on the extent of the resection. The pelvis may be left without reconstruction when a tumor is confined to the pubis, ischium, or iliac wing and the hip joint is preserved. Resection of the hip joint without reconstruction results in a flail and unstable hip, and is associated with significant limb shortening and weakness despite prolonged rehabilitation. Restoration of the disrupted pelvic ring or reconstruction of the hip joint yield better function than no reconstruction; however, too few cases have been reported of any one reconstruction method to demonstrate the superiority of one method over another. Periacetabular resections can be reconstructed with a large segmental pelvic allograft/hip prosthesis composite implant, pelvifemoral arthrodesis, or prosthetic spacer.

Enthusiasm for maximizing function by pelvis and hip reconstruction must be tempered by the high complication rates reported to be associated with this complex surgery. The overall complication rates have ranged between 40% and 65% in several reported large series [78–81]. Infection is the most frequently observed complication. Judicious soft tissue dissection, preservation of flap vascularity, and liberal use of local or free muscle flaps are recommended to minimize this complication.

Management of failed limb-sparing surgery

The advent of limb-sparing surgery for osseous malignancies coincided with the introduction of effective chemotherapy in the mid-1970s. The first generation of patients to undergo these reconstructive procedures has now been followed for approximately 20 years. An increasing number of patients are presenting 5 or more years after primary treatment for osteosarcoma or Ewing's sarcoma with a failed reconstruction. Recent reports of long-term follow-up of prosthetic reconstructions following wide bone resection for tumor have determined 5-year survival to be approximately 70–80% and

10-year survival to approach 60–70% [4,82]. Our experience at the M. D. Anderson Cancer Center with approximately 200 prosthetic reconstructions for bone sarcomas indicates that the probability of survival is site dependent and can be expected to approach 80% at 5 years and 60% at 10 years for reconstructions about the knee (A.W. Yasko, unpublished). The probabilities of surviving a prosthesis-related event for the proximal humeral and proximal femoral prosthetic reconstructions approach 95% and 85% at 5 and 10 years, respectively.

The most common mode of late failure for distal femoral and proximal tibial prostheses is aseptic loosening of the implanted stem. The chronic granulomatous response engendered by the presence of polyethylene wear debris has been reported to the putative factor leading to massive endosteal bone loss, posing a major reconstructive challenge to the revision surgeon [83]. In patients who have maintained adequate quadriceps muscle strength, and who present with symptomatic loosening secondary to periprosthetic osteolysis, our approach has been to revise to a new modular prosthetic design with a press-fit stem augmented with a segmental allograft where necessary. The application of a segmental allograft aids in soft tissue reattachment, restores bone stock for possible future revision, and may prevent further osteolysis due to stress shielding [84]. Patients who have inadequate quadriceps function are better served by revision to a knee arthrodesis.

Late failure of reconstruction of the shoulder girdle is relatively uncommon (5% at 5 years and 15% at 10 years in the our series), and when it occurs is most commonly caused by instability or late infection. In these cases, revision to a prosthesis with a larger articulating surface, or to an arthrodesis, are the best surgical options. Malawer and Chou [4] have emphasized the benefit of meticulous soft-tissue reconstruction.

One of the few long-term follow-up studies of patients undergoing revision surgery for failed limb-sparing surgery [85] reported functional results and early survival roughly equivalent to the results following primary limb-sparing surgery. When limb-sparing surgery was first introduced in the 1970s, many oncologists believed that the reconstructions were temporary and that many, if not all, of the patients would eventually require amputation. The data that are gradually accumulating suggest that long-term survival of reconstructions using massive prostheses is common, and that in cases of loosening revision to another prosthesis is a viable alternative to amputation or arthrodesis. Our experience with 18 patients for whom a revision procedure has been performed indicates that survivorship may be similar to the observed survival of the primary reconstruction. We therefore offer revision to all patients who desire maintenance of a mobile joint, and alternatively, arthrodesis.

Methods available to provide adequate soft tissue coverage have been refined and represent a significant advance in limb-sparing surgery. Compromised wound healing and flap necrosis are devastating consequences of the surgical elevation of extensive soft tissue flaps and resection of large segments of bone and surrounding soft tissues. The insertion of a massive prosthesis or allograft and the long duration of the surgical procedures, coupled with the deleterious effects of chemotherapy on soft tissue and bone healing, render the surgical wound vulnerable to vascular compromise, necrosis, and deep infection. The development of these complications during the period of bone marrow suppression associated with adjuvant chemotherapy can place the patient's limb and life at risk, and can lead ultimately to amputation.

The application of transposition muscle flaps and free tissue transfers has been extremely useful to provide a healthy well-vascularized envelope of soft tissue to protect the reconstruction and facilitate wound healing. The liberal use of these methods has significantly reduced the incidence of infections associated with limb-sparing procedures and has reduced the potential limb-threatening consequences of poorly placed or performed surgical biopsies [86]. Moreover, this technology has expanded the options afforded the orthopedic oncologist to address tumors arising in compromised host tissue beds (e.g., previously irradiated localized Ewing's sarcoma or radiation-induced sarcomas) and in anatomic regions for which host soft tissues may be inadequate for successful salvage (e.g., tibial lesions). The utility of muscle flaps has been demonstrated to salvage reconstructions associated with wound-related complications that might otherwise prompt amputation [87].

Guided tissue regeneration

The limitations of current reconstructive methods have prompted an explosion of interest in the investigation of guided tissue regeneration using biocompatible materials, autologous osteogenic cell preparations, and recently characterized recombinant growth factors to form new bone, cartilage, and connective tissues.

The morphogenesis of new bone tissue is dependent on the presence of favorable conditions that will support the processes of osteoconduction (substratum for vascular ingrowth and cell adherence), osteoinduction (differentiation of uncommitted osteoprogenitor cells), and osteogenesis (bone formation). Experience in animals and humans with various osteoconductive substances, such as ceramics (tricalcium phosphate and hydroxyapatite), demineralized bone matrix ertracts, xenogeneic collagen, and synthetic biodegradable polymers, has yielded encouraging results to facilitate new bone formation.

Most of the preparations investigated have been formulated to promote osteoconduction for non–load-bearing applications as particulate graft material to augment or replace autologous cancellous bone. Ceramics, which mimic the inorganic component of bone, have been used solely for this function as they are brittle and have very little tensile strength. They are of little clinical utility for oncologic reconstructions because they cannot withstand the torsional, bending, or sheer stresses required of a large segmental graft and therefore must be shielded from loading forces until bone ingrowth has occurred. They are ideally suited to restore volume in cavitary defects.

Demineralized bone matrix is formed by acid extraction of the mineralized component of bone, resulting in a residue of collagenous and noncollagenous proteins that exhibits enhanced osteoinductive capability over alternative nondemineralized freeze-dried or fresh-frozen allogeneic particulate bone materials. The clinical application of this material is similar to the ceramic preparations and has limited use for major oncologic reconstructions.

Biodegradable polymers offer an exciting alternative to these materials because of their wide range of properties and performance characteristics. Over the past several decades, interest in the development of these polymers for use in nononcologic orthopedic surgical applications has grown. Although there are a number of polymers available that can support new bone formation, the most frequently studied materials have been the poly(α-hydroxy esters). Homopolymers and copolymers of poly(L-lactic acid), poly(glycolic acid), and poly(lactic-co-glycolic acid) have a long history of use as biodegradable surgical sutures and are approved for human use by the Food and Drug Administration. The advantage of these polymeric formulations is that the products of their degradation are molecules that occur naturally in the body. Most recently, load-bearing polymers have been investigated for this purpose [88].

A wide range of properties make biodegradable polymeric materials an attractive candidate for guided bone regeneration. Pore size and porosity can be controlled to optimize tissue ingrowth, and the chemical composition and ratio of constituent homopolymers can be altered to modulate degradation kinetics. These polymers have been shown to support osteogenic cell adherence, proliferation, and expression of the bone cell phenotype in vitro [89].

Osteogenic cell preparations have been isolated from native bone, bone marrow, and periosteum. The determined and inducible cell populations within these tissues are responsible for the new bone formed in response to trauma and result in bone repair. In vitro these stromal cells are capable of differentiation into osteoblasts under favorable culture conditions [90,91]. Marrow-derived mesenchymal stem cells [92] have been isolated successfully, expanded in culture, and experimentally tested from bone marrow derived from chicks, mice, rats, rabbits, goats, and humans [93–99]. The osteogenic potential of these culture-expanded cells has been shown in animal models using composite implants composed of particulate demineralized guanidine-HCI extracted bone matrix [100] and porous calcium phosphate cubes [95,101–104]. Efforts to seed polymeric foams with autologous osteogenic cells have been encouraging [89]. Three-dimensional polymer-cell composites have supported new bone formation and represent possible constructs for large-segment bone regeneration.

These cell populations have been shown to be responsive to endogenous proteins that induce de novo bone formation. Two recombinant human bone morphogenetic proteins (rhBMP) have been shown to induce new bone formation in animal studies, resulting in the healing of segmental defects. The activity of these proteins has been demonstrated to be optimized when delivered with a suitable carrier, such as demineralized bone matrix, collagen, or biodegradable polymers [105–109]. Polymer materials, particularly poly(α-hydroxy acids), in the form of foams or microparticles, have been shown to be extremely effective as controlled delivery vehicles for osteoinductive proteins [105,107]. The addition of rhBMP to osteogenic cell preparations has potentiated new bone formation and in vivo has resulted in healing comparable with that observed with autologous cancellous bone. A synthetic composite graft composed of an osteoinductive protein, osteoconductive matrix, and osteogenic cells holds tremendous promise for the development of guided bone regeneration and a possible solution for the difficult problem of massive bone loss resulting from oncologic resections.

Equally problematic is the regeneration of articular cartilage [110]. Osteoarticular defects that result from the resection of tumors involving the periarticular regions of the long bone and pelvis present a difficult biologic reconstructive challenge. Despite potentially successful efforts to regenerate large segments of bone, long-term function depends on a competent joint (i.e., articular cartilage and ligamentous structures). Several groups have attempted to grow cartilage grafts in vitro for in vivo use utilizing biodegradable polymer scaffolds [111–114]. One approach has been to isolate and implant mature chondrocytes into controlled defects. Pate et al. have demonstrated successful isolation of putative mesenchymal stem cells from skeletal muscle, which can differentiate into chondrogenic cells, and have used these cells for regeneration [115,116].

Similar efforts are directed at tendon and ligament regeneration. Biodegradable polymers are currently being studied for use in soft tissue repair [117], reconstruction [118], and regeneration [119]. Continued efforts to develop suitable systems for directed cell transplantation on biosynthetic substrates and growth factor delivery will be a vital step toward the advancement of the field of directed mesenchymal tissue regeneration and musculoskeletal reconstruction.

References

1. Meyers PA, Heller G, Healey JH, Huvos A, Lane J, Marcove R, Applewhite A, Vlamis V, Rosen G. Chemotherapy for nonmetastatic osteogenic sarcoma: The MSK experience. J Clin Oncol 10:5–15, 1992.
2. Hudson M, Jaffe MR, Jaffe N, Ayala A, Raymond AK, Carrasco H, Wallace S, Murray JA, Robertson R. Pediatric osteosarcoma: Therapeutic strategies, results and prognostic factors derived from a 10-year experience. J Clin Oncol 8:1988–1997, 1990.
3. Horowitz SM, Glasser DB, Lane JM, Healey JH. Prosthetic and extremity survivorship after limb salvage for sarcoma. How long do the reconstructions last? Clin Orthop Rel Res 293:280–286, 1993.
4. Malawar MM, Chou LB. Prosthetic survival and clinical results with use of large-segment

replacements in the treatment of high-grade bone sarcomas. J Bone Joint Surg 77A:1154–1165, 1995.

5. McManus AP, Gusterson BA, Pinkerton CR, Shipley JM. Diagnosis of Ewing's sarcoma and related tumours by detection of chromosome 22q12 translocations using fluorescence in situ hybridization on tumour touch imprints. J Pathol 176:137–142, 1995.

6. Barr FG, Chatten J, D'Cruz CM, Wilson AE, Navta LE, Nycum LM, Biegel JA, Womer RB. Molecular assays for chromosomal translocations in the diagnosis of pediatric soft tissue sarcomas. JAMA 273:553–557, 1995.

7. Dockhorn-Dworniczak B, Schafer KL, Dantcheva R, et al. Diagnostic value of the molecular genetic detection of the t(11;22) translocation in Ewing's tumours. Virchows Arch 425:107–112, 1994.

8. Sorensen PH, Liu XF, Delattre O, Rowland JM, Biggs CA, Thomas G, Triche TJ. Reverse transcriptase PCR amplification of EWS/FLI-1 fusion transcripts as a diagnostic test for peripheral primitive neuroectodermal tumors of childhood. Diagn Mol Pathol 2:147–157, 1993.

9. Fellinger EJ, Garin-Chesa P, Triche TJ, Huvos AG, Rettig WJ. Immunohistochemical analysis of Ewing's sarcoma. Immunohistochemical analysis of Ewing's sarcoma cell surface antigen p30/32MIC2. Am J Pathol 139:317–325, 1991.

10. Fellinger EJ, Garin-Chesa P, Su SL, DeAngelis P, Lane JM, Rettig WJ. Biochemical and genetic characterization of the HBA71 Ewing's sarcoma. Cancer Res 51:336–340, 1991.

11. Perlman EJ, Dickman PS, Askin FB, Grier HE, Miser JS, Link MP. Ewing's sarcoma — routine diagnostic utilization of MIC2 analysis: A Pediatric Oncology Group/Children's Cancer Group intergroup study. Hum Pathol 25:304–307, 1994.

12. Ladanyi M, Lewis R, Garin-Chesa P, Rettig WJ, Huvos AG, Healey JH, Jhanwar SC. EWS rearrangement in Ewing's sarcoma and peripheral neuroectodermal tumor. Molecular detection and correlation with cytogenetic analysis and MIC2 expression. Diagn Mol Pathol 2:141–146, 1993.

13. Li FP, Fraumeni JF Jr. Soft-tissue sarcomas, breast cancer, and other neoplasms. A familial syndrome? Ann Intern Med 71:747–752, 1969.

14. Malkin D, Li FP, Strong LC, et al. Germ line p53 mutations in a familial syndrome of breast cancer, sarcomas, and other neoplasms. Science 250:1233–1238, 1990.

15. Levine A, Momand J, Finlay C. The p53 tumor suppressor gene. Nature 351:453–456, 1991.

16. Holstein M, Sidransky D, Vogelstein B, Harris CC. P53 mutations in human cancer. Science 253:49–53, 1991.

17. Nigro JM, Baker S, Preisinger AC, et al. Mutations in the p53 gene occur in diverse tumour types. Nature 342:705–707, 1989.

18. McIntyre JF, Smith-Sorensen B, Friend SH, et al. Germline mutations of the p53 tumor suppressor gene in children with osteosarcoma. J Clin Oncol 12:925–930, 1994.

19. Masuda H, Miller C, Koeffler HP, Bahifora H, Cline MJ. Rearrangement of the p53 gene in human osteogenic sarcomas. Proc Natl Acad Sci USA 84:7716–7719, 1987.

20. Wadayama B, Toguchida J, Yamaguchi T, Sasaki MS, Yamamuro T. P53 expression and its relationship to DNA alterations in bone and soft tissue sarcomas. Br J Cancer 68:1134–1139, 1993.

21. Iavarone A, Matthay KK, Steinkirchner TM, Israel MA. Germ-line and somatic p53 mutations in multifocal osteogenic sarcoma. Proc Natl Acad Sci USA 89:4207–4209, 1992.

22. Abramson DH, Ellsworth RM, Kitchin FD, Tung G. Second nonocular tumors in retinoblastoma survivors. Are they radiation-induced? Ophthalmology 91:1351–1355, 1984.

23. Horowitz JM, Yandell DW, Park S-H, Canning S, Whyte P, Buchkovich K, Harlow E, Weinberg RA, Dryja TP. Point mutational inactivation of the retinoblastoma antioncogene. Science 243:937–939, 1989.

24. Huang H-J, Yee J-K, Shew J-Y, Chen PL, Bookstein R, Friedmann T, Lee EY, Lee WH. Suppression of the neoplastic phenotype by replacement of the RB gene in human cancer cells. Science 242:1563–1566, 1988.

142

25. Toguchida J, Ishizaki K, Sasaki MS, Ikenaga M, Sugimoto M, Kotoura Y, Yamamuro T. Chromosomal reorganization for the expression of recessive mutation of retinoblastoma susceptibility gene in the development of osteosarcoma. Cancer Res 48:3939–3943, 1988.

26. Reissmann PT, Simon MA, Lee W-H, Slamon DJ. Studies of the retinoblatoma gene in human sarcomas. Oncogene 4:839–843, 1989.

27. Araki N, Uchida A, Kimura T, Yoshikawa H, Aoki Y, Ueda T, Takai S, Miki T, Ono K. Involvement of the retinoblastoma gene in primary osteosarcomas and other bone and soft-tissue tumors. Clin Orthop 270:271–277, 1991.

28. Wunder JS, Czitrom AA, Kandel R, Andrulis IL. Analysis of alterations in the retinoblastoma gene and tumor grade in bone and soft-tissue sarcomas. J Natl Cancer Inst 83:194–201, 1991.

29. Wadayama B, Toguchida J, Shimizu T, Ishizaki K, Sasaki MS, Kotoura Y, Yamamuro T. Mutation spectrum of the retinoblastoma gene in osteosarcomas. Cancer Res 54:3042–3048, 1994.

30. Stein U, Walther W, Wunderlich V. Point mutations in the mdr1 promoter of human osteosarcomas are associated with in vitro responsiveness to multidrug resistance relevant drugs. Eur J Cancer 30A:1541–1545, 1994.

31. Bodey B, Psenko V, Young L, et al. Immunocytochemical detection of the multidrug resistance (MDR) protein, p170 overexpression in human osteosarcoma (OS) cells. Proc Ann Meet Am Assoc Cancer Res 35:A2811, 1994.

32. Imanishi T, Abe Y, Suto R, Higaki S, Ueyama Y, Nakamura M, Tamaoki N, Fukuda H, Imai N. Expression of the human multidrug resistance gene (MDR1) and prognostic correlation in human osteogenic sarcoma. Tokai J Exp Clin Med 19:39–46, 1994.

33. Gebhardt MC, Kusuzaki K, Mankin HJ, Springfield DS. An assay to measure Adriamycin binding in osteosarcoma cells. J Orthop Res 12:621–627, 1994.

34. Yoshikawa H, Takaoka K, Masuhara K, Ono K, Sakamoto Y. Prognostic significance of bone morphogenetic activity in osteosarcoma tissue. Cancer 61:569–573, 1988.

35. Ferracini R, Di Renzo MF, Scotlandi K, Baldini N, Olivero M, Lollini P, Cremona O, Campanacci M, Comoglio PM. The Met/HGF receptor is over-expressed in human osteosarcomas and is activated by either a paracrine or an autocrine circuit. Oncogene 10:739–749, 1995.

36. Wu JX, Carpenter PM, Gresens C, Keh R, Niman H, Morvis JW, Mercoila D. The proto-oncogene c-fos is over-expressed in the majority of human osteosarcomas. Oncogene 5:989–1000, 1990.

37. Antillon-Klussmann F, Garcia-Delgado M, Villa-Elizaga I, Sierrasesumaga L. Mutational activation of ras genes is absent in pediatric osteosarcomas. Cancer Genet Cytogenet 79:49–53, 1994.

38. Ladanyi M, Park CK, Lewis R, Jhanwar SC, Healey JH, Huvos AG. Sporadic amplification of the MYC gene in human osteosarcomas. Diagn Mol Pathol 2:163–167, 1993.

39. Hinrichs SH, Jaramillo MA, Gumerlock PH, Gardner MB, Lewis JP, Freeman AE. Myxoid chondrosarcoma with a translocation involving chromosomes 9 and 22. Cancer Genet Cytogenet 14:219–226, 1985.

40. Turc-Carel C, Dal Cin P, Rao U, Karakousis L, Sandberg AA. Recurrent breakpoints at 9q31 and 22q12.2 in extraskeletal myxoid chondrosarcoma. Cancer Genet Cytogenet 30:145–150, 1988.

41. Stenman G, Andersson H, Mandahl N, Meis-Kindblom JM, Kindblom LG. Translocation t(9;22)(q22;q12) is a primary cytogenetic abnormality in extraskeletal myxoid chondrosarcoma. Int J Cancer 62:398–402, 1995.

42. Mandahl N, Heim S, Arheden K, Rydholm A, Willen H, Mitelman F. Chromosomal rearrangements in chondromatous tumors. Cancer 65:242–248, 1990.

43. Coughlan B, Feliz A, Ishida T, Czerniak B, Dorfman HD. P53 expression and DNA ploidy of cartilage lesions. Hum Pathol 26:620–624, 1995.

143

44. Yasko AW, Coupe K, Murphy LA, Ayala AG, Murray JA. Cost effectiveness of percutaneous needle biopsy for bone neoplasms. Orthop Trans 18:1130, 1994.
45. Ayala AG, Raymond AK, Ro Y, Carassco CH, Fanning CV, Murray JA. Needle biopsy of primary bone lesions. M.D. Anderson Experience. Pathol Ann 24:219–251, 1989.
46. Mankin HJ, Lange TA, Spanier SS. The hazards of biopsy in patients with malignant primary bone and soft-tissue tumors. J Bone Joint Surg 64A:1121–1127, 1982.
47. Andreo MA, Yasko AW, Ayala AG, Murray JA. Excision of the needle biopsy tract: Is it necessary? Orthop Trans 19:294, 1995.
48. Malawar MM, Meller I, Dunham WK. Shoulder girdle resections for bone and soft tissue tumors: Analysis of 39 patients and presentation of a unified classification system. In Yamamuro T (ed). New Development for Limb Salvage in Musculoskeletal Tumors. Tokyo: Springer-Verlag, 1989, pp 519–530.
49. Jensen KL, Johnston JO. Proximal humeral reconstruction after excision of a primary sarcoma. Clin Orthop 311:164–175, 1995.
50. Ferruzzi A, Ruggiere P, Capanna R, Campanacci M. Prosthetic replacement of the proximal humerus: Update of cases presented in 1981. In Brown KLB (ed). Complications of Limb Salvage. Prevention, Management and Outcome. Montreal: Isols, 1991, pp 473–477.
51. Rock MG, Chao EYS, Shi LY, Sim FH, Sanjay B. Osteoarticular allografts for reconstruction after tumor excision about the knee. In Brown KLB (ed). Complications of Limb Salvage. Prevention, Management and Outcome. Montreal: Isols, 1991, pp 17–25.
52. Samek V, Kotz R, Engel A, Petschnig R, Salzer-Kuntschik M, Windhager R. Ten-year results with a custom-made tumor endoprosthesis of the knee in primary malignant bone tumors. In Brown KLB (ed). Complications of Limb Salvage. Prevention, Management and Outcome. Montreal: Isols, 1991, pp 17–25.
53. Ward WG, Eckardt JJ, Johnston-Jones KS, Eilber FR, Namba R, Dorey FJ, Mirra J, Kabo JM. Five to ten year results of custom endoprosthetic replacement for tumors of the distal femur. In Brown KLB (ed). Complications of Limb Salvage. Prevention, Management and Outcome. Montreal: Isols, 1991, pp 17–25.
54. Sim FH, Beauchamp CP, Chao EYS. Reconstruction of musculoskeletal defects about the knee for tumors. Clin Orthop 221:188–201, 1987.
55. Lord CF, Gebhardt MC, Tomford WW, Mankin HJ. Infection in bone allografts. Incidence, nature and treatment. J Bone Joint Surg 70A:369–376, 1988.
56. Berrey BH Jr, Lord CF, Gebhardt MC. Fractures of allografts: Frequency, treatment and end-results. J Bone Joint Surg 72A:825–833, 1990.
57. Gebhardt MC, Flugstad DI, Springfield DS, Mankin HJ. The use of bone allografts for limb salvage in high-grade extremity osteosarcoma. Clin Orthop 270:181–196, 1991.
58. DuBousset J, Missenard G. Limb salvage for malignant tumours in children — reconstruction with allograft: Critical appraisal of long term follow-up. In Tan SK (ed). Limb Salvage — Current Trends. Montreal: ISOLS, 1993.
59. Manfrini M, Capanna R, Ceruso M, et al. Vascularised fibula autograft as medial support of massive allografts after femur resections for bone tumours (preliminary results). In Tan SK (ed). Limb Salvage — Current Trends. Montreal: ISOLS, 1993.
60. Alman BA, De Bari A, Krajbich JI. Massive allografts in the treatment of osteosarcoma and Ewing sarcoma in children and adolescents. J Bone Joint Surg 77A:54–64, 1995.
61. Kotz R, Salzer M. Rotationplasty for childhood osteosarcoma of the distal part of the femur. J Bone Joint Surg 64A:959–966, 1982.
62. Winkelmann W. Hip rotationplasty for malignant tumours of the proximal part of the femur. J Bone Joint Surg 68A:362–368, 1986.
63. Knahr K, Kristen H, Ritschl P, Sekera J, Salzer M. Prosthetic management and functional evaluation of patients with resection of the distal femur and rotationplasty. Orthopaedics 10:1241–1247, 1987.
64. Murray MP, Jacobs PA, Gore DR, Gardner GM, Mollinger LA. Functional performance after tibial rotationplasty. J Bone Joint Surg 67A:392–399, 1985.

144

65. Krajbich JI. Van Nes rotationplasty in skeletally immature patients with malignant sarcoma of the lower extremity. In Langlais F, Tomeno B (eds). Limb Salvage — Major Reconstructions in Oncologic and Nontumoral Conditions. Berlin: Springer-Verlag, 1991, pp 527–529.

66. Capanna R, Manfrini M, Donati D, et al. Arthrodeses after malignant bone tumor resection in children. In Langlais F, Tomeno B (eds). Limb Salvage — Major Reconstructions in Oncologic and Nontumoral Conditions. Berlin: Springer-Verlag, 1991, pp 543–551.

67. Said GZ, El-Sharif EK. Resection-shortening-distraction for malignant bone tumours: A report of two cases. J Bone Joint Surg 77B:185–188, 1995.

68. Sneath RS, Carter SR, Grimer RJ. Growing endoprosthetic replacements for malignant tumours. In Langlais F, Tomeno B (eds). Limb Salvage — Major Reconstructions in Oncologic and Nontumoral Conditions. Berlin: Springer-Verlag, 1991, pp 573–578.

69. Kenan S, Lewis MM. Limb salvage in pediatric surgery: The use of the expandable prosthesis. Orthop Clin North Am 22:121–131, 1991.

70. Schiller C, Windhager R, Fellinger EJ, Salzer-Kuntschik M, Kaider A, Kotz R. Extendable tumour endoprostheses for the leg in children. J Bone Joint Surg 77B:608–614, 1995.

71. Anderson M, Green WT, Messner MB. Growth and predictions of growth in the lower extremities. J Bone Joint Surg 45A:1, 1963.

72. Moseley CF. A straight-line graph for leg-length discrepancies. J Bone Joint Surg 59A:174–179, 1977.

73. Glasser DB, Duane K, Lane JM, Healey JH, Caparros-Sison B. The effect of chemotherapy on growth in the skeletally immature individual. Clin Orthop 262:93–100, 1991.

74. Safran MR, Eckardt JJ, Kabo JM, Oppenheim WL. Continued growth of the proximal part of the tibia after prosthetic reconstruction of the skeletally immature knee. J Bone Joint Surg 74A:1172–1179, 1992.

75. Eckardt JJ, Eilber FR, Rosen G, et al. Expandable endoprostheses for the skeletally immature: The initial UCLA experience. In Langlais F, Tomeno B (eds). Limb Salvage — Major Reconstructions in Oncologic and Nontumoral Conditions. Berlin: Springer-Verlag, 1991, pp 585–590.

76. Verkerke GJ, van den Kroonenberg HH, Grootenboer HJ, et al. In vitro and in vivo experiments of a lengthening element for a modular femur endoprosthetic system. In Langlais F, Tomeno B (eds). Limb Salvage — Major Reconstructions in Oncologic and Nontumoral Conditions. Berlin: Springer-Verlag, 1991, pp 609–612.

77. Windhager R, Schiller CH, Gisinger B, Kotz R. Expandable prostheses in children. J Bone Joint Surg 74B(Suppl II):178, 1992.

78. Healey JH, Lane JM, Marcove RC, Duane K, Otis JC. Resection and reconstruction of periacetabular malignant and aggressive tumors. In Yamamuro T (ed). New Developments for Limb Salvage in Musculoskeletal Tumors. Tokyo: Springer-Verlag, 1989, pp 443–450.

79. Ritschl P, Kickinger W, Feldner-Busztin H, Windhager R, Kotz R. Pelvic and sacrum resections. In Yamamuro T (ed). New Developments for Limb Salvage in Musculoskeletal Tumors. Tokyo: Springer-Verlag, 1989, pp 491–502.

80. Tomeno B, Languepin A. Innominate bone resection for tumors with limb preservation. In Yamamuro T (ed). New Developments for Limb Salvage in Musculoskeletal Tumors. Tokyo: Springer-Verlag, 1989, pp 459–463.

81. Campanacci M, Capanna R. Pelvic resections: The Rizzoli Institute experience. Orthop Clin North Am 22:65–86, 1991.

82. Turcotte RE, Sim FH, Pritchard DJ, et al. Long-term follow-up of Walldius hinged total knee arthroplasties. In Langlais F, Tomeno B (eds). Limb Salvage — Major Reconstructions in Oncologic and Nontumoral Conditions. Berlin: Springer-Verlag, 1991, pp 277–284.

83. Horowitz SM, Rapuano BP, Lane JM, Burstein AH. The interaction of the macrophage and the osteoblast in the pathophysiology of aseptic loosening of joint replacements. Calcif Tissue Int 54:320–324, 1994.

84. Langlais F, Delepine G, Dubousset JF, Missenard G. Composite prostheses in malignant

tumors: Rationale and preliminary results of 42 cases. In Langlais F, Tomeno B (eds). Limb Salvage — Major Reconstructions in Oncologic and Nontumoral Conditions. Berlin: Springer-Verlag, 1991, pp 387–394.

85. Hsu RWW, Sim FH, Chao EYS. Reoperation of failed prosthetic replacement for limb salvage. In Langlais F, Tomeno B (eds). Limb Salvage — Major Reconstructions in Oncologic and Nontumoral Conditions. Berlin: Springer-Verlag, 1991, pp 449–455.

86. Horowitz SM, Lane JM, Healey JH. Soft-tissue management with prosthetic replacement for sarcomas around the knee. Clin Orthop 275:226–231, 1992.

87. Eckhardt JJ, Lesavoy MA, Dubrow TJ, Wackym PA. Exposed endoprosthesis: Management protocol using muscle and myocutaneous flap coverage. Clin Orthop 251:220–229, 1990.

88. Yaszemski MJ, Payne RG, Hayes WC, Langer RS, Aufdemorte TB, Mikos AG. The in-growth of new bone tissue and initial mechanical properties of a degrading polymeric composite scaffold. Tissue Eng 1:41–52, 1995.

89. Ishaug SL, Yaszemski MJ, Bizios R, Mikos AG. Osteoblast function on synthetic biodegradable polymers. J Biomed Mater Res 28:1445–1453, 1994.

90. Beresford JN, Graves SE, Smoothy CA. Formation of mineralized nodules by bone derived cells in vitro: A model of bone formation? Am J Med Genet 45:163–178, 1993.

91. Maniatopoulos C, Sodek J, Melcher. Bone formation in vitro by stromal cells obtained from bone marrow of young adult rats. Cell Tissue Res 254:317–330, 1988.

92. Caplan AI. Mesenchymal stem cells. J Orthop Res 9:641–650, 1991.

93. Benayahu D, Kletter Y, Zipori DS, Wientroub. Bone marrow-derived stromal cell line expressing osteoblastic phenotype in vitro and osteogenic capacity in vivo. J Cell Physiol 140:1–7, 1989.

94. Bruder SP, Gazit D, Passi-Even L, Bab I, Caplan AI. Osteochondral differentiation and the emergence of stage-specific osteogenic cell-surface molecules by bone marrow cells in diffusion chambers. Bone Miner 11:141–151, 1990.

95. Goshima J, Goldberg VM, Caplan AI. The osteogenic potential of culture-expanded rat marrow mesenchymal cells assayed in vivo in calcium phosphate ceramic blocks. Clin Orthop 262:298–311, 1991.

96. Goshima J, Goldberg VM, Caplan AI. The origin of bone formed in composite grafts of porous calcium phosphate ceramic loaded with marrow cells. Clin Orthop Rel Res 269:274–283, 1991.

97. Lane JM, Tomin M, Fellinger E, Bockman R, Gross J. In vitro augmentation of bone marrow osteoprogenitor cells. Trans Orthop Res Soc 16:417, 1991.

98. Dennis JE, Haynesworth SE, Young RG, Caplan AI. Osteogenesis in marrow-derived mesenchymal cell porous ceramic composites transplanted subcutaneously: Effect of fibronectin and laminin on cell retention and rate of osteogenic expression. Cell Transplant 1:23–32, 1992.

99. Dennis JE, Caplan JE. Porous ceramic vehicles for rat-marrow-derived (*Rattus norvegicus*) osteogenic cell delivery: Effects of pre-treatment with fibronectin or laminin. Oral Implantol 19:106–115, 1993.

100. Tomin E, Browne MG, Lane JM, Gee C, Yasko AW. Stem cell differentiation inhibits osteogenesis. Trans Orthop Res Soc 18:490, 1993.

101. Ohgushi H, Goldberg VM, Caplan AI. Repair of bone defects with marrow cells and porous ceramic. Experiments in rats. Acta Orthop Scand 60:334–339, 1989.

102. Nakamura H, Goldberg VM, Caplan AI. Culture-expanded periosteal-derived cells exhibit osteochondrogenic potential in porous calcium phosphate ceramics in vivo. Clin Orthop Rel Res 276:291–298, 1992.

103. Haynesworth SE, Baber MA, Caplin AI. Cell surface antigens on human marrow-derived mesenchymal cells are detected by monoclonal antibodies. Bone 13:69–80, 1992.

104. Haynesworth SE, Goshima J, Goldberg VM, Caplan AI. Characterization of cells with osteogenic potential from human marrow. 13:81–88, 1992.

105. Yasko AW, Lane JM, Fellinger EJ, Rosen V, Wozney JM, Wang EA. The healing of

146

segmental bone defects, induced by recombinant human bone morphogenetic protein (rhBMP-2). J Bone Joint Surg 74A:659–671, 1992.

106. Heckman JD, Boyan BD, Aufdemorte TB, Abbott JT. The use of bone morphogenetic protein in the treatment of non-union in a canine model. J Bone Joint Surg 73A:750–764, 1991.

107. Lee SC, Shea M, Battle MA, Kozita K, Ron E, Turek T, Schaub RG, Hayes WC. Healing of large segmental defects in rat femurs is aided by rhBMP-2 in PLGA matrix. J Biomed Mater Res 28:1149–1156, 1994.

108. Muschler GF, Lane JM, Werntz J, Gebhart M, Sandu H, Piergentili C, Nottebaert M, Baker C, Burstein A. Segmental femoral defect model in the rat. In Aebi M, Regazzoni P (eds). Bone Transplantation. Berlin: Springer-Verlag, 1989.

109. Cook SD, Wolfe MW, Salkeld SL, Rueger DC. Effect of recombinant human osteogenic protein-1 on healing of segmental defects in non-human primates. J Bone Joint Surg 77A:734–750, 1995.

110. Paige KT, Vacanti CA. Engineering new tissue: Formation of neocartilage. Tissue Eng 1:97–106, 1995.

111. Vacanti CA, Kim W, Schloo B, Upton J, Vacanti JP. Joint resurfacing with cartilage grown in situ from cell-polymer structures. Am J Sport Med 22:485–488, 1994.

112. Vacanti CA, Langer R, Schloo B, Vacanti JB. Synthetic polymers seeded with chondrocytes provide a template for new cartilage formation. Plast Reconstr Surg 88:53–75, 1991.

113. Freed LE, Grande DA, Emmanual J, Marquis JC, Lingbint Z, Langer R. Joint resurfacing using allograft chondrocytes and synthetic biodegradable polymer scaffolds. J Biomed Mater Res 28:891–899, 1994.

114. Freed LE, Marquis JC, Norhia A, Emmanual J, Mikos A, Langer R. Neocartilage formation in vitro and in vivo using cells cultured on synthetic biodegradable polymers. J Biomed Mater Res 27:11–23, 1993.

115. Pate DW, Southerland SS, Grande DA, Young HE, Lucas PA. Isolation and differentiation of mesenchymal stem cells from rabbit muscle. Surg Forum 44:587, 1993.

116. Grande DA, Southerland SS, Manji R, Pate DW, Schwartz RE, Lucas PA. Repair of articular cartilage defects using mesenchymal stem cells. Tissue Eng 1:345–352, 1995.

117. Speer KP, Warren RF. Arthroscopic shoulder stabilization: A role for biodegradable materials. Clin Orthop 291:67–74, 1993.

118. Laitinen O, Tormala P, Taurio R, Skutnabb K, Saarelainum K, Iivonen T, Vainlonpaa S. Mechanical properties of biodegradable ligament augmentation device of poly(L-lactate) in vitro and in vivo. Biomaterials 3:359–364, 1992.

119. Howard CB, McKibbin B, Ralis ZA. The use of dexon as a replacement for the calcaneal tendon in sheep. J Bone Joint Surg 67B:313–316, 1985.

8. Thyroid carcinoma

Ann M. Gillenwater and Randal S. Weber

Introduction

The surgical technique of thyroidectomy has not changed significantly since Kocher performed his first procedure for benign goiter in 1872. Since that time, however, considerable advances have been made toward understanding the physiology and pathology of the thyroid gland. The past decade has witnessed an explosion in our knowledge of the molecular events involved in the development and progression of thyroid carcinoma.

Thyroid cancer is a relatively rare disease, with incidence rates ranging from approximately 0.2 to 6 cases per 100,000 per year in most world populations [1]. Compared with other forms of cancer, the low overall mortality rates reflect the relatively favorable prognosis of thyroid tumors. There are wide variations in the degree of malignancy of thyroid neoplasms, however, ranging from extremely aggressive to almost benign.

Despite its rarity, a considerable amount of literature has been written regarding the management of patients with thyroid cancer. Nevertheless, many of the controversies that have plagued thyroid surgeons during the past century remain unresolved. Issues include: (1) the management of a thyroid nodule; (2) the optimal surgical procedure for small, well-encapsulated tumors (Lobectomy and isthmusectomy or total thyroidectomy); (3) the surgical management of widely invasive thyroid masses; and (4) the most appropriate management of unresectable disease. Resolution of these controversies may await new discoveries in the molecular events leading to the initiation and promotion of thyroid cancer.

Well-differentiated carcinoma

Etiology, molecular carcinogenesis, and prognostic factors

The etiology and natural history of carcinoma of the thyroid gland remain uncertain. In some patients, the development of a well-differentiated carcinoma is strongly correlated with a history of external radiation [2].

Raphael E. Pollock (ed.), SURGICAL ONCOLOGY. Copyright © 1997. Kluwer Academic Publishers. ISBN 0-7923-9900-5. All rights reserved.

Iodine deficiency has been linked to the development of thyroid malignancy as well as goiter; it appears to be important for inciting the development of follicular and anaplastic carcinoma rather than papillary carcinoma. In certain geographic areas where iodine deficiencies were endemic, following the initiation of iodine prophylaxis a decrease in the prevalence of follicular and anaplastic carcinomas and an increase in papillary carcinomas were noted [1].

From clinical and epidemiologic studies of patients with well-differentiated thyroid carcinoma, several factors have been identified that correlate with prognosis and presumably progression of this disease entity toward a more aggressive phenotype. Since they were first introduced, the AMES [3] and AGES [4] classification systems have gained wide acceptance. Based on clinical parameters such as patient age, size and extent of tumor, metastases, and histology, these systems are used to classify patients into high-risk and low-risk groups.

The prognostic importance of these clinical variables has been confirmed in recent univariate and multivariate analyses of patients with well-differentiated carcinoma of the thyroid [5–7]. An evaluation of 2282 patients by Cunningham et al. identified five favorable prognostic indicators: age <50 years, female gender, white race, low-stage tumor, and postoperative thyroid suppression or ablation [6]. Shah et al. found that prognosis correlated with patient age, gender, tumor size, presence of distant metastasis, and histologic grade [5]; following further analysis of this group of patients, Shaha et al. recommended the addition of an intermediate-risk group to the classification scheme [8]. This intermediate-risk group consisted of two sets of patients: those <45 years with high-risk tumor factors such as tumor size >4 cm, follicular or high-grade histology, and presence of metastases; and those >45 years with no high-risk tumor features. The 5- and 20-year survival rates for the intermediate-risk group were 96% and 85%, respectively, compared with 99% and 99%, respectively, for the low-risk group, and 72% and 57%, respectively, for the high-risk group [8]. Many investigators are now attempting to further refine these classifications systems by analyzing other factors, such as tumor suppressor genes, oncogenes, growth factors, and DNA status. These analyses may provide new and important prognostic information.

Cytogenetics

Damage to DNA, including specific mutations or chromosomal rearrangements, is likely to be involved in both radiation-induced and spontaneous carcinogenesis in thyroid cells. During the past few years much progress has been made in delineating the cytogenetic and molecular abnormalities associated with the development and progression of well-differentiated thyroid carcinoma.

Chromosomal abnormalities have been detected in thyroid tissue as early as

150

during the follicular adenoma stage. Cytogenetic studies of follicular adenomas suggest that there is a subset of lesions that contain additional copies of chromosomes, particularly chromosomes 5, 7, and 12 [9,10]. Recurrent breakpoints at 19q13 have also been described in several case reports [11], suggesting the importance of this region of chromosome 19 in the development of follicular adenomas. Loss of heterozygosity (LOH) at 11q13 has also been noted in follicular adenomas [12], as have translocations involving chromosomal regions 2q12–13 and 3p24–25 [13]. The presence of chromosomal abnormalities in adenomas implies that DNA damage is a very early step in the process of thyroid carcinogenesis. Structural abnormalities and LOH involving the short arm of chromosome 3 have been detected in cases of follicular carcinoma [13]; this suggests the possibility that a tumor suppressor gene important for the tumorigenesis of follicular carcinoma is located in chromosomal region 3p. Further investigation may identify the specific genetic mutations involved in the progression from thyroid hyperplasia to invasive follicular carcinoma. In the future this information may be used clinically to predict individual patient prognosis or to develop novel treatment strategies.

Several recent important discoveries have elucidated the mechanisms involved in the development of papillary thyroid carcinoma. Cytogenetic analyses revealed frequent, nonrandom abnormalities in chromosomal region 10q [14,15]. Further molecular investigations of the region 10q have determined that transforming sequences involve the *ret* protooncogene are important in the tumorigenesis of papillary thyroid carcinoma; this oncogene is localized to chromosomal region 10q11.2.

Chimeric oncogenes are formed by the fusion of various DNA sequences upstream from the *ret* protooncogene, resulting in fusion proteins with constitutive tyrosine kinase activities [16]. The oncogene designated *ret*/PTC1, which is frequently found in papillary thyroid carcinoma specimens, is formed by a chromosomal inversion that places the DNA sequence D10S170 located on chromosome 10q21 adjacent to the *ret* protooncogene [17]. A second oncogene found in papillary carcinomas, *ret*/PTC2, is formed by the fusion of the tyrosine kinase domain of *ret* with part of the regulatory subunit R1α of protein kinase A [18]. A newly identified *ret* oncogene, *ret*/PTC3 [16], causes constitutive activation of the RET tyrosine kinase [18]. The *ret*/PTC3 oncogene is formed by a cytogenetically undetectable rearrangement within the DNA sequences around 10q11.2 — the fusion of the *ele1*/*rfg* gene with *ret* [19]. Other chromosomal rearrangements that may be important involve chromosome 1, with the fusion of *ntrk1* and *tpm3* [15].

Identification of the genetic mutations that may be responsible for the initiation of papillary carcinoma represents a major breakthrough in the understanding of the mechanisms of tumor development. Further investigations may lead to improvements in our ability to predict the biologic behavior of tumors, and to the development of novel treatment strategies.

Tumor suppressor genes

Mutations of the tumor suppressor gene *p53* are through to play a role in the progression of many types of malignancies, including lung, head and neck, liver, and colon. The protein product of the *p53* gene appears to be important for cell cycle regulation, particularly the mediation of growth-inhibition signals at the G1-S transition in response to cellular stress and damage. The *p53* protein initiates programmed cell death; its mutation allows progression of damaged cells through the cell cycle. Dobashi et al. [20] evaluated 110 cases of thyroid carcinoma immunohistochemically for overexpression of the *p53* protein. They detected an increased incidence of protein overexpression in undifferentiated carcinomas as compared with well-differentiated papillary and follicular carcinomas. Further analysis of the cases of overexpression revealed point mutations between exons 5 and 3 in two of six (33%) poorly differentiated tumors and in four of six (67%) undifferentiated tumors. While this finding suggests that *p53* mutation and overexpression plays a role in more aggressive lesions [21], no correlation with patient outcomes was attempted. The failure to detect *p53* mutations in the specimens of well-differentiated carcinomas is consistent with earlier studies in which *p53* mutations were found only in undifferentiated thyroid tumors [22–24]. However, Zou et al. did find evidence of *p53* mutations in specimens of well-differentiated thyroid carcinoma [25]. It could be concluded from these findings that *p53* mutations are a late step in thyroid oncogenesis, and they may thus be a useful marker for predicting which patients have more aggressive tumors.

Through its role in regulating cell cycle progression, the retinoblastoma (*Rb*) gene functions as a tumor suppressor gene [26]. In one study, evidence for *Rb* gene mutations was found in 55% of the carcinoma specimens analyzed; no *Rb* mutations were detected in benign thyroid tumors, while the incidence of the mutations in well-differentiated carcinomas was similar to that in undifferentiated tumors [27]. Further evaluation of the gene's role in thyroid carcinogenesis will be necessary to determine if detection of tumor expression of the *Rb* gene could be useful as a prognostic indicator.

Oncogenes

Abnormalities in the *ras* signaling pathway have been detected in all types of thyroid tumors [27]. Three *ras* genes encode four proteins — H-, N-, K4A-, and K4B-Ras — which play critical roles in the regulation of cell growth and the cell cycle [28]. Mutations at residues 12, 13, and 61 in all three *ras* protooncogenes have been implicated in the tumorigenesis of many tumor types. For example, in thyroid tumors point mutations at residue 61 of both the H-*ras* and the N-*ras* genes have been documented [29–31]. In addition, Hara et al. [29] showed that the presence of point mutations at residue 61 of the N-*ras* protooncogene in specimens of papillary thyroid carcinoma was associated with advanced-stage lesions, decreased survival rates, and increased recurrence rates. Multivariate analysis indicated that the N-*ras* mutation was an independent prognostic factor. An increased incidence of N-*ras* mutations in aggressive lesions was also found by Goretzki et al. [32], but in other series this correlation was not evident [30,33]. Interestingly, K-*ras* mutations appear to be specific for radiation-induced thyroid carcinomas [34]. To determine the prognostic significance of mutations in the *ras* protooncogenes in patients with thyroid malignancies, evaluation of larger numbers of patient specimens of thyroid carcinomas will be necessary.

The exact function and mechanism of action of the proteins encoded by the *ras* oncogenes has not yet been fully clarified. These proteins operate in concert with several other protein families to mediate signals in response to extracellular stimuli. The G proteins, a family of GTP-binding proteins, are closely interconnected with the Ras proteins in these signaling pathways. The G proteins mediate signals from membrane receptors, such as the TSH receptor, to downstream second messengers, such as adenylate cyclase, which in turn activates the cAMP cycle. There are both stimulatory and inhibitory G proteins [27,28]. Mutations involving the α-subunit encoded by the *gsp* gene have been identified in thyroid carcinomas; they may be associated with more aggressive lesions [32]. Determination of the clinical importance of *gsp* mutations and the potential interactions with *ras* mutations requires further investigation.

Other oncogenes may also be important in the progression of thyroid carcinomas. Amplification of the *met* oncogene was detected in 70% of papillary and poorly differentiated carcinomas and in 25% of follicular carcinomas; it was not detected in benign tumors nor in normal thyroid tissue [35]. The *ret/PTC* oncogenes may be important for the progression as well as the initiation of thyroid carcinomas [36].

Growth factors and proliferation status

Several groups are investigating the role of growth factors in the progression of thyroid carcinoma. EGF and the EGF receptor were detected immunohistochemically in thyroid carcinoma specimens, but both were undetectable in normal tissue and benign tumors [37]. The level of mRNA transcripts of c-*erbB1* and c-*erbB2/neu*, which encode the EGF receptor and an analog, were higher in papillary carcinomas and in one adenoma [38]. In a study by Di Carlo et al. [39], the level of EGF receptor detected was highest in specimens of anaplastic carcinoma as compared with other benign and malignant thyroid lesions. Furthermore, the patients whose tumors expressed increased levels of EGF had a higher tumor recurrence rate [37], as did the group with increased c-*erbB1* and c-*erbB2/neu* mRNA levels [38]. These studies indicate that abnormalities in the regulation of EGF and the EGF receptor may be important in the progression of thyroid carcinomas and therefore may be useful as indicators of biologic aggressiveness. Other factors that may also play a role include TGF-α, IGF-1, and TGF-β.

The proliferative activity of cancer cells has been used in several tumor types as a measure of aggressiveness. Recent investigations have assessed the prognostic value of proliferating cell nuclear antigen (PCNA) staining in thyroid tumors. In two studies [40,41], poorly differentiated and anaplastic carcinoma specimens had greater PCNA staining than did well-differentiated tumors or benign lesions; there was no significant difference, however, between the level of PCNA staining in well-differentiated tumors and in benign lesions. In a similar study, Tateyama et al. [42] subdivided both oxyphilic and non-oxyphilic follicular thyroid tumors into four subgroups: benign tumors, indeterminate tumors, encapsulated carcinomas, and widely invasive carcinomas. The percentage of PCNA-positive cells was highest in the widely invasive carcinoma subgroup, next highest in the encapsulated carcinoma group, and lowest in the benign tumor subgroup. These investigations suggest that evaluating the proliferative activity of thyroid tumors using PCNA staining may be useful for clinical staging.

Monitoring the expression of various molecular factors may prove important for predicting the biologic behavior of tumors in individual patients. While the number of potentially clinically applicable markers has increased during the past few years, to date there has been no successful attempt to assimilate these molecular markers into a prognostic classification scheme for thyroid carcinoma patients.

Diagnosis

Most often, thyroid malignancy is first detected as a nodule or mass within the thyroid; other patients, particularly young persons, initially present with lymph node metastases. The majority of thyroid nodules are benign, however, and contain little or no malignant potential. The difficulty in discriminating between benign and malignant nodules remains one of the greatest challenges faced by physicians who treat patients with thyroid disease. This dilemma has not yet been resolved, although several new diagnostic tests are now being developed that will increase a physician's ability to predict which patients require surgical intervention. New technologies are also increasing the physician's ability to detect recurrences and distant metastases in patients with thyroid carcinomas.

In addition to a thorough history and physical examination, fine-needle aspiration (FNA) biopsy has become the single most useful diagnostic procedure for determining the need for surgical extirpation in patients with thyroid nodules. Several recent series have confirmed the reliability and cost effectiveness of FNA biopsies using standard cytopathologic criteria to discriminate between benign and neoplastic lesions. For example, Piromalli et al. [43] evaluated a series of almost 800 patients who underwent FNA for thyroid nodules. The cytologic diagnosis was compared with the surgical pathology in 216 patients undergoing thyroidectomy. After excluding the nondiagnostic biopsies, the researchers determined the sensitivity and specificity of FNA to be 95% and 97.5%, respectively [43]. A similar study in which 394 patients were evaluated by FNA biopsy at a major cancer center reported the sensitivity and specificity for detecting malignancy of 93% and 91%, respectively [44].

In up to 20% of patients, however, a cytological diagnosis cannot be made [45]. For example, a major limitation of FNA biopsy lies in its inability to distinguish benign from malignant follicular neoplasms when follicular cells are seen in the aspirate. Tyler et al. [45] reviewed a series of 81 patients to determine if clinical risk factors could be used to improve the predictive ability of indeterminate aspiration biopsies. Indeterminate diagnoses were grouped as (1) suspicious for papillary carcinoma, (2) follicular neoplasm, (3) Hürthle cell neoplasm, and (4) hypercellular follicular aspirates with colloid. Patients with a cytological diagnosis suspicious for papillary carcinoma (9 out of 10, or 90%), and those with a diagnosis consistent with either follicular or Hürthle cell neoplasms who were also >50 years of age (9 out of 20 or 45%), had a significantly high risk of invasive malignancy.

The advent of new antibodies may further increase the predictive value of cytology. DeMicco et al. [46] evaluated the use of thyroid peroxidase immunocytochemistry with monoclonal antibody 47 for improving diagnostic accuracy in follicular neoplasms. One hundred benign adenomas and nine follicular carcinomas were stained with thyroid peroxidase and scored. There were 32% false-positive results, but there were no false-negative results. The authors concluded that the addition of this antibody staining to cytologic evaluation could reduce the number of unnecessary surgeries without increasing the risk of leaving a malignancy untreated.

A dilemma often arises during surgery for follicular neoplasms. Because the diagnosis of malignancy requires evidence of vascular or capsular invasion, multiple histologic sections are required to ensure a correct diagnosis. Discrimination between a benign follicular neoplasm and a malignant follicular neoplasm, therefore, often requires waiting several days to obtain a permanent section analysis of the specimen. Russell et al. [47] have investigated a novel technology to assist in the diagnosis of follicular nodules. They analyzed 53 thyroid specimens, which had been removed for solitary nodules, by using proton magnetic resonance spectrophotometry (^{1}HMRS) in vitro. For this technique, the tissue specimens were placed in a test tube and analyzed with a spectrophotometer. Russell et al. found a consistent and reproducible difference in the ^{1}HMRS spectra obtained from normal thyroid tissue as compared with papillary, medullary, and anaplastic carcinomas. Furthermore, they were able to separate benign follicular neoplasms into two separate groups — those with a benign tissue appearance and those with a malignant tissue appearance. The negative predictive value of magnetic resonance spectra was 100%, and the specificity was 52%. Although still in its infancy, this diagnostic technology may become useful to help differentiate benign follicular neoplasms from malignant follicular neoplasms in real time.

New imaging technologies, particularly positron emission tomography

(PET) scanning, are being evaluated as diagnostic tools for new and recurrent thyroid malignancies. Conventional imaging methods make use of the ability of thyroid cells to preferentially take up and retain radioactively labeled iodine (^{131}I). However, some neoplasms, particularly recurrent lesions, have lost their ability to sequester sufficient iodine to be imaged by scanning devices. Another problem is that patients must abstain from taking thyroid-suppressive therapy prior to these studies. As an alternative, scanning with thallium-201 (^{201}TI) has been investigated. Van Sorge-Van Boxtel et al. [48] recently evaluated the use of ^{201}TI scintigraphy, ^{131}I scintigraphy, and serum thyroglobulin (Tg) levels for the follow-up of patients with well-differentiated thyroid carcinomas. They found that serum Tg levels were the most sensitive (97%) and specific (100%) markers for tumor recurrence or metastases; the sensitivity of ^{131}I and ^{201}TI was only 57% and 55%, respectively. The combination of serum Tg and ^{131}I scintigraphy however, had a sensitivity of 100% and a specificity of 98%. They also found that the use of ^{201}TI scanning could add important localization information. Another study, performed by Ramanna et al. [49], showed that ^{201}TI scanning was more sensitive than ^{131}I scintigraphy for detecting recurrent differentiated thyroid carcinoma. These results may be misleading, however, because many of the presumed recurrences did not undergo pathologic or other confirmation.

Several centers throughout the country have evaluated the use of PET imaging for the diagnosis and follow-up of cancers. Sisson et al. [50] compared the ability of PET imaging of 18-fluoro-2-deoxy-D-glucose (FDG) with ^{131}I imaging and ^{201}TI scintigraphy for the detection of thyroid metastases in one patient. They found that the PET image of a lung metastasis had sharper resolution than either the ^{201}TI image or the ^{131}I image. Furthermore, the intensity of the PET image using FDG correlated with the level of metabolic activity of the tumor, showing a decrease after thyroid suppressive therapy was resumed. The authors concluded that PET imaging using FDG may be useful for the detection of occult metastases in thyroid carcinoma and for monitoring the response to systemic therapy for this disease. Further investigation will be required to determine the efficacy and cost effectiveness of this imaging modality for the diagnosis and follow-up of patients with thyroid cancer.

Treatment

Controversy regarding the most appropriate management for early well-differentiated carcinomas of the thyroid remains unresolved, despite the publication of many articles on the subject during the past half-century. Problems arise because of physicians' inability to predict the biological behavior of thyroid carcinomas in individual patients. While the majority of such tumors will take a benign course, a small percentage will demonstrate aggressive malignant behavior. Proponents of conservative therapy emphasize the benign nature of the disease process in the majority of patients and the increased

156

potential for morbidity associated with total thyroidectomy. Advocates of aggressive surgical management, on the other hand, point out the increased morbidity and mortality associated with local recurrence and second operative procedures, the increased efficacy of ^{131}I imaging and treatment following total thyroidectomy, and the low surgical complication rate for total thyroidectomy by experienced physicians. Comparisons of clinical series reviewing outcomes in patients with well-differentiated thyroid carcinomas are hampered by the tendency for recurrences to develop up to 30 years after the initial diagnosis. The long-term randomized prospective trial required to answer the question of the most appropriate management for early intrathyroidal well-differentiated carcinoma will probably never be performed.

Several recent studies have attempted to resolve this issue by analyzing the contralateral thyroid lobes in patients undergoing completion thyroidectomy for evidence of residual carcinoma. DeJong et al. [51] reviewed 100 specimens from patients undergoing completion thyroidectomy for papillary or follicular carcinoma. In 47% of patients with papillary carcinoma and in 33% of patients with follicular carcinoma, they found that one or more foci of carcinoma were detected in the specimen. Pasieka et al. [52] noted that of 47 patients diagnosed with unilateral well-differentiated thyroid carcinoma, 43% were found to have a tumor in the opposite lobe following completion thyroidectomy. They also found that evidence of multifocal disease in the first lobe was associated with a higher percentage of cancer in the contralateral lobe. Because of the relatively high risk of contralateral lobe carcinoma that was identified, both DeJong et al. and Pasieke et al. recommended total thyroidectomy.

While there is now general agreement on the use of radioactive iodine (RAI) for the treatment of metastatic disease and unresectable tumors, the use of postoperative RAI therapy for ablation of residual normal thyroid tissue is more controversial. This is due to uncertainties regarding its effectiveness in decreasing patient morbidity or mortality. Discussion is primarily concerned with which subset of patients would most benefit from this treatment; several clinical reviews with long follow-up have shed some light on the issue. Mazzaferri and Jhiang [53] reported on a series of 1355 patients with well-differentiated thyroid carcinoma with a median follow-up of almost 16 years. Of the 1152 patients with stage II or III tumors, 350 (30%) were treated with RAI either to ablate normal thyroid tissue or for suspected residual disease. A significant decrease in both local recurrence and mortality rates was found in patients treated with RAI. The researchers also found that low doses (29–50 mCi) were as effective as higher doses (51–200 mCi) for the control of local disease. These results extend the findings of an earlier study by Samaan et al. [54] in which the use of RAI was also found to be a significant factor in decreased local recurrence and mortality rates. It should be noted that in both series the patients were treated with thyroid hormone suppression as well as with RAI. Results suggest that the routine use of RAI with thyroid hormone suppression in patients with primary tumors >1.5 cm may be beneficial for reducing local recurrence and mortality rates from well-differentiated thyroid carcinoma.

Patients with extensive locally invasive disease present yet another therapeutic dilemma. Many studies have been published during the past few years, but there is yet no general consensus regarding the optimal management of patients with well-differentiated thyroid carcinoma invading the midline structures — the larynx, trachea, pharynx, and esophagus. Retrospective clinical reviews suffer from several factors — the limitations posed by small numbers of patients and difficulties in evaluating exact tumor extent and completeness of surgical resection. The conservative school recommends preservation of midline structures by 'shaving' the tumor from the larynx and trachea, potentially leaving behind microscopic disease. Proponents of aggressive therapy, in comparison, recommend extensive en-bloc resection of tumor, including partial or total laryngectomy, pharyngectomy, or tracheal resection, as needed, to obtain clear margins.

Friedman et al. [55] retrospectively evaluated 34 patients who underwent surgical resection for differentiated thyroid carcinoma invading the airway. They divided the patients into four groups, based on their operative reports: Group 1 patients had complete tumor resection, group 2 patients had incomplete resection with microscopic residual tumor, group 3 patients had resections with unclear margins, and group 4 patients had gross tumor remaining. The researchers revealed a statistically significant increase in survival for patients in group 1 compared with group 2; that is, those patients with complete tumor resection had longer survival rates than those with microscopic amounts of tumor remaining. However, no significant difference was found in local control rates between the two groups. Based on their results as well as on a thorough review of the literature, Freidman et al. recommended complete tumor removal in patients with invasive thyroid carcinoma.

McCaffrey et al. [56] reviewed the Mayo Clinic experience with patients presenting with invasive thyroid carcinoma over a 50-year period. They retrospectively evaluated 260 previously untreated patients with papillary carcinoma with extrathyroidal invasion. These patients were divided into three groups: Group 1 had received complete excisions, group 2 had received shave excisions with microscopic residual tumors, and group 3 had received incomplete excisions with gross tumor remaining after surgery. No significant survival difference was found between groups 1 and 2, but group 3 had a decreased survival rate. Based on their results, the authors recommended conservative removal of gross disease with the sacrifice of aerodigestive tract structures only if necessary to eradicate all gross tumor.

Comparison between these two series is difficult because of the different grouping criteria. Freidman et al. separated their patients into four groups, while McCaffrey et al. divided theirs into three groups. Both studies, however, support the concept of resecting all gross tumor whenever possible. Any intraoperative decision to leave microscopic disease or to sacrifice major structures must be determined individually, based on the patient's and the surgeon's willingness to accept a potentially higher level of morbidity, the presence of regional and metastatic disease, and the overall mental and physical status of the patient.

Radiation therapy as an adjunct modality should be considered in patients with invasive carcinoma of the thyroid. In all patients with symptomatic surgically unresectable disease, radiation therapy may offer palliation. Indications for postoperative adjuvant external-beam radiation therapy (XRT) in patients with well-differentiated thyroid carcinoma, however, are more controversial. O'Connell et al. [57] reported a series of 113 such patients who received XRT. For patients with residual microscopic disease, the local recurrence rate was 19% and the overall 5-year survival rate was 85%. For patients with gross disease, complete regression was obtained in 37.5% and the 5-year survival rate was 27%. Reasonable indications for postoperative XRT in patients with well-differentiated thyroid carcinomas that do not concentrate RAI include recurrent local disease, direct invasion of adjacent structures, and incomplete resection when no further surgery is contemplated [58].

The progress made during the past few years in our understanding of the basic molecular events involved in the development and progression of differentiated thyroid carcinoma, as well as the availability of new technologic advances in diagnostic modalities, have failed to resolve some of the basic controversies concerning the management of patients with this disease entity. Nevertheless, the information provided through these investigations may soon allow us to improve our predictions of prognosis in individual patients and to tailor treatment strategies accordingly.

Medullary carcinoma of the thyroid

Medullary carcinoma of the thyroid (MCT) was first identified as a distinct thyroid malignancy by Hazard et al. in 1959 [59]. Sipple [60] first reported a patient with bilateral pheochromocytomas associated with thyroid malignancy in 1961, but it was not until 1968 that the terminology multiple endocrine neoplasia (MEN) type II was proposed for the familial syndrome of MCT, pheochromocytoma, and hyperparathyroidism [61]. The RET protooncogene located on chromosome 10 was identified as the gene responsible for MEN IIA and familial MCT in 1993 [62,63].

Diagnosis

MCT occurs both in sporadic and in hereditary forms. Patients with the sporadic type usually present with a neck mass; the diagnosis of medullary carcinoma is made by FNA. Patients with MEN IIB — pheochromocytoma, multiple mucosal neuromas, intestinal ganglioneuromas, and marfanoid habitus — are usually diagnosed by physical examination alone. MEN IIA requires more complex diagnosis. Patients with MEN IIA and familial MCT are often diagnosed through screening for elevated serum calcitonin levels in family members at risk for the disease; by the time this type of tumor becomes clinically palpable, there is high likelihood of lymph node metastases or even of distant metastases. Most experts, therefore, recommend at least annual screening of family members by pentagastrin stimulation and serum calcitonin testing.

With the recent identification of the RET protooncogene as the gene responsible for MCT, genomic DNA analysis is now being used to identify family members with the inherited genetic mutation. Feldman et al. [64] analyzed DNA from persons with MEN IIA. A specific mutation in the RET protooncogene was identified in 12 of 17 families (71%). After each specific mutation was detected, genomic DNA from 95 at-risk family members was screened for the presence of disease. The diagnosis of MCT was confirmed with this technique in 39 patients. More importantly, in 56 family members at risk for the disease, 15 had inherited the RET protooncogene mutation, while 41 were found to be noncarriers. The noncarriers, who pose no risk for transmitting the syndrome to their offspring, will no longer require surveillance for the development of medullary carcinoma. The methodology of Feldman et al. holds great promise for the screening and early detection of patients with hereditable MCT.

Prognostic indicators

The clinical course of patients with MCT is variable, ranging from indolent to extremely aggressive. The identification of prognostic indicators has important ramifications for the management of this disease entity. Schröder et al. [65] retrospectively evaluated a battery of pathological and clinical parameters of prognostic significance to 45 patients with MCT. They found that only patient age, sex, and tumor stage correlated with survival; morphologic features and immunocytochemical staining, including calcitonin and carcinoembryonic antigen scores, revealed no prognostic significance. Patients whose tumors had diploid DNA content demonstrated a trend toward better outcomes.

A retrospective analysis of 65 patients by Pyke et al. [66] identified calcitonin staining as well as age, sex, and tumor stage as significant predictors of survival. DNA ploidy status was not found to be a significant prognostic factor. But Ekman et al. [67] found both DNA ploidy status and total DNA content to have prognostic relevance in their analysis of 231 patients with MCT. In the future, DNA analysis may provide useful prognostic information.

Serum calcitonin and carcinoembryonic antigen (CEA) levels have been suggested as possible prognostic markers for MCT. An elevated preoperative stimulated calcitonin level ($>10,000$ pg/ml) was found to be associated with not only greater extent of disease at presentation but also poorer prognosis [68]. Both calcitonin and CEA levels are higher in patients with disseminated disease [69].

160

Several molecular markers are being investigated as potential prognostic indicators. Thirty-three cases of MCT were analyzed for expression of the *bcl*-2 protooncogene, another gene that functions to block programmed cell death. Lack of *bcl*-2 immunoreactivity was a negative prognostic indicator [70]. In a multivariate analysis, Roncalli et al. [71] found that patients with tumors containing >10% of cells that stain for N-*myc* had poorer survival. They also found that the level of PCNA immunostaining, an indication of tumor cell proliferation, did not correlate with the patient's clinical outcome. This finding contradicted an earlier study of 11 MCT patients in whom PCNA staining correlated positively with tumor stage, grade, and disease progression [72].

Another potential marker for aggressive phenotype in MCT is CD15 (LeuMI), which has been shown to correlate positively both with local recurrence and with death [68,73]. Clearly, molecular markers with potential prognostic relevance will need further evaluation and then incorporation into standard staging systems to improve our ability to predict outcome for patients presenting with MCT.

Treatment

Surgery is considered to be the only curative treatment modality for MCT. While the extent of the surgical procedure recommended varies from institution to institution, such procedures have changed little during the past three decades. At the M.D. Anderson Cancer Center in Houston, total thyroidectomy with a central compartment nodal dissection is performed for palpable primary tumors. In patients with clinically evident metastases, an ipsilateral or bilateral neck dissection is performed. For C-cell hyperplasia or occult disease, a total thyroidectomy without neck dissection is appropriate.

The role of XRT for MCT is more controversial. As of early 1996, no large prospective randomized trial had yet been conducted to answer this question. Samaan et al. [74] reviewed the outcome of 202 patients treated for MCT. Of these patients, 57 (28%) received postoperative XRT when the surgeons believed that there might be microscopic residual disease in the neck. Patients receiving XRT were matched with controls for age, extent of disease, and surgical procedure. Those who received the treatment fared worse than the patients who did not. The researchers concluded that adjuvant XRT failed to provide additional clinical benefit. The effects of XRT on local disease control, however, were not addressed in the Samaan study.

Other retrospective reviews have reported increased survival rates with postoperative XRT [75]. Nguyen et al. [76], reporting the results of postoperative XRT in 59 patients, determined that this modality provided increased local control but no improvement in survival when compared with historical controls treated with surgery alone. They speculated that local control in MCT may not influence survival rates. XRT is currently recommended as an adjunct to surgery in patients with incomplete resections, direct extrathyroidal invasion, recurrent disease, extensive nodal disease, or persistently elevated calcitonin levels without demonstrable distant metastases [58].

The role of systemic chemotherapy in MCT remains unclear. Because of the indolent nature of the disease and the long survival of many patients despite the presence of distant metastases, chemotherapy is usually only recommended for those patients with progressive distant metastases. Doxorubicin has been the most frequently used agent for disseminated MCT, with reported response rates averaging approximately 30% [77]. New regimens currently in clinical trials include combinations of cyclophosphamide, vincristine, and dacarbazine [77]; 5-FU (fluorouracil) and dacarbazine [78]; and 5-FU with dacarbazine and streptozocin [79].

Management of occult disease

Several diagnostic modalities for detecting recurrent or residual disease are currently being evaluated. Serum calcitonin and CEA levels have been shown to be useful for monitoring disease status in patients with MCT. Elevated serum calcitonin and CEA levels indicate the presence of persistent disease. Interestingly, elevations in serum CEA levels may correlate more closely with progression of disease than alterations in calcitonin levels [80,81].

Various scintigraphy techniques have been evaluated for effectiveness at localizing persistent disease in patients with elevated serum calcitonin levels. Small series have used radioisotopic techniques — technetium phosphate (^{99m}Tc phosphate) and ^{99m}Tc sulphur colloid — to localize metastatic medullary thyroid carcinoma; results suggest that these techniques may be successful in some patients with elevated calcitonin levels [82].

Another technique used to help localize the site of persistent MCT is selective venous sampling. In one series of 19 patients with persistent hypercalcitoninemia who underwent catheterization for selective venous sampling, 13 of the patients subsequently had surgical procedures. In all but one patient, tumor was located at the site of the elevated calcitonin gradient [83]. Another localization method was reported by Waddington et al. [84]. A case of recurrent MCT was detected preoperatively with an indium-111 pentetreotide scan and was localized intraoperatively using a nuclear surgical probe.

A strategy is being developed to image as well as to potentially treat metastatic MCT by radiolabeling monoclonal antibodies against CEA. Juweid et al. [85] evaluated 19 patients with MCT using ^{131}I-anti-CEA monoclonal antibodies. They found that this technique was sensitive for detecting both known and occult lesions in all 19 patients; the overall lesion sensitivity was 91%. While this technology is still in the experimental stage, it appears to have definite potential for the detection of occult lesions.

Continued improvements in the various imaging modalities may someday solve the therapeutic problems encountered when patients manifest elevated plasma calcitonin and/or CEA levels without detectable residual or metastatic disease. The optimum management of these patients was addressed by Tisell et al. [86] in a study of 11 patients with elevated stimulated plasma calcitonin levels following surgical therapy of MCT. Cervical and mediastinal lymph node dissection was performed on all of the patients; normal plasma calcitonin levels were achieved in four (36%) of the patients and reduced calcitonin levels in other four (36%). The effect of reoperation on locoregional control and overall survival, however, has not yet been established.

Buhr et al. [87] performed neck dissections in 53 patients with elevated calcitonin levels from 1 month to 13 years following their primary thyroidectomy. The postoperative basal serum calcitonin levels normalized in 41 (77%) of the patients. In eight (15%) of these patients the calcitonin levels remained normal following pentigastric stimulation; during the follow-up period, with a median of 38 months, no tumor recurrence was detected. Buhr et al. reported three permanent complications out of a total of 77 neck dissections — 2 recurrent laryngeal nerve paralyses and 1 case of hypoparathyroidism. Longer follow-up periods will be required to determine whether normalization of calcitonin levels facilitates increased survival.

Van Heerden et al. [88] approached this problem differently. They presented data that suggested an aggressive surgical approach for asymptomatic metastatic MCT is not indicated. Thirty-one patients with elevated plasma calcitonin levels, in the absence of clinically or radiographically demonstrable disease, were followed from 1.3 to 16.8 years. Eleven (36%) of these patients had an additional surgical procedure during the follow-up period after they developed clinically or radiographically demonstrable disease. The overall 5- and 10-year survival rates were 90% and 86%, respectively. Van Heerden et al. argue that observing patients with elevated calcitonin levels in presumed occult metastatic disease, and deferring surgical therapy until demonstrable disease develops does not decrease overall survival. Further clinical studies with longer follow-up periods are required to determine the optimum management of patients with occult metastatic MCT.

Anaplastic thyroid carcinoma

Anaplastic carcinoma of the thyroid has an extremely poor prognosis, and there has been very little improvement in survival rates during the past few decades; only patients presenting with a discrete, well-localized lesion amenable to surgical resection and postoperative radiation therapy have a viable chance for cure. Recent retrospective clinical reviews have confirmed these poor survival rates [89–92]. Tumor size and gender were reported to be significant prognostic factors [91]. A significant percentage of patients reported in these series had a history of prior thyroid disease, which suggests that the anaplastic carcinoma may be arising through dedifferentiation of either benign or well-differentiated thyroid tumors. The molecular data on the stepwise progression of differentiated thyroid carcinoma presented earlier also supports the theory of dedifferentiation as a possible etiology of anaplastic thyroid carcinoma.

The results of two clinical trials of combined modality treatment have been recently reported. Schlumberger et al. [93] reported 20 patients treated with chemotherapy and XRT. Eight (40%) of the 20 patients had undergone complete or nearly complete surgical therapy prior to the clinical trial, and nine had distant metastases at the time of presentation. Patients <65 years were treated with a combination of doxorubicin and cisplatinum; older patients received mitoxantrone. All patients received XRT consisting of 17.5 Gy in seven fractions to the neck and superior mediastinum. Five patients had a complete local response to the treatment regimen, but all of those patients with distant metastases had progression of these tumors. Schlumberger et al. concluded that this protocol is promising as a means of preventing the severe symptomatology associated with local tumor growth, despite the presence of relatively high acute toxicity levels.

Tennvall et al. [94] reported a second treatment regimen for patients with anaplastic carcinoma of the thyroid, consisting of doxorubicin with concomitant hyperfractionated radiotherapy and debulking surgery when possible. Of the 33 evaluable patients, the tumors of 23 (70%) were amenable to debulking surgery. In 48% of the patients no signs of local recurrence were detected; death secondary to local failure occurred in 24% of the patients. Four (12%) of the patients survived for more than 2 years with no evidence of disease. The researchers considered this treatment regimen to be effective, with acceptable toxicities.

The aggressive multimodality treatment regimens have shown some promise toward improvement in local control. Survival rates for patients with anaplastic carcinoma of the thyroid, however, remain low.

Summary

During the past years advances have been made in the understanding of the molecular mechanisms involved in the initiation and progression of thyroid carcinoma. Mutations in tumor suppressor genes such as *p53* and oncogenes such as N-*ras* may be important for progression of well-differentiated thyroid carcinomas. Activation of the *ret* protooncogene located on chromosomal region 10q11.2 has been identified as a key factor in the initiation of papillary and medullary carcinoma. Integration of these discoveries into a prognostic classification scheme may allow us to better predict the biologic behavior of tumors in individual patients.

Despite the recent advances in our understanding of the molecular events occurring during thyroid carcinogenesis, major questions persist regarding aspects of patient management. New diagnostic modalities may enable us to noninvasively discriminate between benign and malignant thyroid nodules, and to detect recurrent disease earlier. Although the optimal surgical procedure for well-encapsulated tumors is still debated, recent clinical studies have shown that for those patients with tumors >1.5 cm, the routine use of RAI and

164

hormone suppression can improve local control and survival rates. Findings in two recent reviews suggest that patients with widely invasive thyroid masses benefit from the surgical removal of all gross tumor. Further investigation is required to define the role of adjuvant radiotherapy and the most appropriate management of unresectable disease.

Incorporation of prognostic markers into clinical staging systems should allow surgeons to better tailor their treatment plans for each patient. Translation of recent basic science advances into the clinical arena may also aid in the development of novel treatment strategies for patients with aggressive tumors.

References

1. Franceschi S, Boyle P, Maisonneuve P, et al. The epidemiology of thyroid carcinoma. Crit Rev Oncogen 4:25–52, 1993.
2. Ron E, Modan B, Preston D, Alfandary E, Stovall M, Boice JD, Jr. Thyroid neoplasia following low-dose radiation in childhood. Radiat Res 120:516–531, 1989.
3. Cady B, Sedgwick CE, Meissner WA, Salzman FA, Werber J. Risk factor analysis in differentiated thyroid cancer. Cancer 43:810–819, 1979.
4. Hay ID, Grant CS, Taylor WF, McConahey WM. Ipsilateral lobectomy versus bilateral lobar resection in papillary thyroid carcinoma: A retrospective analysis of surgical outcome using a novel prognostic scoring system. Surgery 102:1088–1095, 1987.
5. Shah JP, Loree TR, Dharker D, Strong EW, Begg C, Vlamis V. Prognostic factors in well differentiated carcinoma of the thyroid gland. Am J Surg 164:658–661, 1992.
6. Cunningham MP, Duda RB, Recant W, Chmiel JS, Sylvester JA, Fremgen A. Survival discriminants for differentiated thyroid cancer. Am J Surg 160:344–347, 1990.
7. Ruiz do Almodovar JM, Ruiz-Garcia J, Olea N, Villalobos M, Pedraza V. Analysis of risk of death from differentiated thyroid cancer. Radiother Oncol 31:207–212, 1994.
8. Shaha AR, Loree TR, Shah JP. Intermediate-risk group for differentiated carcinoma of thyroid. Surgery 116:1036–1040, 1994.
9. Roque L, Castedo S, Clode A, Soares J. Deletion of 3p25 pter in a primary follicular thyroid carcinoma and its metastasis. Genes Chromosom Cancer 8:199–203, 1993.
10. Antonini P, Levy N, Caillou B, et al. Numerical aberrations, including trisomy 22 as the sole anomaly, are recurrent in follicular thyroid adenomas. Genes Chromosom Cancer 8:63–66, 1993.
11. Dal Cin P, Sneyers W, Sayed Aly M, et al. Involvement of 19q13 in follicular thyroid adenoma. Cancer Genet Cytogenet 60:99–101, 1992.
12. Matsuo K, Tang S-H, Fagin JA. Allelotype of human thyroid tumors: Loss of chromosome 11q13 sequences in follicular neoplasms. Mol Endocrinol 5:1873–1879, 1991.
13. Roque L, Castedo S, Gomes P, Soaraes P, Clode A, Soares J. Cytogenetic findings in 18 follicular thyroid adenomas. Cancer Genet Cytogenet 67:1–6, 1993.
14. Antonini P, Venuat A-M, Caillou B, et al. Cytogenetic studies on 19 papillary carcinomas. Genes Chromosom Cancer 5:206–211, 1992.
15. Sozzi G, Bongarzone I, Miozzo M, et al. Cytogenetic and molecular genetic characterization of papillary thyroid carcinomas. Genes Chromosom Cancer 5:212–218, 1992.
16. Bongarzone I, Butti MG, Coronelli S, et al. Frequent activation of *ret* protooncogene by fusion with a new activating gene in papillary thryoid carcinomas. Cancer Res 54:2979–2985, 1994.
17. Pierotti MA, Santoro M, Jenkins RB, et al. Characterization of an inversion on the long arm of chromosome 10 juxtaposing D10S170 and *ret* and creating the oncogenic sequence *ret/ptc*. Proc Natl Acad Sci USA 89:1616–1620, 1992.

18. Sozzi G, Bongarzone I, Miozzo M, et al. A t(10;17) translocation creates the *ret*/ptc2 chimeric transforming sequence in papillary thyroid carcinoma. Genes Chromosom Cancer 9:244–250, 1994.
19. Minoletti F, Butti MG, Coronelli S, et al. The two genes generating RET/PTC3 are localized in chromosomal band 10q11.2. Genes Chromosom Cancer 11:51–57, 1994.
20. Dobashi Y, Sugimura H, Sakamoto A, et al. Overexpression of p53 as a possible prognostic factor in human thyroid carcinoma. Am J Surg Pathol 17:375–381, 1993.
21. Dobashi Y, Sugimura H, Sakamoto A, et al. Stepwise participation of p53 gene mutation during dedifferentiation of human thyroid carcinomas. Diagn Mol Pathol 3:9–14, 1994.
22. Ito T, Seyama T, Mizuno T, et al. Unique association of p53 mutations with undifferentiated but not with differentiated carcinomas of the thyroid gland. Cancer Res 52:1369–1371, 1992.
23. Nakamura T, Yana I, Kobayashi T, et al. p53 gene mutation associated with anaplastic transformation of human thyroid carcinomas. Jpn J Cancer Res 83:1293–1298, 1992.
24. Donghi R, Longoni A, Pilotti S, Michieli P, Della Porta G, Pierotti MA. Gene p53 mutations are restricted to poorly differentiated and undifferentiated carcinomas of the thyroid gland. J Clin Invest 91:1753–1760, 1993.
25. Zou M, Shi Y, Farid NR. p53 mutations in all stages of thyroid carcinomas. J Clin Endocrinol Metab 77:1054–1058, 1993.
26. Ewen ME. The cell cycle and the retinoblastoma protein family. Cancer Metastasis Rev 13:45–66, 1994.
27. Farid NR, Shi Y, Zou M. Molecular basis of thyroid cancer. Endocr Rev 15:202–232, 1994.
28. Khosravi-Far R, Der CJ. The ras signal transduction pathway. Cancer Metastasis Rev 13:67–89, 1994.
29. Hara H, Fulton N, Yashiro T, Ito K, DeGroot LJ, Kaplan EL. N-ras mutation an independent prognostic factor for aggressiveness of papillary thyroid carcinoma. Surgery 116:1010–1016, 1994.
30. Shi YF, Zou MJ, Schmidt H, et al. High rates of ras codon 61 mutation in thyroid tumors in an iodide-deficient area. Cancer Res 51:2690–2693, 1991.
31. Karga H, Lee JK, Vickery AL, Jr., Thor A, Gaz RD, Jameson JL. Ras oncogene mutations in benign and malignant thyroid neoplasms. J Clin Endocrinol Metab 73:415–418, 1991.
32. Goretzki PE, Lyons J, Stacy-Phipps S, et al. Mutational activation of RAS and GSP oncogenes in differentiated thyroid cancer and their biological implications. World J Surg 16:576–582, 1992.
33. Namba H, Rubin SA, Fagin JA. Point mutations of ras oncogenes are an early event in thyroid tumorigenesis. Mol Endocrinol 4:1474–1479, 1990.
34. Wright PA, Williams ED, Lemoine DR, Wynford-Thomas D. Radiation-associated and 'spontaneous' human thyroid carcinomas show a different pattern of ras oncogene mutation. Oncogene 6:471–473, 1991.
35. Di Renzo MF, Olivero M, Fero S, et al. Overexpression of the c-MET/HGF receptor gene in human thyroid carcinomas. Oncogene 7:2549–2553, 1992.
36. Jhiang SM, Caruso DR, Gilmore E, et al. Detection of the PTC/ret TPC oncogene in human thyroid cancer. Oncogene 7:1331–1337, 1992.
37. Mizukami Y, Nonomura A, Hashimoto T, et al. Immunohistochemical demonstration of epidermal growth factor and c-*myc* oncogene product in normal benign and malignant thyroid tissues. Histopathology 18:11–18, 1991.
38. Assland A. Expression of oncogenes in thyroid tumors: Coexpression of c-erbB2/neu and c-erbB. Br J Cancer 57:358–363, 1988.
39. Di Carlo A, Mariano A, Pisano G, Parmeggiani V, Beguinot L, Macchia V. Epidermal growth factor receptor and thyrotropin response in human tissue. J Endocrinol Invest 13:293–299, 1990.
40. Shimizu T, Usuda N, Yamanda T, Sujenoya A, Iida F. Proliferative activity of human thyroid tumors evaluated by proliferative cell nuclear antigen/cyclin immunhistochemical studies. Cancer 71:2807–2812, 1993.

166

41. Soares P, Sobrinho-Simões M. Proliferative activity of human thyroid tumors evaluated by proliferating cell nuclear antigen/cyclin immunhistochemical studies. Cancer 73:2880–2881, 1994.

42. Tateyama H, Yang Y-P, Eimoto T, et al. Proliferative cell nuclear antigen expression in follicular tumours of the thyroid with special reference to oxyphilic cell lesions. Virchows Arch 424:533–537, 1994.

43. Piromalli D, Martelli G, Del Prato I, Collini P, Pilotti S. The role of fine-needle aspiration in diagnosis of thyroid nodules: Analysis of 795 consecutive cases. J Surg Oncol 50:247–250, 1992.

44. Caraway NP, Sneige N, Samaan NA. Diagnostic pitfalls in thyroid fine-needle aspiration: A review of 394 cases. Diagn Cytopathol 9:345–350, 1993.

45. Tyler DS, Winchester DJ, Caraway NP, Hickey RC, Evans DB. Indeterminate fine-needle aspiration biopsy of the thyroid: Identification of subgroups at high risk for invasive carcinoma. Surgery 116:1054–1160, 1994.

46. DeMicco C, Vasko V, Garcia S, Zoro P, Denizot A, Henry JF. Fine-needle aspiration of thyroid follicular neoplasm: Diagnostic use of thyroid peroxidase immunocytochemistry with monoconal antibody Surgery 116:1031–1035, 1994.

47. Russell P, Lean CL, Delbridge L, May GL, Dowd S, Mountford CE. Proton magnetic resonance and hyman thyroid neoplasia 1: Discrimination between benign and malignant neoplasms. Am J Med 96:383–388, 1994.

48. Van Sorge-Van Boxtel RAJ, Van Eck-Smit BLF, Goslings BM. Comparison of serum thyrogobulin, ^{131}I and ^{201}Tl scintigraphy in the postoperative follow-up of differentiated thyroid cancer. Nucl Med Commun 14:365–372, 1993.

49. Ramanna L, Waxaman A, Braunstein G. Thallium-210 scintigraphy in differentiated thyroid cancer: Comparison with radioiodine scintigraphy and serum thyroglobulin determinations. J Nucl Med 32:441–446, 1991.

50. Sisson JC, Ackermann RJ, Meyer MA, Wahl RL. Uptake of 18-fluoro-2-deoxy-D-glucose by thyroid cancer: Implications for diagnosis and therapy. J Clin Endocrinol Metab 77:1090–1094, 1993.

51. DeJong SA, Demeter JG, Lawrence AN, Palowan E. Necessity and safety of completion thyroidectomy for differentiated thyroid carcinoma. Surgery 112:734–739, 1992.

52. Pasieka JL, Thompson NW, McLeod MK, Burney RE, Macha M. The incidence of bilateral well-differentiated thyroid cancer found at completion thyroidectomy. World J Surg 16:711–717, 1992.

53. Mazzaferri EL, Jhiang SM. Long-term impact of initial surgical and medical therapy on papillary and follicular thyroid cancer. Am J Med 97:418–428, 1994.

54. Samaan NA, Schultz PN, Hickey RC, et al. The results of various modalities of treatment of well-differentiated thyroid carcinoma: A retrospective review of 1599 patients. J Clin Endocrinol Metab 75:714–720, 1992.

55. Friedman M, Danielzadeh JA, Caldarelli DD. Treatment of patients with carcinoma of the thyroid invading the airway. Arch Otolaryngol Head Neck Surg 120:1377–1381, 1994.

56. McCaffrey TV, Bergstralh EJ, Hay ID. Locally invasive papillary thyroid carcinoma: 1940–1990. Head Neck 16:165–172, 1994.

57. O'Connell MEA, A'Hern RP, Harmer CL, et al. Results of external beam radiotherapy indifferentiated thyroid carcinoma: A respective study from the Royal Marsden Hospital. Eur J Cancer 30A:733–739, 1994.

58. Ang KK, Kaanders JHAM, Peters LJ. Radiotherapy for head and neck cancers: Indications & techniques. Malvern, PA: Lea & Febiger, 1994, p 119.

59. Hazard JB, Hawk WA, Crile G Jr. Medullary (solid) carcinoma of the thyroid — A clinicopathologic entity. J Clin Endocrinol Metab 19:152–161, 1959.

60. Sipple JH. The association of pheochromocytoma with carcinoma of the thyroid gland. Am J Med 31:163–166, 1961.

61. Steiner AL, Goodman AD, Powers SR. Study of a kindred with pheochromocytoma,

medullary thyroid carcinoma, hyperparathyroidism, and Cushing's disease: Multiple endocrine neoplasia, Type II. Medicine 47:371–409, 1968.

62. Mulligan LM, Kwok LBJ, Healey CS, et al. Germ-line mutations of the RET proto-oncogene and multiple endocrine neoplasia type IIA. Nature 363:458–460, 1993.

63. Donis-Keller H, Dou S, GC HID, et al. Mutations in the RET proto-oncogene are associated with MEN IIA and FMTC. Hum Mol Genet 851–856, 1993.

64. Feldman GL, Kambouris M, Talpos GB, Mulligan LM, Ponder BAJ, Jackson CE. Clinical value of direct DNA analysis of the RET proto-oncogene in families with multiple endocrine neoplasia type IIA. Surgery 116:1042–1047, 1994.

65. Schröder S, Schwarz W, Rehpenning W, Dralle H, Bay V, Böcker W. Leu-M1 immunoreactivity and prognosis in medullary carcinomas of the thyroid gland. J Cancer Res Clin Oncol 114:291–296, 1988.

66. Pyke CM, Hay ID, Goellner JR, Bergstralh EJ, van Heerden JA, Grant CS. Prognostic significance of calcitonin immunoreactivity, amyloid staining, and flow cytometric DNA measurements in medullary thyroid carcinoma. Surgery 110:964–971, 1991.

67. Ekman ET, Bergholm U, Bäckdahl M, et al. and the Swedish Medullary Thyroid Study Group. Nuclear DNA content and survival in medullary thyroid carcinoma. Cancer 65:511–517, 1990.

68. Wells S, Baylin S, Leight G, Dale JK, Dilley WG, Farndon JR. The importance of early diagnosis in patients with heritary medullary thyroid carcinoma. Ann Surg 195:595, 1982.

69. Wells SA Jr., Haagensen DE, Linehan WM, Farrell RE, Dilley WG. The detection of elevated plasmal levels of carcinoembryonic antigen in patients with suspected or established medullary thyroid carcinoma. Cancer 42:1498–1503, 1978.

70. Viale G, Roncalli M, Grimelius L, et al. Prognostic value of bcl-2 immunoreactivity in medullary thyroid carcinoma. Hum Pathol 26:945–950, 1995.

71. Roncalli M, Viale G, Grimelius L, et al. Prognostic value of N-MYC immunoreactivity in medullary thyroid carcinoma. Cancer 74:134–141, 1994.

72. Skopelitou A, Korkolopoulou P, Papanikolaou A, Hadjiyannakis M. Proliferating cell nuclear antigen (PCNA) in medullary thyroid carcinoma. J Cancer Res Clin Oncol 119:379–381, 1993.

73. Längle F, Soliman T, Neuhold N, et al. Study Group on Multiple Endocrine Neoplasia of Austria. CD15 (LeuM1) immunoreactivity: Prognostic factor for sporadic and hereditary medullary thyroid cancer? World J Surg 18:583–587, 1994.

74. Samaan NA, Schultz PN, Hickey RC. Medullary thyroid carcinoma: Prognosis familial versus sporadic disease in the role of radiotherapy. J Clin Endocrinol Metab 67:801–805, 1988.

75. Sarrazin D, Fontaine F, Rougier P, et al. Role of radiotherapy in the treatment of medullary cancer of the thyroid. Bull Cancer 71:200–208, 1984.

76. Nguyen TD, Chassard JL, Lagarde P, et al. Results of postoperative radiation therapy in medullary carcinoma of the thyroid: A retrospective study by the French Federation of Cancer Institutes — The Radiotherapy Cooperative Group. Radiother Oncol 23:1–5, 1992.

77. Wu L-T, Averbuch SD, Ball DW, de Bustros A, Baylin SB, McGuire III WP. Treatment of advanced medullary thyroid carcinoma with a combination of cyclophosphamide, vincristine, and dacarbazine. Cancer 73:432–435, 1994.

78. Orlandi F, Caraci P, Berruti A, et al. Chemotherapy with dacarbazine and 5-fluorouracil in advanced medullary thyroid cancer. Ann Oncol 5:763–765, 1994.

79. Schlumberger M, Abdelmoumene N, Delisle MJ, Couette JE, and the Groupe d'Etude des Tumeurs á Calcitonine (GETC). Treatment of advanced medullary thyroid cancer with an alternating combination of 5FU-streptozocin and 5-FU-dacarbazine. Br J Cancer 71:363–365, 1995.

80. Rougier P, Calmettes C, Laplanche A, et al. The values of calcitonin and carcinoembryonic antigen in the treatment and management of non-familial medullary thyroid carcinoma. Cancer 51:885–862, 1983.

81. Saad MF, Fritsche HA, Jr., Samaan NA. Diagnostic and prognostic values of

168

carcinoembryonic antigen in medullary carcinoma of the thyroid. J Clin Endocrinol Metab 58:889–894, 1984.

82. Johnson DG, Coleman RE, McCook TA, Dale JK, Wells SA. Bone and liver images in medullary carcinoma of the thyroid gland: Concise communication. J Nucl Med 25:419–422, 1984.

83. Abdelmoumene N, Schlumberger M, Gardet P, et al. Selective venous sampling catheterization for localisation of persisting medullary thyroid carcinoma. Br J Cancer 69:1141–1144, 1994.

84. Waddington WA, Kettle AG, Heddle RM, Coakley AJ. Intraoperative localization of recurrent medullary carcinoma of the thyroid using indium-111 pentetreotide and a nuclear surgical probe. Eur J Nucl Med 21:363–364, 1994.

85. Juweid M, Sharkey RM, Behr T, et al. Targeting and initial radio-immunotherapy of medullary thyroid carcinoma with [131I]-labeled monoclonal antibodies to carcinoembryonic antigen. Cancer Res 55(Suppl M):5946s–5951s, 1995.

86. Tisell LE, Hansson G, Jansson S, Salander H. Re-operation in the treatment of asymptomatic metastizing medullary thyroid carcinoma. Surgery 99:60–66, 1986.

87. Buhr HJ, Kallinowski F, Raue F, Frank-Raue K, Herfarth C. Microsurgical neck dissection for metastisizing medullary thyroid carcinoma. Eur J Surg Oncol 21:195–197, 1995.

88. Van Heerden JA, Grant CS, Gharib H, Hay ID, Ilstrup DM. Long-term course of patients with persistent hypercalcitoninemia after apparent curative primary surgery for medullary thyroid carcinoma. Ann Surg 212:395–401, 1990.

89. Junor EJ, Paul J, Reed NS. Anaplastic thyroid carcinoma: 91 patients treated by surgery and radiotherapy. Eur J Surg Oncol 18:83–88, 1992.

90. Demeter JG, De Jong SA, Lawrence AM, Paloyan E. Anaplastic thyroid carcinoma: Risk factors and outcome. Surgery 110:956–963, 1991.

91. Tan RK, Finley RK III, Driscoll D, Bakamjian V, Hicks WL, Shedd DP. Anaplastic carcinoma of the thyroid: A 24-year experience. Head Neck 17:41–48, 1995.

92. Venkatesh YSS, Ordonez NG, Schultz PN, Hickey RC, Goepfert H, Samaan NG. Anaplastic carcinoma of the thyroid. A clinical pathologic study of 1 to 1 cases. Cancer 66:321–330, 1990.

93. Schlumberger M, Parmentier C, Delisle M-J, Couette J-E, Droz J-P, Sarrazin D. Combination therapy for anaplastic giant cell thyroid carcinoma. Cancer 67:564–566, 1991.

94. Tennvall J, Lundell G, Hallquist A, Wahlberg P, Wallin G, Tibblin S and the Swedish Anaplastic Thyroid Cancer Group. Combined doxorubicin, hyperfractionated radiotherapy, and surgery in anaplastic thyroid carcinoma. Cancer 74:1348–1354, 1994.

9. Changing trends in the diagnosis and treatment of early breast cancer

Kelly K. Hunt and Merrick I. Ross

Introduction

Breast cancer is the most frequently diagnosed malignancy and the second leading cause of cancer-related deaths in American women today. It is estimated that 180,200 cases will be diagnosed and 43,900 women will die in 1997 alone [1]. Although the incidence rate for breast cancer has been steadily increasing at a rate of 1–2% per year since the 1960s, the mortality rates have remained stable. This is due in part to effective screening programs and the detection of an increasing proportion of early invasive breast cancers and ductal carcinoma in situ [2].

Over the past decade, the management of early invasive cancers has changed. The current emphasis is placed on less invasive diagnostic methods, less radical surgical approaches, and more liberal use of aggressive systemic therapies. In clinical practice, for example, surgical treatments have evolved from the standard Halsted radical mastectomy to lumpectomy, axillary dissection, and postoperative radiotherapy. These breast-conserving therapies have become more widely accepted both by patients and physicians because several large, randomized studies have documented similar survival rates regardless of the local therapy employed (i.e., mastectomy alone vs. lumpectomy and radiation therapy) [3,4].

Furthermore, improved understanding of the biology of breast cancer has led to the belief that breast cancer is often systemic, even in its early stages, and that relapses are a result of occult micrometastases. Therefore, even though lesser surgical procedures provide effective locoregional control, multidisciplinary approaches using systemic therapies need to be incorporated into the management of higher risk patients for systemic disease control. This chapter reviews the current status of diagnostic techniques, treatment strategies, and prognostic factors in the management of early stage breast cancer and discusses the contemporary controversies.

Staging

Current guidelines for the clinical and pathologic staging of breast cancer are listed in Tables 1 and 2 [5]. This staging system depends on information

Raphael E. Pollock (ed.), SURGICAL ONCOLOGY. Copyright © 1997. Kluwer Academic Publishers. ISBN 0-7923-9900-5. All rights reserved.

Table 1. TNM staging of breast cancer

Primary tumor (T)	
TX	Primary tumor cannot be assessed
T0	No evidence or primary tumor
Tis	Carcinoma in situ or Paget's disease of the nipple
T1	Tumor ≤ 2 cm in greatest dimension
	T1a ≤ 0.5 cm in greatest dimension
	T1b >0.5 cm but not >1 cm
	T1c >1 cm but not >2 cm
T2	Tumor >2 cm but not >5 cm
T3	Tumor >5 cm in greatest dimension
T4	Tumor of any size with direct extension of chest wall or skin
Regional Lymph Node (N)	
NX	Regional lymph nodes cannot be assessed
N0	No regional lymph node metastasis
N1	Metastasis to movable ipsilateral axillary lymph node or nodes
N2	Metastasis to ipsilateral axillary lymph node(s) fixed to one another or to other structures
N3	Metastasis to ipsilateral internal mammary lymph node(s)
Distant Metastasis (M)	
MX	Presence of distant metastasis cannot be assessed
M0	No evidence of distant metastasis
M1	Distant metastasis (includes metastasis to ipsilateral supraclavicular lymph nodes(s)

Adapted from the American Joint Committee on Cancer [5].

Table 2. Stage grouping for breast cancer using TNM criteria

Stage	T	N	M
0	Tis	N0	M0
I	T1	N0	M0
IIA	T0	N1	M0
	T1	N1	M0
	T2	N0	M0
IIB	T2	N1	M0
	T3	N0	M0
IIIA	T0	N2	M0
	T1	N2	M0
	T2	N2	M0
	T3	N1,N2	M0
IIIB	T4	Any N	M0
	Any T	N3	M0
IV	Any T	Any N	M1

concerning the primary tumor (T), regional lymph nodes (N), and distant metastases (M) (see Table 1). Important changes from the previous staging system include the classification of carcinoma in situ as stage 0 and the subclassification of T1 tumors as T1a, T1b, and T1c. While definitions may vary in the literature, early breast cancer generally includes stages 0, I, and II [6]. The stage grouping based on TNM classification is listed in Table 2 [5].

Imaging

Mammography, the best imaging technique available for the detection and diagnosis of breast cancer, is also important in the surveillance of breast cancer patients who have been treated with conservation therapy [7]. Technology continues to improve; however, up to 15% of newly diagnosed palpable breast cancers are not detected on mammograms, and the sensitivity of surveillance mammography in the post-treatment breast may be diminished [8]. In addition, there are limitations related to the density of the breast and the experience of the observer. These factors have led to a search for new techniques of imaging the breast. Some of the areas that show promise are breast ultrasonography, magnetic resonance imaging (MRI), digital mammography, computer-aided diagnosis, positron-emission tomography (PET), and single-photon emission planar CT imaging (SPECT).

Breast ultrasonography

Breast ultrasonography is often used in the evaluation of breast abnormalities noted on physical examination or mammography; however, it has not been shown to be useful as a screening examination [9]. Ultrasonography is most helpful in distinguishing solid from cystic lesions and can distinguish a simple cyst from one that is complex and therefore requires further investigation with pneumocystogram or surgical biopsy [9]. Ultrasonography may be useful in the dense breast; in lactating women, in whom mammography is often limited; or during pregnancy, when ionizing radiation should be avoided. It is difficult to image microcalcifications using breast ultrasonography unless they are associated with a mass lesion. Breast carcinomas are typically seen in ultrasonography studies as ill-defined, hypoechoic masses with posterior acoustic shadows [10].

MRI

Early attempts to use MRI to study the breast were limited by poor resolution and difficulty distinguishing between benign and malignant processes [11]. The development of contrast-enhanced MRI using gadopentetate dimeglumine (Gd- DTPA), fast-scan sequences, and fat-suppression methods has greatly improved the images obtained [12]. The reported sensitivity of MRI of the breast for malignant processes ranges from 88% to 100% [12–16]. The reported specificity of MRI in the diagnosis of breast cancer is much more variable, ranging from 30% to 97% [14,16–17]. These wide ranges are in part due to the fact that study methods and imaging techniques are not standardized and are still in the investigational phase. There are specific areas where MRI is emerging as an important tool, including the evaluation of patients with silicone breast prostheses, follow-up after breast-conservation therapy, and cases of indeterminant findings on routine mammography.

173

More studies with pathologic correlation of MRI-detected abnormalities are needed before the technique can be widely used. MRI is also limited by inadequate systems for MRI-guided biopsies. Currently, the biopsy needles employed are conventional ferromagnetic needles that produce significant artifacts on MRI studies [11]. Overall, MRI of the breast appears to be very sensitive but is not specific enough to be routinely applied to current practice. In addition, this imaging modality requires an experienced radiologist who is familiar with both image acquisition and interpretation.

Digital mammography and computer-aided diagnosis

Digital mammography allows for wider variation in exposures and amplification of contrast differences between tissues [12]. Digital images can also be transmitted to distant sites, which may facilitate mammography screening efforts. As with other imaging systems, there is some variability in results based on the radiologist's experience with the technique [18]. The digital system is also limited by spatial resolution; the field of view is limited, and this may make it difficult to visualize some calcifications and soft tissue masses [19].

Computer-aided diagnosis (CAD) is a logical outgrowth of available digital technology. In this system, computers are programmed to detect calcifications, masses, and spiculations and to classify mammograms as having fatty or dense tissue patterns [12]. Investigators have also developed artificial neural networks for recognition of microcalcifications with increased sensitivity and reduction in false-positive detections [20]. CAD will become more useful as digital technology improves and as radiologists develop more experience with the technology.

Positron emission tomography and SPECT scanning

The role of PET in the imaging of primary and metastatic breast cancer remains unclear. The technique uses specific metabolic tracers labeled with positron emitters to detect cancer cells, which have altered metabolism compared with normal tissues [12]. The most commonly used tracer is fluorodeoxyglucose (FDG), which is a structural analogue of glucose. Other tracers with sensitivity for the estrogen receptor have been developed, but these are of limited use in estrogen receptor–negative tumors. The method provides better than 90% accuracy in diagnosis of tumors greater than 1 cm, but some false-negative results are seen when pathologic evaluation is compared with the results of PET images. PET scanning does appear to be a good indicator of tumor response to therapy and therefore may be useful in assessing treatment efficacy. Preliminary studies have also shown PET scanning to be useful in the noninvasive staging of axillary lymph nodes [12,21–23]. The major disadvantages of this imaging modality are the limited availability of radiopharmaceuticals and the cost of the scanners [12].

Single-photon emission planar CT imaging, or SPECT scanning, may be a more viable alternative of nuclear medicine imaging than PET scanning because it uses more standard radiopharmaceuticals, such as thallium 201 (^{201}Tl) and technetium 99 (^{99m}Tc) [12]. The most common agent employed for imaging breast lesions is ^{99m}Tc-sestamibi (sestamibi scanning). Initial studies reported a sensitivity of greater than 95% and a specificity of 87% [12]. More experience with these imaging methods is needed before their role can be defined in the imaging of primary and metastatic breast cancer.

Diagnosis

Palpable and nonpalpable breast abnormalities have traditionally been diagnosed by examining excisional breast biopsy specimens. Histologic examination of these biopsy specimens shows benign tissue in 70–80% of cases [24]. Several methods have been introduced to establish a more selective use of excisional breast biopsy in the management of patients with palpable and occult breast lesions. These methods include fine-needle aspiration biopsy (FNA), stereotactic FNA, core needle biopsy, and ultrasound-guided FNA. Excisional breast biopsy is still important when the results from these less invasive techniques are nondiagnostic or when the diagnosis is discordant with the clinical picture.

Fine-needle aspiration biopsy

Fine-needle aspiration biopsy is now widely used in the management of breast abnormalities. It has several advantages in that it is highly sensitive, fairly inexpensive, and easily tolerated by patients with minimal discomfort and low morbidity. FNA biopsy results can be interpreted in a relatively short period of time and therefore provides the patient and physician with an opportunity to plan definitive treatment. FNA results provides a cytology-based diagnosis that requires an experienced cytopathologist for accurate interpretation.

It has been shown that the accuracy of diagnoses made from FNA biopsy results improves when the cytopathologist performs the biopsy and then immediately interprets the material to assess the quality of the specimen [25–27]. With an FNA biopsy, an experienced aspirator can achieve low false-negative rates (which range from 1% to 31% in the literature) and avoid false-positive results (0–4.1%) by obtaining adequate specimens and adhering to cytologic criteria [25]. The major difficulties in sampling errors are encountered with small masses of less than 1 cm and large masses with a significant necrotic component. In these cases, ultrasound-guided FNA can be helpful in placing the needle and confirming that the appropriate area has been sampled [28].

Because FNA biopsy results provide a cytologic diagnosis, that is, evaluation of single cells, the technique cannot be used to distinguish between in situ and invasive carcinomas. If segmental mastectomy is performed based on the results of FNA and no gross lesion is found for confirmation by frozen section, patients may require a separate procedure for axillary lymph node dissection at a later date should the lesion ultimately prove to be invasive on permanent histologic examination [29]. Patients who are candidates for tumor downstaging with preoperative chemotherapy also require histologic confirmation of invasive carcinoma before therapy is begun. These examples illustrate drawbacks to FNA biopsy in that an additional biopsy may be needed depending on the clinical scenario. The final interpretation of FNA biopsy results requires correlation with clinical findings, and an open biopsy (or needle core biopsy) should be done when there is discordance between clinical and cytologic findings. Figure 1 provides an algorithm for the diagnosis of palpable breast masses. FNA is the first procedure; it can easily distinguish between solid and cystic masses.

Ultrasound-guided FNA is recommended for patients with breast implants because of the risk of damage to the implant with palpation-guided procedures. Fornage et al. reported results of ultrasound-guided FNA both in reconstructed breasts and augmented breasts [30]. The diagnosis was confirmed by surgical excision and was correct in 21 of 22 cases (95%). There were no complications related to the biopsy procedure, even when the mass was directly adjacent to the prosthesis. However, the material obtained from ultrasound-guided or stereotactic-guided FNA is limited to cytologic interpretation and therefore will not distinguish between in situ and invasive carcinomas.

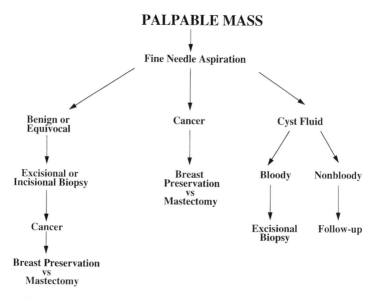

Figure 1. Algorithm for the diagnosis of palpable breast masses.

Core needle biopsy

Stereotactic core needle biopsy (SCNB) is the most recent addition to the myriad of minimally invasive biopsy techniques. The technology for stereotactic localization has been available since 1977; however, the initial studies used fine-needle aspiration, which provided only cytologic analysis (individual cells) of breast lesions [31,32]. The major advantage afforded by SCNB over stereotactic FNA is that it provides a histologic diagnosis (tissue architecture) of the mammographic abnormality. SCNB is a much less invasive means of obtaining a tissue diagnosis than open surgical biopsy, and because many of the abnormalities identified by screening mammography are benign, this offers an attractive alternative. The appropriate use of SCNB for cases of mammographic abnormalities requires an understanding of the accuracy of the technique and its limitations.

SCNB is most commonly performed with the patient in the prone position. An automated 'biopsy gun' with a 14-gauge needle and a 23-mm throw is used [33,34]. The number of core biopsy specimens needed is dependent on the type of mammographic abnormality being targeted. Liberman et al. reported a 99% diagnostic yield with five core biopsy specimens of mammographically identified masses [35]. When calcifications were the indication for biopsy, the diagnostic accuracy was reduced to 87%. Six biopsy specimens for mammographic calcifications improved the diagnostic accuracy to 92%. It is important to make radiographs of the core specimens to confirm the presence of calcifications prior to histologic evaluation. Agreement between core biopsy specimens and surgical biopsy specimens is also an important issue in the accuracy of SCNB. Core needle biopsy may fail to identify small areas of invasion in cases of ductal carcinoma in situ (DCIS) with microinvasion or focal areas of invasion [36,37].

When mammographic abnormalities are highly suspect for carcinoma, SCNB can be employed for diagnosis and may reduce the number of surgical procedures necessary for definitive treatment [33,38]. However, if used inappropriately, core biopsy may actually increase the cost of a diagnostic workup by introducing another test when the clinician knows the results of the core biopsy will not change the treatment plan.

Specimens obtained from core biopsies can provide tissue for diagnosis and reliable flow cytometric measurements of ploidy and S-phase fractions. Other prognostic factors can be examined as well using the paraffin-embedded tissue sections [39]. While mammography-detected calcifications can be accurately evaluated using SCNB, there is a danger of completely removing the calcifications after multiple core biopsies of small clusters of calcifications. This could result in difficulties in planning treatment options because there are no further calcifications to target when lumpectomy is chosen as part of a breast conserving approach. The use of SCNB may be most appropriate in the indeterminate mammographic abnormality. If the radiologic, histologic, and clinical features are concordant, then open surgical biopsy can be avoided. When there is a high likelihood of benign histology based on mammographic features or when the patient will almost certainly require an open biopsy for definitive diagnosis, SCNB should not be employed [34]. Figure 2 provides an algorithm for evaluation of mammographic abnormalities using ultrasonography prior to any biopsy procedure.

Core biopsy is also appropriate under ultrasound guidance depending on the radiologist's experience and whether the abnormality is best visualized using mammography or ultrasonography. When minimally invasive biopsy techniques are not appropriate or are not readily available, mammographic needle localization biopsy or ultrasound-guided localization biopsy are the next step [40]. Just as specimen mammography is important after mammographic localization biopsy, to ensure the index lesion has been removed, specimen ultrasonography should be performed when ultrasound-guided localization biopsy has been used.

Surgical management

Once the diagnosis has been established, surgical options for treatment of early breast cancer include mastectomy with or without reconstruction and breast conservation. The ultimate decision regarding the type of surgery is multifactorial and is dependent on the patient's desires, the surgeon's ability to provide effective locoregional control with breast conservation, the need for radiation therapy and/or axillary dissection, and whether the tumor process is invasive or noninvasive.

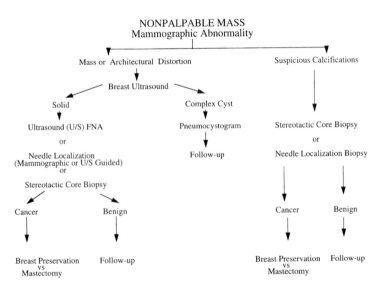

Figure 2. Algorithm for the evaluation of mammographic or nonpalpable breast abnormalities.

178

Because of widespread screening mammography, the average size of invasive tumors has decreased, and the incidence of noninvasive breast carcinoma has increased. At least half of the patients presenting with breast cancer will have localized disease that should be amenable to breast-preserving procedures. Patients who are not appropriate candidates for breast conservation are those with a history of previous radiation in the planned field that would preclude additional radiation therapy after surgical excision, women with collagen vascular diseases, and patients with evidence of multicentric disease in the breast [41,42]. Many other issues may be important in decision making, including the risk of local recurrence, the ability to achieve a satisfactory cosmetic result, and the psychological impact of breast preservation or mastectomy.

Clearly, the most important issue in the decision to proceed with breast-conserving therapy is assessing the risk for local recurrence. Factors reported to influence the development of in-breast recurrence after conservation treatment are listed in Table 3. Many series have reported an association between young age and an increased risk of locoregional recurrence after breast conservation [43–48]. The definition of young age in these studies ranges from patients under 35 years to those up to 50 years old, with the most common cutoff being less than 35 years. Other series have not corroborated these findings [49–52]. Harris has pointed out that young age is a risk factor for local recurrence after both breast conservation and mastectomy, and is also associated with distant relapse after any local therapy [53]. With such conflicting data in the literature and a sense that the biology of breast cancer in young women may be different, it would not be reasonable to deny a young patient breast-conservation therapy based on age alone.

The presence of extensive intraductal component (EIC) associated with invasive cancer has been reported as a major risk factor for locoregional recurrence by many groups [43,54–56]. The definition varies with each series, but in initial reports EIC was defined as intraductal carcinoma comprising 25% or more of the primary tumor. Physicians at the Joint Center for Radiation Therapy (JCRT) were among the first to show that EIC increased the risk of local disease recurrence; however, this group did not assess microscopic margins for tumor clearance. A more recent evaluation of 181 patients treated

Table 3. Prognostic factors reported to influence the risk of local disease recurrence after breast conservation

---

Young age
Extensive intraductal component (EIC)
Tumor necrosis
Intralymphatic extension
Vascular invasion
Close or positive histologic margins

---

at the JCRT, with 5 years of follow-up data, revealed local disease recurrence in 12 patients (7%) [57]. The investigators found a higher recurrence rate in EIC-positive tumors; however, when microscopic margins were negative or close (but still negative), there was no local recurrence in patients with EIC-positive tumors. The importance of microscopically negative margins has been confirmed by others [56,58–60], although opinion on the necessary extent of the margin varies markedly. Solin et al. [61] defined negative margins as 2 mm, while Borger and colleagues [43], in the Netherlands required excision of the tumor with 1–2 cm of macroscopically uninvolved tissue. In Solin's study, the radiation dose was escalated depending on the margin status, with the primary site boosted to 65 Gray when the margins were positive. There were no differences between groups of patients with negative, close, or positive margins with respect to locoregional control using this strategy.

Other factors associated with an increased risk of locoregional recurrence after breast-conservation surgery include tumor necrosis, intralymphatic extension of disease, vascular invasion, and high tumor grade [43,62–64]. While these pathologic features may be important in determining local recurrence, none are predictive, and therefore they would not generally be used to exclude patients from the option of conservation treatment. While many factors may influence the risk of local recurrence in the breast, multiple studies have confirmed that overall survival is not influenced by the type of local therapy [3,4,65–67].

In addition to local factors, such as extent of resection and radiation dose, there is emerging evidence that the use of systemic treatments may influence local and regional control after breast conservation as well. Rose et al. reported that premenopausal patients treated with adjuvant chemotherapy after breast conservation had a statistically significant decrease in local failure (5%) at 5 years when compared with women who did not receive adjuvant chemotherapy (17%) [68]. Haffty et al. made a similar observation when they reviewed 548 patients with a median follow-up time of 6.4 years and found that patients who did not receive adjuvant chemotherapy had a higher rate of breast relapse (7%) than did patients who received chemotherapy during or after their radiation therapy (1%) [69]. There was a trend toward decreased breast relapse in patients who received adjuvant hormonal therapy, but this was not statistically significant.

Role of radiotherapy

Radiotherapy is an integral part of breast-preserving treatment for invasive breast cancer. That radiation therapy can decrease the risk of relapse in the breast after lumpectomy has been demonstrated in several large randomized trials [65,67,70,71]. Data from the recent meta-analysis by the Early Breast Cancer Trialists' Collaborative Group of randomized trials of radiotherapy and surgery for early breast cancer showed that the rate of local disease recurrence was three times lower when radiotherapy was added to surgery than when patients were treated with surgery alone [65]. While fewer patients who had radiotherapy died of breast cancer, more patients in this group died of other causes, and therefore no difference in overall survival was observed at 10 years. As a result, many are now questioning the need for routine radiation therapy in all patients undergoing breast-preserving surgery. Multiple factors must be considered, including quality of life issues, expected cosmetic results, cost of radiotherapy, and the time needed (5–6 weeks) for radiation treatment, in the decision process to select patients who are appropriate candidates for conservation surgery without radiation.

Cady et al. recently reported their experience with 130 patients treated in a nonconventional fashion [72]. Ninety patients were treated without axillary dissection and 45 patients without radiotherapy following segmental resection of the primary tumor. Radiotherapy was avoided because of small tumor size in 18 patients, low histologic grade in 6 patients, advanced age or confounding medical problems in 14 patients, patient refusal in 4 patients, and the need for subsequent mastectomy in 2 patients. There were fewer failures in the patients who had radiotherapy after surgery than there were in patients who did not receive radiotherapy. However, the only statistically significant difference was an increased incidence of nodal failure in the nonirradiated group. In four of the patients with locoregional recurrences, aggressive local disease developed and three out of four developed metastatic disease.

Hermann et al. treated 620 patients from 1975 to 1988 with partial mastectomy without adjuvant radiation therapy [73]. Patients had routine axillary lymph node dissection as part of their surgical management. When evaluating patients for recurrence after 4–8 years of follow-up, they found a significant increase in local recurrence in patients who did not receive radiotherapy compared with those treated with surgery and radiotherapy. At 12 years of follow-up, the recurrence rates in the two groups are similar. However, in patients with stage II disease there was a local recurrence rate at 10 years of 21.6% in unirradiated patients versus a rate of 10.3% in those who received radiation ($p = 0.01$). The rate of salvage or type of treatment following locoregional recurrence was not reported; however, disease-free survival rates were similar regardless of the local therapy.

The above-mentioned studies illustrate some of the difficulties with nonrandomized studies. First, the patients selected for nonconventional treatment may not be comparable with those in the standard treatment group. Second, these series contain relatively small numbers of patients; therefore, it may be difficult to show that the small differences observed are statistically significant. The report by Hermann et al. suggests that local failure rates are similar in stage 0 and I patients, whether or not they received postoperative radiation therapy, but that the timing of recurrence is different. When postoperative radiation is omitted, patients will manifest local recurrence earlier in the course of their disease. If this is true, two important questions arise: (1) Does the increase in ipsilateral breast recurrences without radiotherapy lead to a higher incidence of distant relapse. (2) Can patients who relapse after conservative surgery without radiation be salvaged for eventual locoregional control?

Recht and Houlihan reviewed distant failure rates in randomized trials comparing conservative surgery with or without radiotherapy to determine the relative risk in each treatment group [74]. They found that the relative reduction in risk of distant metastasis was 17–23% in patients who received postoperative radiation compared with those treated with surgery alone. However, there were no differences in overall survival rates in any of these randomized studies. Fisher et al. evaluated 9-year follow-up data from the NSABP B-06 trial to examine the relationship between ipsilateral breast recurrence and the risk of development of distant disease [75]. These investigators found that the risk of distant metastases was 3.41 times higher in patients who developed an in-breast recurrence; however, there was no difference in distant disease-free survival among the treatment groups. Fisher and colleagues proposed from their analysis that ipsilateral breast tumor recurrence is a marker and not a cause for the development of distant metastatic disease.

With the widespread use of screening mammography allowing detection of smaller invasive tumors and the increasing number of in situ carcinomas, more physicians will question the need for adjuvant radiation therapy after primary tumor excision. Although proponents of selective treatment algorithms quote excessive morbidity with radiation therapy, including osteonecrosis of bone, cardiomyopathy, neuropathy, leukemia, and postradiation sarcomas, the incidence of these complications has significantly decreased as radiotherapy techniques have improved and radiation doses have been standardized [76]. Nevertheless, if specific factors can be identified that clearly define a subset of patients who will not benefit from radiation therapy, significant cost reduction, a shorter treatment period, and improved quality of life might be gained for those patients. The NSABP trial B-21 is an ongoing, multi-institutional trial that randomizes patients with small primary tumors (≤ 1 cm) to postoperative radiotherapy, versus tamoxifen, versus tamoxifen and radiotherapy. The B-21 trial will undoubtedly provide additional information that can be used to define the appropriate role for radiotherapy in the postsurgical treatment of small primary breast cancers.

Role of lymph node dissection and lymphatic mapping

Just as the need for radiation therapy after breast-conserving surgery has been questioned for patients with early-stage disease, the necessity of axillary lymph node dissection for every patient with invasive breast cancer is the subject of ongoing debate in the literature [77–79]. The reasons to include axillary lymph node dissection as a standard part of the surgical management of patients with breast cancer are as follows: (1) Patients who have small breast cancers and axillary lymph node metastases can be identified and therefore offered systemic therapy. (2) Locoregional control can be optimized. (3) The number of involved lymph nodes may indicate changes to the systemic regimen. (4) The information gained from examination of the lymph nodes is necessary for accurate disease staging. (5) It is the most discriminating prognostic factor available.

Patients with small palpable tumors or mammographically detected nonpalpable tumors undergoing breast-conservation therapy are really at the center of this debate. Because patients with tumors smaller than 1–1.5 cm generally would not be offered systemic treatment, it is important to identify such patients whose nodal metastases in fact would indicate the need for systemic therapy. Table 4 lists published series of patients with tumors that were ≤1 cm in size and the corresponding incidence of nodal metastases; the incidence of nodal involvement ranges from 5% to 21%. The EORTC trial correlated the incidence of nodal involvement by clinical examination and pathologic examination, and found that there was a 15% false-negative rate and a 51.5% false-positive rate [80]. In the patients who had proven metastases on pathologic examination, 69% had a normal clinical examination. This study and others confirm that there is a significant incidence of nodal metastases in small invasive tumors and that clinical examination of the axilla is unreliable in determining which patients harbor nodal metastases [81]. This is an argument in favor of axillary dissection for accurate staging.

The issue of axillary failure is difficult to resolve because patients who have breast-conserving surgery and postoperative breast irradiation will receive some radiation therapy to the axilla, and patients who are treated with total mastectomy often have a variable number of level I lymph nodes removed when the axillary tail is removed. To compare the aforementioned patients with patients having formal axillary treatment will introduce some error. The National Surgical Adjuvant Breast and Bowel Project (NSABP) B-04 trial randomized patients to axillary dissection, axillary radiation, or no treatment if there was no clinical evidence of nodal involvement at the time of initial evaluation [82]. Of the patients with clinically negative lymph nodes, 17.8% had histologic evidence of nodal involvement at delayed axillary dissection.

Table 4. Incidence of nodal metastases in patients with primary tumors less than 1 cm in size

Series	Dates	Number of patients	Incidence of positive nodes (%)
SEER	1972–1982	1335	21
Östergötland	1978–1985	310	12
Uppsala	1977–1988	74	19
Vienna	1969–1989	138	12
Linköping	1988–1990	284	14
Kopparberg-Östergötland	1977–1990	272	5
Beth Israel, NY	1990–1991	99	15
EORTC	1989–1992	164	16
M.D. Anderson	1985–1992	39	12
Van Nuys	1979–1994	336	13

Adapted from Recht and Houlihan [74], with permission.

This is in contrast to histologic nodal involvement in 40% of patients treated by radical mastectomy (with axillary dissection). This study has been criticized because some patients treated with mastectomy alone did indeed have lymph nodes removed at surgery, and axillary failures occurring after other sites of relapse were not recorded as locoregional failures [79]. Despite these criticisms, there was no difference in the overall survival rate of patients who had either immediate or delayed treatment of the axillary nodes, and radiotherapy appeared to control the axilla as well as surgery.

Cady et al. reviewed their recent experience with 90 patients whose breast cancer treatment did not include axillary lymph node dissection [72]. In this group, the median tumor diameter was 1 cm and the most common reason for avoiding axillary dissection was small tumor size. Eight patients (9%) developed recurrence in the axillary nodes, and in all of these patients local or distant disease developed at the same time as the axillary recurrence. This rate of axillary recurrence is much lower than those reported in series that did not include axillary treatment, which ranged from 19% to 21% [83,84]. Because a number of these patients were treated with postoperative breast irradiation, the lower axilla was included in the radiation fields and therefore the axilla was not completely excluded from treatment. Indeed, there was a significantly lower nodal failure rate in the group who received postoperative radiation than there was in the group that did not undergo radiation. There are several other series that report a similarly low nodal failure rate when patients undergo postoperative breast radiotherapy [85,86]. Clearly, the results of selective axillary treatment depend not only on whether the axilla is dissected or not but also on postoperative treatments such as radiation and systemic therapy, which may also decrease axillary failure rates.

In summary, there are many reasons not to perform routine axillary lymph node dissection: (1) The primary tumor may have features that indicate a need for systemic therapy. (2) The survival rate of patients is the same whether dissection is performed initially or when the patient develops clinically evident lymph node metastases (NSABP). (3) A lumpectomy without axillary dissection can be done under local anesthesia on an outpatient basis. (4) There is significant morbidity associated with axillary node dissection, even when the nodes do not contain metastatic disease. (5) Locoregional control can be preserved with radiotherapy alone to the axilla. (6) The incidence of axillary nodal metastases is low in mammographically detected cancers. (7) Patients with medial quadrant tumors may drain exclusively to the internal mammary lymph nodes, and therefore axillary lymphadenectomy would not provide accurate staging information or impact on locoregional control in those individuals.

Lymphatic mapping

Several 'less invasive' surgical methods have been used in the past for axillary staging; these include axillary sampling and intraoperative palpation of the axilla with removal of abnormal-appearing nodes. These techniques failed to provide an accurate assessment of axillary nodal involvement. Physical examination has also been shown to be unreliable in axillary staging. As yet, there is no radiologic study that can accurately stage the axilla, especially in the case of micrometastases. A surgical technique that has been introduced for minimally invasive nodal basin evaluation is lymphatic mapping and sentinel lymph node biopsy. First introduced by Morton and colleagues in 1992 for the evaluation of patients with early stage melanoma, the technique has since been extended to several other disease sites, including carcinoma of the breast and carcinoma of the vulva [87–91]. This approach is based on the observation that specific regions of the skin and breast parenchyma drain to one lymph node or one group of nodes, called the sentinel node(s), within a nodal basin.

Figure 3 illustrates how tumors in different quadrants of the breast and the lymphatic vessels could drain from the tumor into the sentinel lymph node. Early studies with lymphatic mapping injected 3–5 ml of a blue dye, 1% isosulfan blue (Lymphazurin), into and around the tumor, which then passes through afferent lymphatics to the sentinel lymph node(s) [92]. Figure 4 illustrates intraoperative lymphatic mapping of a sentinel lymph node and afferent lymphatic after Lymphazurin was injected into a breast tumor. A palpable tumor can be injected directly by the surgeon in the operating room. A nonpalpable tumor can be injected using ultrasound guidance in the operating room. Five to 10 minutes after the tumor is injected, a small incision is made in the nodal basin to identify the sentinel node. Subsequent studies used a technetium sulphur colloid alone or with Lymphazurin, and had more success in identification of the sentinel node [88,93].

Giuliano et al. reported their experience with 174 lymphatic mapping procedures in which sentinel lymph node biopsy was followed by formal axillary lymphadenectomy and pathologic examination [92]. It was possible to identify the sentinel node in 114 (65.5%) of 174 cases, and this procedure accurately predicted the status of the nodal basin 95.6% (109/114) of the time. As previously noted by Morton et al., there is a learning curve with the procedure, and the accuracy improves with experience of the surgeon [87]. In fact, Giuliano and colleagues reported five false-negative sentinel nodes in their first 87 cases and none in the second half of their study (an additional 87 cases) [92]. In a follow-up study, Giuliano et al. compared a group of patients undergoing standard axillary lymph node dissection with a second group having sentinel lymph node biopsy followed by complete node dissection [94]. Multiple histologic sections were made of each sentinel node, and examinations were then performed with standard hematoxylin and eosin staining, in addition to immunohistochemical studies using antibodies to cytokeratin. They found that 26 (38.2%) of 68 patients who had sentinel lymph node biopsy had micrometastases, compared with only 4 (10.3%) of 39 patients who had axillary lymph node dissection without sentinel node biopsy. The authors concluded that in patients with small primary tumors who are expected to have a lower rate of axillary nodal metastases, sentinel lymph node biopsy can pro-

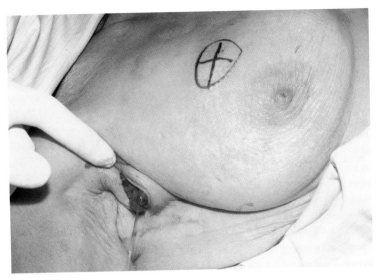

Figure 3. Illustration of tumors in different quadrants of the breast and potential lymphatic drainage patterns.

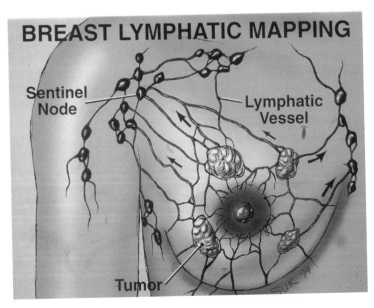

Figure 4. Successful lymphatic mapping with demonstration of the sentinel lymph node (blue node) and afferent lymphatic channel.

vide a more discriminating method of examining the nodal basin because the pathologist can perform more intensive studies on one or two sentinel nodes than would be feasible on all nodes retrieved from the dissection.

Lymphatic mapping for breast cancer is technically more difficult than it is for melanoma. In patients with breast cancer, there is a higher incidence of more than one sentinel node, and tumors may drain directly to level II nodes and 'skip' nodes in level I [92]. The use of a technetium sulphur colloid and a handheld gamma probe (neoprobe) was reported by Albertini and colleagues; the sentinel lymph node was successfully identified in 20 (95%) of 21 patients [93]. This group did not encounter any false-negative events. Krag et al. were able to identify the sentinel node in 18 of 22 patients with breast cancer when they used the technetium sulphur colloid and neoprobe [88]. They found that the sentinel lymph node was positive for metastases in seven (100%) out of seven patients who had metastatic disease to the axilla.

Because radiation therapy can provide effective control of the axillary nodal basin, the major advantage to axillary lymphadenectomy in cases of small primary breast cancers is to identify patients with micrometastases who would then be candidates for systemic therapy programs. Lymphatic mapping and sentinel lymph node biopsy can provide that information. The technique selects patients with metastases to the sentinel node who can then have complete axillary dissection. In addition, the pathologist can focus their attention on one or two sentinel nodes with molecular and immunohistochemical studies, which may allow a more accurate assessment of the nodal basin. At this time, however, axillary node dissection remains the standard of care and should be provided for patients who are not candidates for clinical protocols of selective axillary management using lymphatic mapping, axillary radiation, or other techniques for axillary control. We are hopeful that the ongoing trials of lymphatic mapping and sentinel node biopsy with concomitant formal axillary dissection will demonstrate that sentinel node biopsy is an accurate assessment of the nodal basin and therefore establish selective lymphadenectomy as the standard.

Outpatient breast surgery

As surgical procedures for the treatment of breast cancer have changed, the need for extended hospital stays has decreased [95]. When definitive surgery for breast cancer does not include immediate reconstruction, most procedures can be performed on an outpatient basis with a short observation period. Feig et al. reviewed the experience of The University of Texas M. D. Anderson Cancer Center with 23-hour observation in 187 patients undergoing breast surgery and found that all hemorrhagic complications (2.7%) were identified within 8 hours of surgery [96]. In this study from the M. D. Anderson Cancer Center, even patients who required reoperation for postoperative hemorrage were able to be discharged within the 23-hour observation period. The authors concluded that 23 hours was a safe period of time and that a shorter period of observation may be even more cost effective while still being medically safe.

Several investigators have evaluated patient acceptance of short-stay policies and found that more than 80% of patients feel that early discharge is a good idea [97,98]. When patients and families receive preoperative teaching on drain and incision care and what to expect in the short-stay setting, postoperative adjustment is much easier. Patients in the M. D. Anderson 23-hour observation program were interviewed as to their perceptions of the program, and more than 85% felt that they were ready for discharge 1 day after surgery [99]. The institution of short-stay programs has also led to a significant reduction in costs per patient, largely by reducing hospital charges [100–102]. When patients and care partners are given preoperative or even postoperative teaching, most do not require home health care nursing visits or numerous outpatient clinic visits. While outpatient care is less expensive, many of the home health delivery systems can still be a significant economic burden for patients and their families. Many centers are now shifting to outpatient care centers for patients who require breast cancer surgery with the knowledge that outpatient care is safe, accepted by patients, and more cost effective.

Treatment of noninvasive carcinoma

The incidence of noninvasive breast cancer, also called ductal carcinoma in situ (DCIS), has increased from about 5% of breast cancers diagnosed 20 years ago to a current rate of up to 40% of all breast cancers detected with screening mammography [103]. Significant controversy currently exists regarding the appropriate management of DCIS. Treatment ranges from total mastectomy to segmental mastectomy plus irradiation to wide local excision alone. Page et al. have provided information on the natural history of DCIS through follow-up of 28 women with DCIS who were treated with excisional biopsy only [104]. Within 10 years of the initial biopsy, invasive breast cancer developed in 7 of the 28 women. Carcinoma developed on subsequent follow-up in three additional patients, two with invasive tumors 23 and 31 years after biopsy, and one with extensive DCIS 25 years after biopsy. Five of the 28 patients died of breast cancer. Although these women were found to have DCIS in the 1970s, the pathology slides have been extensively reviewed; all showed low-grade DCIS and none qualified as comedo type. This information suggests that patients with low-grade DCIS are just as likely to recur as patients with high-grade or comedo-type DCIS, but the time interval to recurrence may be much longer.

Lagios et al. reported on 79 patients with mammographically detected DCIS measuring 25 mm or less on histologic examination whose treatment consisted of segmental mastectomy alone [105]. These patients were carefully evaluated for complete excision in a process that included histologic examination of margins, postoperative mammography, and radiographic and pathologic correlation. Lagios et al. noted a recurrence rate of 10.1% at 48 months of follow-up; 50% of the recurrences were invasive disease. After exclusion of three patients whose margins were not adequately analyzed or

188

who did not have postoperative mammography confirming no residual disease, the recurrence rate decreased to 6.5%. In this early study, Lagios and colleagues noted that the histologic subtype was important in determining the incidence and time interval to recurrence. Patients with comedo-type DCIS (high nuclear grade) and/or necrosis had a higher recurrence rate and a shorter time interval to recurrence.

Silverstein et al. recently developed a prognostic classification for predicting local recurrence in patients with DCIS; it is designated the Van Nuys classification [106]. This classification system defines three subgroups based on the presence or absence of high nuclear grade and comedo-type necrosis. Group 3 includes all patients with high nuclear grade DCIS, group 2 includes patients with non–high-grade DCIS with necrosis, and group 1 includes patients with non–high-grade DCIS without necrosis. The authors reported results in patients classified with the Van Nuys system who underwent mastectomy or breast-conservation surgery. There was no difference in the disease-free survival rate in group 2 patients who were treated with excision plus radiotherapy (66 patients) or with excision alone (24 patients). In group 3 patients, however, there was a significantly lower disease-free survival rate in patients treated with excision only (31 patients). They concluded from this series that patients who are classified as group 2 DCIS may not require postoperative radiotherapy in all cases and that patients in group 3 may not be good candidates for breast-conservation surgery. Of note is that a cutoff of 1 mm was used as the definition of a negative margin and, in addition, 30 of the 31 local recurrences in patients with breast conservation occurred near or at the site of the original primary tumor. This suggests that a margin greater than 1 mm may be necessary to achieve local control in patients with DCIS.

The only published multiinstitutional, randomized trial designed to study the role of postoperative radiotherapy in patients with DCIS is the NSABP B-17 trial [103]. Patients treated with lumpectomy alone had an ipsilateral breast recurrence rate of 16.4% at 5 years, whereas women treated with lumpectomy and radiotherapy had a recurrence rate of 7% at 5 years. There was a significant reduction in the number of invasive cancers in the patients who received radiotherapy. Some of the criticisms of this study include the high local recurrence rate and the failure to define margins. There was also a higher than expected rate of second primary cancers in other locations of the breast remote from the primary tumor.

The NSABP B-17 trial demonstrated a significant reduction in the rate of local recurrence in patients who had radiotherapy after excision of localized DCIS. However, with careful margin assessment and histologic assessment of the primary tumor, appropriate candidates may be identified who do not require postoperative radiotherapy. Axillary lymph node dissection is not currently recommended for patients with DCIS unless the patient has a large palpable breast tumor that carries a higher risk of microinvasion. Numerous series have examined the question of microinvasion and axillary nodal metastases [105,108–111]. The definition of microinvasion has varied with different series. However, the reported incidence of axillary nodal metastases in patients with microinvasion is low and ranges from 0% to 3%. The debate on axillary dissection for invasive cancer probably applies to patients with DCIS and microinvasion because the ability to identify patients will nodal metastases would change the treatment (systemic therapy) they receive and therefore may have an impact on survival.

As a follow-up to B-17, the NSABP trial B-24 was designed to determine whether tamoxifen could prevent subsequent ipsilateral or contralateral breast cancers following lumpectomy and postoperative radiotherapy in patients with DCIS. This study, which completed accrual in April 1994, did not require negative margins after surgical excision and did not stratify patients based on nuclear grade or size of the tumor. Over 80% of the patients accrued to B-24 had tumors <1.0 cm in size. In clinical practice, patients with DCIS cover a wide spectrum and standardization of treatment is difficult. At the present time, treatment of DCIS is tailored to the individual patient, and the decision to perform breast conservation or mastectomy is made using all of the available information, including nuclear grade, tumor size, and ability to achieve negative margins.

Prognostic factors

As more is learned about the biology of breast cancer, physicians have searched for markers to predict which patients will develop systemic disease and may therefore benefit from systemic treatment programs, even in the earliest stages of disease. The size of the primary tumor and involvement of the axillary lymph nodes are the two most important prognostic factors that are currently available through standard surgical treatment and disease staging [112]. Because primary tumors can metastasize to distant sites without detectable axillary nodal disease and approximately 30% of patients with negative nodes will experience disease recurrence and die of metastatic disease, factors other than tumor size and nodal status are important guides in determining the need for systemic therapy. We discuss new prognostic factors in addition to histologic features of the primary tumor, DNA flow cytometry studies, and hormone receptors, which have become more routine facets of tumor evaluation.

Histologic features and DNA flow cytometry studies

Numerous histologic features of the primary tumor, including nuclear grade, tumor necrosis, vascular invasion, and lymphatic invasion, have been reported to be important predictors of disease-free survival rates in node-negative patients [113–115]. Some of these factors are difficult to quantitate, and analysis may vary depending on the pathologist's interpretation. Evaluation of the tumor using standard DNA flow cytometry studies provides an assessment of

190

DNA content and cell cycle characteristics (proliferative capacity) that may predict the biologic behavior. Dressler et al. reported their analysis of 1331 tumors for ploidy and S-phase fraction [116]. They found that 57% of the evaluable tumors were aneuploid and that the median S-phase fraction was significantly higher in aneuploid tumors. Subsequent studies have shown that DNA analysis from paraffin-embedded tissue specimens correlates well with information obtained from frozen sections [117]. While aneuploid, hypertetraploid, and hypodiploid amounts of DNA may be associated with a worse prognosis, the S-phase fraction appears to be a more reliable predictor of disease-free and overall survival rates [117–119]. There is some variability in reporting S-phase fraction, depending on the laboratory. However, a value of 8% is generally used as the cutoff between low and high S-phase. Isola et al. reported results of S-phase studies in 213 patients with node-negative breast cancer and found a relative risk of death of 3.8 when the S-phase fraction was greater than 8% [120]. Clark et al. found that a cutoff point of 6.7 for S-phase fraction was highly significant in predicting the survival rate in their analysis of 851 patients with node-positive breast cancer [121]. In a study of patients with positive or negative nodes who did not receive adjuvant chemotherapy, the NSABP B-04 trial showed improved disease-free and overall survival rates in patients whose tumors had a low S-phase fraction [122].

Hormone receptors

Estrogen receptor (ER) and progesterone receptor (PR) status have been reported as significant determinants of prognosis by many investigators [113,123–125]. The survival rate in patients with ER-positive tumors who received no additional therapy after surgical treatment is generally reported to be 8–12% higher than that of patients with ER-negative tumors [126]. The ability to detect smaller primary tumors has necessitated the development of other assay techniques to determine receptor status in addition to the standard dextran-coated charcoal assay. Immunohistochemical assays have been used to evaluate hormone receptor status on both frozen tumor sections and paraffin-embedded tissues. Andersen et al. looked specifically at the issue of different techniques for measuring ER status in 130 breast cancer specimens from postmenopausal women in the Danish Breast Cancer Cooperative Group [127]. Immunohistochemical assays on either frozen or paraffin-embedded tissues were less sensitive than the standard dextran-coated charcoal assays; however, they did maintain prognostic value and were equivalent in predicting response to endocrine treatment.

Biochemical and genetic markers

Numerous biochemical and genetic markers have been reported as potential prognostic factors in breast cancer. These include oncogenes, tumor suppressor genes, hormones, growth factor receptors, and determinants of tumor cell growth and cell survival. The most extensively studied group is the type 1 family of growth factor receptors, which includes the epidermal growth factor receptor (EGFR or c-*erb* B-1), c-*erb* B-2 (Her-2/*neu* oncogene), c-*erb* B-3, and c-*erb* B-4 [128]. Both EGFR and c-*erb* B-2 are overexpressed in breast cancer, in addition to several other related growth factors, such as transforming growth factor α, amphiregulin, and cripto-1 [129]. The biological function of these growth factors has not been fully elucidated; however, they do appear to be involved in the pathogenesis of breast cancer. Overexpression of Her-2/*neu* was shown to correlate with poorer survival rates in patients with node-positive and node-negative breast cancer [130–132]. In addition, patients in whom Her-2/*neu* is overexpressed have a higher risk of relapse after receiving traditional systemic therapies [133]. This background has prompted the development of clinical trials using the Her-2/*neu* oncogene as a target for therapy in patients with breast cancer and Her-2/*neu* overexpression. Both basic science and clinical studies with the Her-2/*neu* oncogene are discussed in detail elsewhere in this book.

Changes in three tumor suppressor genes — *p53*, *nm23*, and the retinoblastoma gene (*Rb*) — have been found in human primary breast cancers. The *p53* gene has been found to be mutated in 15–20% of breast cancers. It encodes for the nuclear phosphoprotein TP53 and is considered to play an important role in a number of human malignancies. Loss of normal *p53* tumor suppressor function or overexpression of mutant, oncogenic *p53* are important steps in carcinogenesis [134]. Thor et al. found the accumulation of mutant *p53* protein to be an independent predictor of poorer survival in patients with sporadic breast cancer and familial breast cancer syndromes [135]. Germ-line mutations in *p53* have been found in families with hereditary breast and ovarian cancer syndromes distinct from mutations of other breast cancer susceptibility genes (BRCA1 and BRCA2) and may account for up to 10% of hereditary breast cancers [136,137].

Other investigators have evaluated the relationship between *p53* gene expression and DNA content or proliferative rate to provide a combination of factors that may predict survival rate. Cunningham et al. reported that patients with positive nodes and diploid tumors had significantly shorter relapse-free and overall survival times if their tumors were positive for mutant *p53* expression [138]. This significance remained when multivariate analysis was performed with other standard prognostic factors. Of interest, this study did not identify any relationship between *p53* expression and aneuploid or tetraploid tumors, and tumor samples from only 39 (16%) of the 247 patients in the study were positive for *p53* expression. In a study of 289 node-negative breast cancer cases, Isola et al. reported *p53* immunoreaction in 80 (27.7%) tumors [120]. Overexpression of *p53* was seen in 41 tumors, and these were more commonly ER-negative tumors with a high histologic grade and S-phase fraction and overexpression of c-*erb* B-2. In a Cox regression analysis, *p53* overexpression was not an independent predictor of survival when S-phase fraction was included. These studies identify subsets of patients in whom *p53* overexpression in combination with other established prognostic factors may predict shorter survival times.

Angiogenesis and breast cancer

An emerging area of interest is tumor angiogenesis and how it correlates with invasion and metastasis in breast cancer. In an initial study of 49 patients with breast cancer, Weidner et al. tested their hypothesis that the extent of angiogenesis correlates with the occurrence of metastasis [139]. Investigators evaluated tumors for microvessel count and density grade without prior knowledge of the patient's clinical outcome. They found that microvessel counts and density grades were significantly higher in patients with both regional lymph node involvement and distant metastases. Subsequent studies have confirmed the findings of this early work and in addition found that microvessel density is a highly significant and independent predictor for over-all and relapse-free survival rates in patients with early-stage disease [140]. Microvessel density was a significant predictor of the overall survival rate in node-negative patients but did not correlate with the relapse-free survival rate in that subset. The authors concluded that measurement of microvessel density may be a useful factor in identifying node-negative patients who are candidates for adjuvant therapy programs.

Many of the newer prognostic factors, such as oncogene amplification and measurement of tumor angiogenesis, show promise as useful tools in the management of patients with breast cancer. Additional studies are needed with long-term follow-up and correlation with established prognostic factors. It may be that a combination of factors will best predict patients at risk for relapse and that a different set of factors will define subsets of patients whose response to traditional adjuvant therapy regimens is unlikely.

Conclusions

Because of mammographic screening programs, an increasing number of early-stage invasive and noninvasive breast cancers are being detected. This fact, combined with an increasing understanding of the biology of breast cancer, has led to a shift in treatment strategies from radical surgical procedures to multidisciplinary treatment strategies embracing breast-conserving approaches in combination with systemic chemotherapy and hormonal therapy. Lumpectomy and postoperative radiotherapy are proven acceptable alternatives to mastectomy. Controversy remains, however, regarding the need for routine use of axillary node dissection and postoperative radiotherapy. Lymphatic mapping and sentinel node biopsy offer a more selective approach to the axilla and may prove to be an important method of identifying early breast cancers with occult nodal metastases. In addition, this technique may allow us to revisit the issue of internal mammary nodal staging for medial quadrant lesions that do not drain to the axilla.

The management of noninvasive breast cancer also remains controversial. Mastectomy was the standard of care in the past but may not be necessary for small and localized in situ carcinomas with a low nuclear grade and no evidence of multifocality. The role of postoperative radiotherapy after lumpectomy for noninvasive disease is still being defined. Despite these changes, surgical therapy continues to be the mainstay of locoregional control in early breast cancer.

The variety of breast imaging techniques now includes not only improved mammographic techniques but also breast ultrasonography, MRI, PET scanning, and other sensitive nuclear medicine studies. While some of these imaging methods remain investigational, others such as MRI are now part of the diagnostic workup of the augmented breast and the follow-up of the post-treatment breast. Methods for pathologic diagnosis have also improved, and physicians now rely on fine-needle aspiration biopsy and core needle biopsy. These procedures can be performed on palpable masses or on nonpalpable abnormalities under mammographic or ultrasound guidance. The use of excisional or open biopsies is now reserved for diagnostic dilemmas or for definitive treatment once the diagnosis is established with a less invasive method.

Several potential prognostic factors were introduced over the past decade to supplement the more established factors, such as tumor size, nuclear grade, lymph node status, and hormone receptor status. The clinical use of oncogene amplification, mutated tumor suppressor genes, and measurements of tumor angiogenesis are less well defined. These techniques may help to identify patients whose response to traditional systemic regimens is less likely and who therefore could be spared the attendant toxicity or offered alternative investigational approaches.

References

1. Parker SL, Tong T, Bolden S, Wingo PA. Cancer Statistics, 1997. CA Cancer J Clin 47:5–27, 1997.
2. Miller BA, Feuer EJ, Hankey BF. Recent incidence trends for breast cancer in women and the relevance of early detection: An update. CA Cancer J Clin 43:27–41, 1993.
3. Fisher B, Redmond C, Poisson R, Margolese R, Wolmark N, Wickerham L, Fisher E, Deutsch M, Caplan R, Pilch Y, Glass A, Shibata H, Lerner H, Terz J, Sidorovich L. Eight-year results of a randomized clinical trial comparing total mastectomy and lumpectomy with or without irradiation in the treatment of breast cancer. N Engl J Med 320:882–828, 1989.
4. Veronesi U, Banfi A, Salvadori B, Luini A, Saccozzi R, Zucali R, Marubini E, Del Vecchio M, Boracchi P, Marchini S, Merson M, Sacchini V, Riboldi G, Santoro G. Breast conservation is the treatment of choice in small breast cancer: Long-term results of a randomized trial. Eur J Cancer 26:668–670, 1990.

5. American Joint Committee on Cancer. Manual for Staging of Cancer, 4th ed. Philadelphia: J.B. Lippincott, 1992, pp. 149–154.

6. Balch CM, Singletary SE, Bland KI. Clinical decision-making in early breast cancer. Ann Surg 217:207–225, 1993.

7. Mendelson EB. Evaluation of the postoperative breast. Radiol Clin North Am 30:107–138, 1992.

8. Bird R, Wallace T, Yankaskas B. Analysis of cancers missed at screening mammography. Radiology 184:613–617, 1992.

9. Jokich PM, Monticciolo DL, Adler YT. Breast ultrasonograpy. Radiol Clin North Am 30:993–1009, 1992.

10. Feig SA. Breast masses: Mammographic and sonographic evaluation. Radiol Clin North Am 30:67–92, 1992.

11. Weinreb JC, Newstead G. MR imaging of the breast. Radiology 196:593–610, 1995.

12. Adler DD, Wahl RL. New methods for imaging the breast: Techniques, findings, and potential. AJR 164:19–30, 1995.

13. Gilles R, Guinebretière J-M, Lucidarme O, Cluzel P, Janaud G, Finet J-F, Tardivon A, Masselot J, Vanel D. Nonpalpable breast tumors: Diagnosis with contrast-enhanced subtraction dynamic MR imaging. Radiology 191:625–631, 1994.

14. Heywang-Köbrunner SH. Contrast-enhanced magnetic resonance imaging of the breast. Invest Radiol 29:94–104, 1994.

15. Lewis-Jones HG, Whitehouse GH, Leinster SJ. The role of magnetic resonance imaging in the assessment of local recurrent breast carcinoma. Clin Radiol 43:197–204, 1991.

16. Harms SE, Flamig DP, Hesley KL, Meiches MD, Jensen RA, Evans WP, Savino DA, Wells RV. MR imaging of the breast with rotating delivery of excitation off resonance: Clinical experience with pathologic correlation. Radiology 187:493–501, 1993.

17. Boetes C, Barentsz JO, Mus RD, van der Sluis RF, van Erning LJTO, Hendriks JHCL, Holland R, Ruys SHJ. MR characterization of suspicious breast lesions with a gadolinium-enhanced Turbo-FLASH subtraction technique. Radiology 193:777–781, 1994.

18. Kimme-Smith C, Gold RH, Bassett LW, Gormley L, Morioka C. Diagnosis of breast calcifications: Comparison of contact, magnified, and television-enhanced images. AJR 153:963–967, 1989.

19. Dershaw DD, Fleischman RC, Liberman L, Deutch B, Abramson AF, Hann L. Use of digital mammography in needle localization procedures. AJR 161:559–562, 1993.

20. Fam BW, Olson SL, Winter PF, Scholz FJ. Algorithm for the detection of five clustered calcifications on film mammograms. Radiology 169:333–337, 1988.

21. Hoh CK, Hawkins RA, Glaspy JA, et al. Cancer detection with whole-body PET using 2-[18F]fluoro-2-deoxy-D-glucose. J Comput Assist Tomogr 17:582–589, 1993.

22. Wahl RL, Cody R, August D. Initial evaluation of FDG PET for the staging of the axilla in newly-diagnosed breast carcinoma patients (abstr). J Nucl Med 32:981, 1991.

23. Tse NY, Hoh CK, Hawkins RA, Zinner MJ, Dahlbom M, Choi Y, Maddahi J, Brunicardi FC, Phelps ME, Glaspy JA. The application of positron emission tomographic imaging with fluorodeoxyglucose to the evaluation of breast disease. Ann Surg 216:27–34, 1992.

24. Layfield LJ, Glasgow BJ, Cramer H. Fine-needle aspiration in the management of breast masses. Pathol Ann 24:23–62, 1989.

25. Silverman JF. Diagnostic accuracy, cost-effectiveness, and triage role of fine-needle aspiration biopsy in the diagnosis of palpable breast lesions. Breast J 1:3–8, 1995.

26. Frable WJ. Needle aspiration biopsy: Past, present, and future. Hum Pathol 20:504–517, 1989.

27. Zarbo RJ, Howanitz PJ, Bachner P. Interinstitutional comparison of performance in breast fine-needle aspiration cytology. Arch Pathol Lab Med 115:743–750, 1991.

28. Fornage BD, Coan JD, David CL. Ultrasound-guided needle biopsy of the breast and other interventional procedures. Radiol Clin North Am 30:167–185, 1992.

29. Sneige N, Singletary SE. Fine-needle aspiration of the breast: Diagnostic problems and approaches to surgical management. Pathol Ann 20:281–301, 1994.

30. Fornage BD, Sneige N, Singletary SE. Masses in breasts with implants: Diagnosis with US-guided fine-needle aspiration biopsy. Radiology 191:339–342, 1994.
31. Bolmgren J, Jacobson B, Nordenström B. Stereotaxic instrument for needle biopsy of the mammogram. AJR 129:121–125, 1977.
32. Nordenström B, Zajicek J. Stereotaxic needle biopsy and preoperative indication of non-palpable mammary lesions. Acta Cytol 21:350–351, 1977.
33. Liberman L, Dershaw DD, Rosen PP, Cohen MA, Hann LE, Abramson AF. Stereotaxic core biopsy of impalpable spiculated breast masses. AJR 165:551–554, 1995.
34. McCombs MM, Bassett LW, Jahan R, Fu YS. Imaging-guided core biopsy of the breast. Breast J 1:9–16, 1995.
35. Liberman L, Dershaw DD, Rosen PP, Abramson AF, Deutch BM, Hann LE. Stereotaxic 14-gauge breast biopsy: How many core biopsy specimens are needed? Radiology 192:793–795, 1994.
36. Jackman RJ, Nowels KW, Shepard MJ, Finkelstein SI, Marzoni FA. Stereotaxic large-core needle biopsy of 450 nonpalpable breast lesions with cancer or atypical hyperplasia. Radiology 193:91–95, 1994.
37. Liberman L, Dershaw DD, Rosen PP, Giess CS, Cohen MA, Abramson AF, Hann LE. Stereotactic core biopsy of breast carcinoma: Accuracy at predicting invasion. Radiology 194:379–381, 1995.
38. Lindfors KK, Rosenquist CJ. Needle core biopsy guided with mammography: A study of cost-effectiveness. Radiology 190:217–222, 1994.
39. Lovin JD, Sinton EB, Burke BJ, Reddy VVB. Stereotaxic core breast biopsy: Value in providing tissue for flow cytometric analysis. AJR 162:609–612, 1994.
40. Fornage BD, Ross MI, Singletary SE, Paulus DD. Localization of impalpable breast masses: Value of sonography in the operating room and scanning of excised specimens. AJR 163:569–573, 1994.
41. Osteen RT. Selection of patients for breast conserving surgery. Cancer 74:366–371, 1994.
42. Fleck R, McNeese MD, Ellerbroek NA, Hunter TA, Holmes FA. Consequences of breast irradiation in patients with pre-existing collagen vascular disease. Int J Radiat Oncol Biol Phys 17:829–833, 1989.
43. Borger J, Kemperman H, Hart A, Peterse H, van Dongen J, Bartelink H. Risk factors in breast-conservation therapy. J Clin Oncol 12:653–660, 1994.
44. Matthews RH, McNeese MD, Montague ED, Oswald MJ. Prognostic implications of age in breast cancer patients treated with tumorectomy and irradiation or with mastectomy. Int J Radiat Oncol Biol Phys 14:659–663, 1988.
45. Haffty BG, Fischer D, Rose M, Beinfield M, McKhann C. Prognostic factors for local recurrence in the conservatively treated breast cancer patient: A cautious interpretation of the data. J Clin Oncol 9:997–1003, 1991.
46. Stotter AT, McNeese MD, Ames FC, Oswald MJ, Ellerbroek NA. Predicting the rate and extent of locoregional failure after breast conservation therapy for early breast cancer. Cancer 64:2217–2225, 1989.
47. Clark RM, McCulloch PB, Levine MN, Lipa M, Wilkinson RH, Mahoney LJ, Basrur VR, Nair BD, McDermot RS, Wong CS, Corbett PJ. Randomized clinical trial to assess the effectiveness of breast irradiation following lumpectomy and axillary dissection for node-negative breast cancer. J Natl Cancer Inst 84:683–689, 1992.
48. Veronesi U, Luini A, Galimberti V, Zurrida S. Conservation approaches for the management of stage I/II carcinoma of the breast: Milan Cancer Institute trials. World J Surg 18:70–75, 1994.
49. Clarke DH, Le MG, Sarrazin D, Lacombe M-J, Fontaine F, Travagli J-P, May-Levin F, Contesso G, Arriagada R. Analysis of local-regional relapses in patients with early breast cancers treated with excision and radiotherapy: Experience of the Institut Gustave-Roussy. Int J Radiat Oncol Biol Phys 11:137–145, 1985.
50. Solin LJ, Fowble B, Schultz DJ, Goodman RL. Age as a prognostic factor for patients treated

with definitive irradiation for early stage breast cancer. Int J Radiat Oncol Biol Phys 16:373–381, 1989.

51. Mate TP, Carter D, Fischer DB, Hartman PV, McKhann C, Merino M, Prosnitz LR, Weissberg JB. A clinical and histopathological analysis of the results of conservation surgery and radiation therapy in stage I and II breast carcinoma. Cancer 58:1995–2002, 1984.

52. van Limbergen E, van den Bogaert W, van der Schueren E, Rijnders A. Tumor excision and radiotherapy as primary treatment of breast cancer. Analysis of patient and treatment parameters and local control. Radiother Oncol 8:1–9, 1987.

53. Harris JR, Gelman R. What have we learned about risk factors for local recurrence after breast-conserving surgery and irradiation? [editorial] J Clin Oncol 12:647–649, 1994.

54. Recht A, Silen W, Schnitt SJ, Connolly JL, Gelman RS, Rose MA, Silver B, Harris JR. Time-course of local recurrence following conservative surgery and radiotherapy for early stage breast cancer. Int J Radiat Oncol Biol Phys 15:255–261, 1988.

55. Vicini FA, Recht A, Abner A, Boyages J, Cady B, Connolly JL, Gelman R, Osteen RT, Schnitt SJ, Silen W, Harris JR. Recurrence in the breast following treatment of patients with early stage breast cancer with conservative surgery and radiation therapy. J Natl Cancer Inst Monogr 11:33–39, 1992.

56. Kurtz JM, Amalric R, Delouche G, Pierquin B, Roth J, Spitalier J-M. The second ten years: Long-term risks of breast conservation in early breast cancer. Int J Radiat Oncol Biol Phys 13:1327–1332, 1987.

57. Schnitt SJ, Abner A, Gelman R, Connolly JL, Recht A, Duda RB, Eberlein TJ, Mayzel K, Silver B, Harris JR. The relationship between microscopic margins of resection and the risk of local recurrence in patients with breast cancer treated with breast-conserving surgery and radiation therapy. Cancer 74:1746–1751, 1994.

58. Veronesi U, Volterrani F, Luini A, Saccozzi R, Del Vecchio M, Zucali R, Galimberti V, Rasponi A, Di Re E, Squicciarini P, Salvadori B. Quadrantectomy versus lumpectomy for small size breast cancer. Eur J Cancer 26:671–673, 1990.

59. Ghossein NA, Alpert S, Barba J, Pressman P, Stacey P, Lorenz E, Shulman M, Sadarangani GJ. Importance of adequate surgical excision prior to radiotherapy in the local control of breast cancer in patients treated conservatively. Arch Surg 127:411–415, 1992.

60. Vicini FA, Eberlein TJ, Connolly JL, Recht A, Abner A, Schnitt SJ, Silen W, Harris JR. The optimal extent of resection for patients with stages I or II breast cancer treated with conservative surgery and radiotherapy. Ann Surg 214:200–205, 1991.

61. Solin LJ, Fowble BL, Schultz DJ, Goodman RL. The significance of the pathology margins of the tumor excision on the outcome of patients treated with definitive irradiation for early stage breast cancer. Int J Radiat Oncol Biol Phys 21:279–287, 1991.

62. Lindley R, Bulman A, Parsons P, Phillips R, Henry K, Ellis H. Histologic features predictive of an increased risk of early local recurrence after treatment of breast cancer by local tumor excision and radical radio-therapy. Surgery 105:13–20, 1989.

63. Fourquet A, Campana F, Zafrani B, Mosseri V, Vielh P, Durand J-C, Vilcoq JR. Prognostic factors of breast recurrence in the conservative management of early breast cancer: A 25-year follow-up. Int J Radiat Oncol Biol Phys 17:719–725, 1989.

64. Fisher ER, Sass R, Fisher B, Gregorio R, Brown R, Wickerham L, Collaborating NSABP Investigators. Pathologic findings from the National Surgical Adjuvant Breast Project (protocol 6): II. Relation of local breast recurrence to multicentricity. Cancer 57:1717–1724, 1986.

65. Early Breast Cancer Trialists' Collaborative Group. Effects of radiotherapy and surgery in early breast cancer. An overview of the randomized trials. N Engl J med 333:1444–1455, 1995.

66. Lichter AS, Lippman ME, Danforth DN, d'Angelo T, Steinberg SM, deMoss E, MacDonald HD, Reichert CM, Merino M, Seain SM, Cowan K, Gerber LH, Bader JL, Findlay PA, Schain W, Gorrell CR, Straus K, Rosenberg SA, Glatstein E. Mastectomy versus breast-conserving therapy in the treatment of stage I and II carcinoma of the breast: A randomized trial at the National Cancer Institute. J Clin Oncol 10:976–983, 1992.

67. Fisher B, Anderson S, Redmond CK, Wolmark N, Wickerham DL, Cronin WM. Reanalysis and results after 12 years of follow-up in a randomized clinical trial comparing total mastectomy with lumpectomy with or without irradiation in the treatment of breast cancer. N Engl J Med 333:1456–1461, 1995.

68. Rose MA, Henderson IC, Gelman R, Boyages J, Gore SM, Come S, Silver B, Recht A, Connolly JL, Schnitt SJ, Coleman CN, Harris JR. Premenopausal breast cancer patients treated with conservative surgery, radiotherapy and adjuvant chemotherapy have a low risk of local failure. Int J Radiat Oncol Biol Phys 17:711–717, 1989.

69. Haffty BG, Wilmarth L, Wilson L, Fischer D, Beinfield, McKhann C. Adjuvant systemic chemotherapy and hormonal therapy. Effect on local recurrence in the conservatively treated breast cancer patient. Cancer 73:2543–2548, 1994.

70. Liljegren G, Holmberg L, Adami H-O, Westman G, Graffman S, Bergh J, Uppsala-Örebro Breast Cancer Study Group. Sector resection with or without postoperative radiotherapy for stage I breast cancer: Five-year results of a randomized trial. J Natl Cancer Inst 86:717–722, 1994.

71. Veronesi U, Luini A, Del Vecchio M, Greco M, Galimberti V, Merson M, Rilke F, Sacchini V, Saccozzi R, Savio T, Zucali R, Zurrida S, Salvadori B. Radiotherapy after breast-preserving surgery in women with localized cancer of the breast. N Engl J Med 328:1587–1591, 1993.

72. Cady B, Stone MD, Wayne J. New therapeutic possibilities in primary invasive breast cancer. Ann Surg 218:338–349, 1993.

73. Hermann RE, Esselstyn CB, Grundfest-Broniatowski S, Steiger E, Vogt DP, Broughan TA, Dowden RV, Hardesty I, Medendorp SV, Boyett JM. Partial mastectomy without radiation is adequate treatment for patients with stages 0 and I carcinoma of the breast. Surg Gynecol Obstet 177:247–253, 1993.

74. Recht A, Houlihan MJ. Conservative surgery without radiotherapy in the treatment of patients with early-stage invasive breast cancer. A review. Ann Surg 222:9–18, 1995.

75. Fisher B, Andeson S, Fisher ER, Redmond C, Wickerham DL, Wolmark N, Mamounas EP, Deutsch M, Margolese R. Significance of ipsilateral breast tumour recurrence after lumpectomy. Lancet 338:327–331, 1991.

76. Wazer DE, DiPetrillo T, Schmidt-Ullrich R, Weld L, Smith TJ, Marchant DJ, Robert NJ. Factors influencing cosmetic outcome and complication risk after conservative surgery and radiotherapy for early-stage breast carcinoma. J Clin Oncol 10:356–363, 1992.

77. Silverstein MJ, Gierson ED, Waisman JR, Senofsky GM, Colburn WJ, Gamagami P. Axillary lymph node dissection for T1a breast carcinoma. Is it indicated? Cancer 73:664–667, 1994.

78. Cady B. The need to reexamine axillary lymph node dissection in invasive breast cancer [editorial]. Cancer 73:505–508, 1994.

79. Recht A, Houlihan MJ. Axillary lymph nodes and breast cancer. A review. Cancer 76:1491–1512, 1995.

80. Ptaszynski A, Van den Bogaert W, Van Glabbeke M, Pierart M, Bartelink H, Horiot JC, Fourquet A, Struikmans H, Hamers H, Müller RP, Hoogenraad WJ, Jager JJ, van der Schueren E. Patient population analysis in EORTC trial 22881/10882 on the role of a booster dose in breast-conserving therapy. Eur J Cancer 30A:2073–2081, 1994.

81. Sacre RA. Clinical evaluation of axillar lymph nodes compared to surgical and pathological findings. Eur J Surg Oncol 12:169–173, 1984.

82. Fisher B, Redmond C, Fisher ER, Bauer M, Wolmark N, Wickerham L, Deutsch M, Montague E, Margolese R, Foster R. Ten-year results of a randomized clinical trial comparing radical mastectomy and total mastectomy with or without radiation. N Engl J Med 312:674–681, 1985.

83. Graversen HP, Blichert-Toft M, Andersen JA, Zedeler K, and the Danish Breast Cancer Cooperative Group. Breast cancer: Risk of axillary recurrence in node-negative patients following partial dissection of the axilla. Eur J Surg Oncol 14:407–412, 1988.

84. Gateley CA, Mansel RE, Owen A, Redford J, Sellwood RA, Howell A. Treatment of the axilla in operable breast cancer (abstr). Br J Surg 78:750, 1991.

85. Halverson KJ, Taylor ME, Perez CA, Garcia DM, Myerson R, Philpott G, Levy J, Simpson JR, Tucker G, Rush C. Regional nodal management and patterns of failure following conservative surgery and radiation therapy for Stage I and II breast cancer. Int J Radiat Oncol Biol Phys 26:593–599, 1993.

86. Hoskin PJ, Rajan B, Ebbs S, Tait D, Milan S, Yarnold JR. Selective avoidance of lymphatic radiotherapy in the conservative management of early breast cancer. Radiother Oncol 25:83–88, 1992.

87. Morton DL, Wen D-R, Wong JH, Economou JS, Cagle LA, Storm FK, Foshag LJ, Cochran AJ. Technical details of intraoperative lymphatic mapping for early stage melanoma. Arch Surg 127:392–399, 1992.

88. Krag DN, Weaver DL, Alex JC, Fairbank JT. Surgical resection and radiolocalization of the sentinel lymph node in breast cancer using a gamma probe. Surg Oncol 2:335–340, 1993.

89. LevenbacK C, Burke TW, Gershenson DM, Morris M, Malpica A, Ross MI. Intraoperative lymphatic mapping for vulvar cancer. Obstet Gynecol 84:163–167, 1994.

90. Ross MI, Reintgen D, Balch CM. Selective lymphadenectomy: Emerging role for lymphatic mapping and sentinel node biopsy in the management of early stage melanoma. Semin Surg Oncol 9:219–223, 1993.

91. Reintgen D, Cruse CW, Wells K, Berman C, Fenske N, Glass F, Schroer K, Heller R, Ross M, Lyman G, Cox C, Rappaport D, Seigler HF, Balch C. The orderly progression of melanoma nodal metastases. Ann Surg 220:759–767, 1994.

92. Giuliano AE, Kirgan DM, Guenther JM, Morton DL. Lymphatic mapping and sentinel lymphadenectomy for breast cancer. Ann Surg 220:391–401, 1994.

93. Albertini J, Cox C, Yeatman T, Smith D, Hutson L, Falcone R, Berman C, Ross M, Reintgen D. Lymphatic mapping and sentinel node biopsy in the breast cancer patient. Proce Ann Meet Am Soc Clin Oncol 14:A99, 1995.

94. Giuliano AE, Dale PS, Turner RR, Morton DL, Evans SW, Krasne DL. Improved axillary staging of breast cancer with sentinel lymphadenectomy. Ann Surg 222:394–401, 1995.

95. Hunt KK, Feig BW, Ames FC. Ambulatory surgery for breast cancer. Cancer Bull 47:292–297, 1995.

96. Feig BW, Singletary SE, Ross MI, Kluger M, Ames FC. 23 hour observation is safe following breast surgery (abstr). Proceedings of the 48th Annual Cancer Symposium of the Society of Surgical Oncology 1995, p. 27.

97. Galante E, Cerrotta A, Martelli G, Del Prato I, Moglia D, Piromalli D. Treatment of breast cancer in elderly women: Retrospective analysis of 111 wide lumpectomies performed in a day hospital regimen between 1982 and 1988. Tumori 78:111–114, 1992.

98. Clark JA, Kent RB. One-day hospitalization following modified radical mastectomy. Am Surg 58:239–242, 1992.

99. Burke CC, Zabka CL, McCarver KJ, Singletary SE. Short stay surgery for breast cancer: Patient perceptions and program evaluation. Oncol Nurs Forum 22:350, 1995.

100. Edwards MJ, Broadwater JR, Bell JL, Ames FC, Balch CM. Economic impact of reducing hospitalization for mastectomy patients. Ann Surg 208:3360–3366, 1988.

101. Capri S, Majno E, Mauri M. The cost of hospital stay for operable breast cancer. Tumori 78:359–362, 1992.

102. Goodman AA, Mendez AL. Definitive surgery for breast cancer performed on an outpatient basis. Arch Surg 128:1149–1152, 1993.

103. Lagios MD. Ductal carcinoma in situ: Controversies in diagnosis, biology, and treatment. Breast J 1:68–78, 1995.

104. Page DL, Dupont WD, Rogers LW, Jensen RA, Schuyler PA. Continued local recurrence of carcinoma 15–25 years after a diagnosis of low grade ductal carcinoma in situ of the breast treated only by biopsy. Cancer 76:1197–1200, 1995.

105. Lagios MD, Margolin FR, Westdahl PR, Rose MR. Mammographically detected duct carci-

noma in situ. Frequency of local recurrence following tylectomy and prognostic effect of nuclear grade on local recurrence. Cancer 63:618–624, 1989.

106. Silverstein MJ, Poller DN, Waisman JR, Colburn WJ, Barth A, Gierson ED, Lewinsky B, Gamagami P, Slamon DJ. Prognostic classification of breast ductal carcinoma-in-situ. Lancet 345:1154–1157, 1995.

107. Fisher B, Costantino J, Redmond C, Fisher E, Margolese R, Dimitrov N, Wolmark N, Wickerham DL, Deutsch M, Ore L, Mamounas E, Poller W, Kavanah M. Lumpectomy compared with lumpectomy and radiation therapy for the treatment of intraductal breast cancer. N Engl J Med 328:1581–1586, 1993.

108. Wong JH, Kopald KH, Morton DL. The impact of microinvasion on axillary node metastases and survival in patients with intraductal breast cancer. Arch Surg 125:1298–1302, 1990.

109. Silverberg SG, Chitale AR. Assessment of significance of proportions of intraductal and infiltrating tumor growth in ductal carcinoma of the breast. Cancer 32:830–837, 1973.

110. Silverstein MJ, Rosser RJ, Gierson ED, Waisman JR, Gamagami P, Hoffman RS, Fingerhut AG, Lewinsky BS, Colburn W, Handel N. Axillary lymph node dissection for intraductal breast carcinoma. Is it indicated? Cancer 59:1819–1824, 1987.

111. Silverstein MJ, Waisman JR, Colburn WJ, Furmanski M, Lewinsky BS, Cohlan BF, Senofsky GM, Gierson ED, Gamagami P. Intraductal breast carcinoma (DCIS) with and without microinvasion (MI): Is there a difference in outcome? Proceedings of ASCO 12:56, 1993.

112. Carter CL, Allen C, Henson DE. Relation of tumor size, lymph node status, and survival in 24,740 breast cancer cases. Cancer 63:181–187, 1989.

113. Fisher B, Redmond C, Fisher ER, Caplan R, and other contributing National Surgical Adjuvant Breast and Bowel Project Investigators. Relative worth of estrogen or progesterone receptor and pathologic characteristics of differentiation as indicators of prognosis in node negative breast cancer patients: Findings from National Surgical Adjuvant Breast and Bowel Project protocol B-06. J Clin Oncol 6:1076–1087, 1988.

114. Gilchrist K, Gray R, Fowble B, Tormey D, Taylor S. Tumor necrosis is a histoprognosticator for early recurrence and death in stage II breast cancer (abstr). Lab Invest 58:34, 1988.

115. Neville AM, Bettelheim R, Gelber RD, Säve-Söderbergh† J, Davis BW, Reed R, Torhorst J, Golouh R, Peterson HF, Price KN, Isley M, Rudenstam C-M, Collins J, Castiglione M, Senn H-J, and Goldhirsch A for the International (Ludwig) Breast Cancer Study Group. Factors predicting treatment responsiveness and prognosis in node-negative breast cancer. J Clin Oncol 10:696–785, 1992.

116. Dressler LG, Seamer LC, Owens MA, Clark GM, McGuire WL. DNA flow cytometry and prognostic factors in 1331 frozen breast cancer specimens. Cancer 61:420–427, 1988.

117. Dressler LG, Duncan MH, Varsa EE, McConnell TS. DNA content measurement can be obtained using archival material for DNA flow cytometry: A comparison with cytogenetic analysis in 56 pediatric solid tumors. Cancer 72:2033–2041, 1993.

118. Hedley DW, Clark GM, Cornelisse CJ, Killander D, Kute T, Merkel D. Consensus review of the clinical utility of DNA cytometry in carcinoma of the breast. Cytometry 14:482–485, 1993.

119. Fernö M, Baldetorp B, Borg A, Olsson H, Sigurdsson H, Killander D. Flow cytometric DNA index and S-phase fraction in breast cancer in relation to other prognostic variables and to clinical outcome. Acta Oncol 31:157–165, 1992.

120. Isola J, Visakorpi T, Holli K, Kallioniemi O-P. Association of overexpression of tumor suppressor protein p53 with rapid cell proliferation and poor prognosis in node-negative breast cancer patients. J Natl Cancer Inst 84:1109–1114, 1992.

121. Clark GM, Wenger CR, Beardslee S, Owens MA, Pounds G, Oldaker T, Vendely P, Pandian MR, Harrington D, McGuire WL. How to integrate steroid hormone receptor, flow cytometric, and other prognostic information in regard to primary breast cancer. Cancer 71:2157–2162, 1993.

122. Fisher B, Gunduz N, Costantino J, Fisher ER, Redmond C, Mamounas EP, Siderits R. DNA flow cytometric analysis of primary operable breast cancer: Relation of ploidy and S-phase

fraction to outcome of patients in NSABP B-04. Cancer 68:1465–1475, 1991.

123. Chevallier B, Heintzmann F, Mosseri V, Dauce JP, Bastit P, Graic Y, Brunelle P, Basuyau JP, Comoz M, Asselain B. Prognostic value of estrogen and progesterone receptors in operable breast cancer: Results of a univariate and multivariate analysis. Cancer 62:2517–2524, 1988.

124. Mason BH, Holdaway IM, Mullins PR, Yee LH, Kay RG. Progesterone and estrogen receptors as prognostic variables in breast cancer. Cancer Res 43:2985–2990, 1983.

125. McGuire WL, Clark GM, Dressler LG, Owens MA. Role of steroid hormone receptors as prognostic factors in primary breast cancer. Natl Cancer Inst Monogr 1:19–23, 1986.

126. Mansour EG, Ravdin PM, Dressler L. Prognostic factors in early breast cancer. Cancer 74:381–400, 1994.

127. Andersen J, Thorpe SM, King WJ, Rose C, Christensen I, Rasmussen BB, Poulsen HS. The prognostic value of immunohistochemical estrogen receptor analysis in paraffin-embedded and frozen sections versus that of steroid-binding assays. Eur J Cancer 26:442–449, 1990.

128. Rajkumar T, Gullick WJ. The type I growth factor receptors in human breast cancer. Breast Cancer Res Treat 29:3–9, 1994.

129. Normanno N, Ciardiello F, Brandt R, Salomon DS. Epidermal growth factor-related peptides in the pathogenesis of human breast cancer. Breast Cancer Res Treat 29:11–27, 1994.

130. Slamon DJ, Clark GM, Wong SG, Levin WJ, Ullrich A, McGuire WL. Human breast cancer: Correlation of relapse and survival with amplification of the Her-2/neu oncogene. Science 235:177–182, 1987.

131. Kallioniemi O-P, Holli K, Visakorpi T, Koivula T, Helin HH, Isola JJ. Association of c-erbB-2 protein over-expression with high rate of cell proliferation, increased risk of visceral metastasis and poor long-term survival in breast cancer. Int J Cancer 49:650–655, 1991.

132. Horiguchi J, Iino Y, Takei H, Yokoe T, Ishida T, Morishita Y. Immunohistochemical study on the expression of c-erbB-2 oncoprotein in breast cancer. Oncology 51:47–51, 1994.

133. Gusterson BA, Gelber RD, Goldhirsch A, Price KN, Säve-Söderborgh J, Anbazhagan R, Styles J, Rudenstam C-M, Golouh R, Reed R, Martinez-Tello F, Tiltman A, Torhorst J, Grigolato P, Bettelheim R, Neville AM, Bürki K, Castiglione M, Collins J, Lindtner J, Seen H-J for the International (Ludwig) Breast Cancer Study Group. Prognostic importance of c-erb B-2 expression in breast cancer. International (Ludwig) Breast Cancer Study Group. J Clin Oncol 10:1049–1056, 1992.

134. Kuerbitz SJ, Plunkett BS, Walsh WV, Kastan MB. Wild-type p53 is a cell cycle checkpoint determinant following irradiation. Proc Natl Acad Sci USA 89:7491–7495, 1992.

135. Thor AD, Moore DH, Edgerton SM, Kawasaki ES, Reihsaus E, Lynch HT, Marcus JN, Schwartz L, Chen L-C, Mayall BH, Smith HS. Accumulation of p53 tumor suppressor gene protein: An independent marker of prognosis in breast cancers. J Natl Cancer Inst 84:845–855, 1992.

136. Jolly KW, Malkin D, Douglass EC, Brown TF, Sinclair AE, Look AT. Splice-site mutation of the p53 gene in a family with hereditary breast-ovarian cancer. Oncogene 9:97–102, 1994.

137. Malkin D, Li FP, Strong LC, Fraumeni JF, Nelson CE, Kim DH, Kassel J, Gryka MA, Bischoff FZ, Tainsky MA, Friend SH. Germ line p53 mutations in a familial syndrome of breast cancer, sarcomas, and other neoplasms. Science 250:1233–1238, 1990.

138. Cunningham JM, Ingle JN, Jung SH, Cha SS, Wold LE, Farr G, Witzig TE, Krook JE, Wieand HS, Kovach JS. p53 gene expression in node-positive breast cancer: Relationship to DNA ploidy and prognosis. J Natl Cancer Inst 86:1871–1873, 1994.

139. Weidner N, Semple JP, Welch WR, Folkman J. Tumor angiogenesis and metastasis-correlation in invasive breast carcinoma. N Engl J Med 324:1–8, 1991.

140. Weidner N, Folkman J, Pozza F, Bevilacqua P, Allred EN, Moore DH, Meli S, Gasparini G. Tumor angiogenesis: A new significant and independent prognostic indicator in early-stage breast carcinoma. J Natl Cancer Inst 84:1875–1887, 1992.

201

10. Classification, staging, and management of non-Hodgkin's lymphomas

Paul F. Mansfield and Kelly K. Hunt

Introduction

The understanding and management of lymphomas have evolved significantly over the past decade. Among the most important changes have been the development of new classification systems that include molecular determinants, identification of etiologic factors for mucosa-associated lymphomas (and their implications for management), demonstration of the importance of T cells in the progression of B-cell lymphomas, development of an international tumor scoring system to better determine prognosis, and establishment of bone marrow transplant as effective therapy in relapsed non-Hodgkin's lymphoma. This chapter explores these issues and their implications for the practicing oncologist.

Lymphoma classification

Perhaps no disease has undergone more modification of its classification system than lymphomas. Table 1 lists the types of lymphoid neoplasms that are currently recognized by the International Lymphoma Study Group [1]. The Working Formulation is the classification system most widely used in the United States today [2]. Table 2 lists the 10 major types of non-Hogkin's lymphomas described by the Working Formulation, including response rates to chemotherapy and 5-year survival rates. This system has some significant flaws, including misuse of the term *grade* and poor applicability to T-cell lymphomas. Grade, as defined in the Working Formulation, relates to clinical course rather than to histologic features, as it is more normally used in other diseases. These problems prompted the International Lymphoma Study Group to propose a new system, called the Revised European-American Lymphoma (REAL) classification [3].

The REAL classification is a comprehensive system incorporating histologic, clinical, molecular, and genetic information. Patients are generally classified as having lymphoid malignancies of the B-cell or T-cell types, or Hodgkin's disease. Within each of these broad groups, there are lymphomas

Raphael E. Pollock (ed.), SURGICAL ONCOLOGY. Copyright © 1997. Kluwer Academic Publishers.
ISBN 0-7923-9900-5. All rights reserved.

Table 1. Lymphoid neoplasms recognized by the International Lymphoma Study Group

B-cell neoplasms
  I.   Precursor B-cell neoplasm: B-lymphoblastic leukemia/lymphoma
  II. Peripheral B-cell neoplasms
       B-cell chronic lymphocytic leukemia/prolymphocytic leukemia/small lymphocytic
         lymphoma
       Lymphoplasmacytoid lymphoma/immunocytoma
       Mantle cell lymphoma
       Follicle center cell lymphoma, follicular
       Marginal zone B-cell lymphoma
       Provisional entity: splenic marginal zone lymphoma
       Hairy cell leukemia
       Plasmacytoma/plasma cell myeloma
       Diffuse large B-cell lymphoma
       Burkitt's lymphoma
       Provisional entity: high-grade B-cell lymphoma, Burkitt-like

T-cell and putative natural killer cell neoplasms
  I.   Precursor T-cell neoplasm: T-lymphoblastic lymphoma/leukemia
       T-cell chronic lymphocytic leukemia/prolymphocytic leukemia
       Large granular lymphocyte leukemia
       Mycosis fungoides/Sézary's syndrome
       Peripheral T-cell lymphomas, unspecified
       Angioimmunoblastic T-cell lymphoma
       Angiocentric lymphoma
       Intestinal T-cell lymphoma
       Adult T-cell lymphoma/leukemia
       Anaplastic large cell lymphoma
       Provisional entity: anaplastic large-cell lymphoma, Hodgkin's-like

Hodgkin's disease
  I.   Lymphocyte predominance
  II.   Nodular sclerosis
  III. Mixed cellularity
  IV.   Lymphocyte depletion
  V.   Provisional entity: lymphocyte-rich classical Hodgkin's disease

Adapted from Harris et al. [1], with permission.

that are distinctive, others that have a provisional classification, and a few remaining malignancies that are designated as unclassified. Longo [3] has suggested that the REAL classification can be translated into a useful clinical schema that divides patients into five clinical disease syndromes: (1) chronic leukemia/lymphoma, (2) nodal or extranodal lymphoma, (3) acute leukemia/ lymphoma, (4) plasma cell disorders, and (5) Hodgkin's disease.

There has been a tremendous expansion of knowledge of the molecular characteristics of lymphomas, including cluster designate (CD) expression and specific gene rearrangements. Despite these advances, most clinical decisions are still based on the histologic classification. Therefore, even though the diagnosis of lymphoma may be made by fine-needle aspirate, for the foreseeable future surgeons will frequently be called upon to provide sufficient tissue for histologic examination.

Table 2. Working formulation for classification of non-Hodgkin's lymphomas

Subtype	Complete response rate (%)	5-year survival rate (%)
Low grade		
Small lymphocytic (A)	61	59
Follicular, small cleaved (B)	73	70
Follicular, mixed cell (C)	65	50
Intermediate grade		
Follicular, large cell (D)	61	45
Diffuse, small cleaved cell (E)	56	33
Diffuse, mixed cell (F)	69	38
Diffuse, large cell (G)	59	35
High grade		
Immunoblastic (H)	53	32
Lymphoblastic (I)	69	26
Small, noncleaved cell (J)	48	23

Adapted from The Non-Hodgkin's Lymphoma Pathologic Classification Project [2], with permission.

International index

One of the major problems with classification and staging systems such as the Working Formulation or REAL system has been the wide discrepancy in prognosis for patients with aggressive non-Hodgkin's lymphomas. Many staging systems have been developed, but the most widely used is the Ann Arbor system. This system, originally designed for Hodgkin's disease and still commonly used in staging non-Hodgkin's lymphomas, correlates poorly with prognosis. Several factors, including age, presence of B symptoms, performance status, extent of disease (i.e., bulk and number of sites), and serum lactate dehydrogenase (LDH) and β-2 microglobulin (β-2M) levels, have been shown to correlate with prognosis in many small studies. The lick of an accurate, cohesive, and simple system for determining prognosis led the International Non-Hodgkin's Lymphoma Prognostic Factors Project to the development of the international index. This index was developed by a systematic analysis of over 2000 patients with aggressive lymphomas from Europe and North America [4].

The investigators from the International Non-Hodgkin's Lymphoma Prognostic Factors Project found five factors that proved to be independent prognostic factors for survival: age (greater than or less than 60 years old), performance status (0 or 1 vs. 2–4), Ann Arbor Stage (I or II vs. III or IV), serum LDH (normal or greater than upper limits of normal), and number of extranodal sites involved (0 or 1 vs. >1). By awarding 1 point for each factor that carried a poorer prognosis, patients were divided into four risk groups: low (0 or 1 points), low intermediate (2 points), high intermediate (3 points), or high (4 or 5 points). This resulted in a prognostic range for 5-year survival from 73% (low-risk group) to 26% (high-risk group). As an example of the inaccuracy of the Ann Arbor Staging system, for this group of patients the 5-year disease-free survival rate was 75% for stage I and 48% for stage IV. The range obtained with the international index is significantly better than the 27 percentage point range found using the Ann Arbor stage alone. This international index also contains an age-adjusted index for patients ≤ 60 years of age. In this setting the 5-year survival rates range from 83% (low risk) to 32% (high risk).

The applicability of the international index to low-grade lymphomas was demonstrated by López-Guillermo et al. [5]. The complete response rates and 10-year overall survival rates were 60% and 73.6% for low risk, 35% and 45% for low-intermediate risk, 23% and 53.5% for high-intermediate, and 21% and 0% for high risk. Thus, while the prognostic value for intermediate-risk patients was marginal, the low- and high-risk designations are clearly predictive of outcome.

A similar system, called the tumor score, has been described by Rodriguez et al. from the M. D. Anderson Cancer Center [6]. In this prognostic system, patients are given 1 point for each unfavorable factor, including Ann Arbor stage III or IV, LDH level greater than 10% above top normal, bulky disease (>7 cm or more than $\frac{2}{3}$ of an organ), presence of B symptoms, and a β-2M level >3.0 mg/l. Using this system, patients with 0, 1, or 2 points had an 83% 3-year relapse-free survival rate, while the rate for patients with a score of 3 or more was 24%. Thus, by using a simple system patients could be separated into two very distinct prognostic groups. In this study there were no 3-year survivors among the patients with 5 points. A significant difference between this system and the international index is the use of β-2M level, which was available for only 6% of patients when the international index was developed and thus could not be adequately evaluated.

There are two important reasons for clinicians to be aware of these scoring systems. First, with the increasing incidence of lymphoma, practicing physicians will be more frequently involved in the management of these patients. A firm grasp of the prognosis for a given patient can aid in treatment planning decisions when consulted for an emergency condition in a lymphoma patient. Second, given the controversy in management that still surrounds some gastrointestinal lymphomas (particularly of the stomach), surgeons in particular must be certain that patients with a similar prognosis are being compared when evaluating the efficacy of a given therapy.

Mucosa-associated lymphoid tissue lymphoma

Since the initial description of mucosa-associated lymphoid tissue (MALT) lymphoma by Isaacson in 1983, the understanding of the etiology and management of this disease has grown enormously [7]. Isaacson found a striking similarity between Mediterranean lymphoma and primary gastrointestinal lymphoma with follicular center cell origin. Mediterranean lymphoma is fairly common in the Middle East and has a known indolent benign phase. Historically, lymphomas of the gastrointestinal tract have been lumped together as extranodal non-Hodgkin's lymphomas in planning treatment and evaluating the response to various therapeutic regimens. These tumors were frequently considered small-cell or low-grade lymphomas, and their underlying favorable prognosis has, in part, led to some of the confusion in the literature as to the optimal management for gastric lymphomas, Isaacson suggested a possible progression of these tumors from a follicular center cell to a plasma cell infiltrate to lymphoma. He also suggested the role of intraluminal antigenic stimulus, probably bacterial in origin, because of reports demonstrating that Mediterranean lymphoma could be treated with antibiotics. (Curiously, in the same year Warren and Marshall first described *Helicobacter pylori* [8].)

Understanding of the correlation of *H. pylori* with lymphoid proliferation, particularly in the stomach, has led to dramatic changes in the management of low-grade MALT lymphomas. Whereas Radaszkiewicz et al. have shown in a large retrospective study that gastrointestinal malignant lymphomas of the MALT type have a high cure rate with radical surgery (particularly early stage lesions confined to the mucosa and submucosa), it has been suggested that these patients may be cured or achieve remission by treatment of the associated *H. pylori* infection alone [9]. Roggero et al. reported that of 26 patients with low-grade MALT lymphoma who were treated for *H. pylori*, 25 had their infection successfully eradicated by antibiotic therapy [10]. After eradication of *H. pylori*, 15 patients (60%) had either a complete disappearance of lymphoid tissue or only a residua of benign lymphoid follicles. Bayerdörffer et al. showed similar results in 33 patients with MALT lymphoma, all of whom had their *H. pylori* infections cleared and 23 (70%) of whom had complete regression of their lymphoma [11]. Despite these encouraging findings, MALT lymphoma can recur with *H. pylori* reinfection [12]. This implies that patients with MALT lymphoma and *H. pylori* infection who have been successfully treated by *H. pylori* eradication require long-term follow-up for *H. pylori* reinfection.

Parsonnet et al. have also provided evidence that *H. pylori* infection not only predates the development of MALT lymphoma but that it also precedes the development of intermediate and high-grade gastric lymphomas [13]. This, coupled with the fact that mixed (large and small) cell lymphomas are frequently found in the gastrointestinal tract, suggests that high-grade gastric lymphoma and low-grade MALT lymphoma are related and may be part of a single disease process [14].

It should be mentioned that not all geographic areas with high *H. pylori* infection rates have commensurately high MALT lymphoma rates. This may be related to the specific strain(s) of *H. pylori* present or possibly to other nutritional or underlying host genetic factors. Hussell et al. demonstrated that proliferation of B cells from MALT lymphomas required both *H. pylori* antigens as well as *H. pylori*–specific T cells [15]. Additionally, certain human leukocyte antigen (HLA) DQA1 alleles have been found to be associated with *H. pylori* infection. HLA-DQA1*0102 is more common in *H. pylori*–negative controls than in those infected with the bacteria, while HLA-DQA1*0301 is strongly associated with both duodenal and gastric ulcers [16]. These findings underscore the complex interactions involved in the gastric lining that may lead to inflammation or malignancy.

Given the high response rates to simple *H. pylori* eradication for MALT-associated low-grade lymphoma, it would seem prudent that a trial of antimicrobial therapy precede any consideration for chemotherapy or surgery in these patients. These more aggressive therapies should be reserved for inter-mediate- or high-grade non-Hodgkin's lymphomas, such as diffuse large cell lymphoma.

In a series of gastric lymphoma patients treated at the M. D. Anderson Cancer Center, with similar international indices, the use of surgery up front did not prolong survival over treatment with chemotherapy along [17]. This is at variance with other reported series, but, given the broad spectrum of patients included in many studies, comparisons between studies are difficult at best. To accurately compare treatment approaches in the future, it is strongly encouraged that patients be identified not only by histology but also by inter-national index. A full discussion of the management of gastric lymphoma is beyond the scope of this chapter.

Mantle cell lymphoma

When mantle cell lymphoma is included in the differential diagnosis after fine-needle aspiration biopsy, an open biopsy is frequently required because a specific diagnosis will impact the recommended therapy. The term *mantle cell lymphoma* was proposed in 1992 to unify various prior descriptions and define the entity [18]. These patients typically have diffuse adenopathy in addition to involvement of the bone marrow, spleen, and gastrointestinal tract. Mantle cell lymphomas typically express CD20 and CD22 (B-cell antigens) and CD5 (T-cell antigen), and 60% express a chromosomal translocation t(11;14) at the *bcl*-1 locus. This results in the overexpression of the *PRAD*1 gene, which codes for cyclin D1. Besides these specific molecular and genetic markers, the morphologic appearance of mantle cell lymphoma is considered characteristic.

In the past, mantle cell lymphomas were designated as intermediately dif-ferentiated lymphocytic lymphomas, but they have a poorer prognosis than the more indolent lymphomas with which they were grouped [19]. In a study by Fisher et al. from the Southwest Oncology Group, 376 patients treated on three trials were reevaluated (all patients were Ann Arbor stage III or IV and Working Formulation A, B, C, D, or E), and in fact 10% had mantle cell lymphomas and 11% had marginal zone lymphomas [19]. The patients with mantle cell lymphoma had 10-year disease-free and overall survival rates of less than 10% while these rates were 25% and 35% respectively, for patients with Working Formulation A–E lymphomas (both p < 0.001). The median disease-free survival duration for patients with mantle cell lymphoma is less than 2 years. This poor prognosis warrants a more aggressive approach in these patients, and thus tissue diagnosis remains important.

Bone marrow transplant has been reported as a salvage therapy for some patients with recurrent mantle cell lymphoma. In nine previously treated patients, Stewart et al. used autologous bone marrow transplant and reported overall and failure-free 2-year survival rates of 34% [20]. This is compared with their experience with up-front chemotherapy with an anthracycline-based regimen, which resulted in a 29% complete response rate and an 8% 5-year failure-free response rate.

Bone marrow transplant

Patients with intermediate-grade, aggressive non-Hodgkin's lymphoma usually respond well to frontline chemotherapy regimens (typically doxorubicin based) and have a 40–45% long-term survival rate [21]. The patients who do not respond to therapy either die quickly or relapse during or shortly after treatment. As one would expect, patients who relapse have a poor prognosis. Despite complete response rates of 30% or more with various salvage regimens, less than 10% of these patients will achieve long-term survival [22].

Because of this poor outcome, and some early promising results with high-dose chemotherapy and autologous bone marrow transplantation, a prospective, randomized, multiinstitutional trial was performed to determine the benefit, if any, of bone marrow transplant for salvage [23]. This study was conducted by the Parma group and included patients from several European universities. Two hundred and fifteen patients were accrued to the study over a 7-year period. All patients had had doxorubicin as part of their previous therapy. Patients received two cycles of dexamethasone, cisplatin, and cytarabine (DHAP), a proven effective salvage regimen, and had bone marrow harvested between the first and second courses if their disease did not progress. One hundred and twenty-five patients (58%) had a response to DHAP. Sixteen patients were excluded for various reasons; thus, 109 patients were randomized to receive high-dose chemotherapy, irradiation, and autologous bone marrow transplant or four additional cycles of DHAP (standard therapy). Both 5-year event-free survival (46% vs. 12%, p = 0.001) and overall survival (53% vs. 32%, p = 0.038) rates were improved with transplantation. This study clearly demonstrated the potential benefit of bone marrow transplantation for this group of patients.

Several points should be noted from this recent Parma group study. The overall response rate was 84% in the transplant group and only 44% for the standard treatment group. The treatment-related mortality rate, however, was 8% for the transplant group, while there were no treatment-related deaths in the standard therapy group. The timing of relapse either after or during prior therapy was an important factor. Whereas 64% of patients responded to DHAP if their relapse occurred after therapy, only 21% responded if the relapse occurred during the doxorubicin-based therapy.

Diespite the increased treatment-related mortality rate, autologous bone marrow transplantation is now accepted as the treatment of choice for chemotherapy-sensitive, relapsed, intermediate- or high-grade, aggressive non-Hodgkin's lymphoma. Further improvements in this area may arise by (1) the application of peripheral blood stem cell harvest, (2) the use of multidrug-resistance gene-reversing drugs or altered treatment regimens, and (3) the use of hematopoietic growth factors. The use of bone marrow transplant may soon be frontline therapy for patients with non-Hodgkin's lymphoma who are at high risk for relapse [24].

References

1. Harris NL, Jaffe ES, Stein H, Banks PM, Chan JKC, Cleary ML, Delsol G, De Wolf-Peeters C, Falini B, Gatter KC, Grogan TM, Isaacson PG, Knowles DM, Mason DY, Muller-Hermelink H-K, Pileri SA, Piris MA, Ralfkiaer E, Warnke RA. A revised European-American classification of lymphoid neoplasms: A proposal from the International Lymphoma Study Group. Blood 84:1361–1392, 1994.
2. The Non-Hodgkin's Lymphoma Pathologic Classification Project. National Cancer Institute sponsored study of classifications of Non-Hodgkin's lymphomas. Summary and description of a Working Formulation for clinical usage. Cancer 49:2112–2135, 1982.
3. Longo DL. The REAL classification of lymphoid neoplasms: One clinician's view. Principles Pract Oncol Update 9:1–12, 1995.
4. The International Non-Hodgkin's Lymphoma Prognostic Factors Project. A predictive model for aggressive non-Hodgkin's lymphoma. N Engl J Med 329:987–994, 1993.
5. López-Guillermo A, Montserrat E, Bosch F, Terol M, Campo E, Rozman C. Applicability of the international index for aggressive lymphomas to patients with low-grade lymphoma. J Clin Oncol 12:1343–1348, 1994.
6. Rodriguez J, Cabanillas F, McLaughlin P, Swan F, Rodriguez M, Hagemeister F, Romaguera J. A proposal for a simple staging system for intermediate grade lymphoma and immunoblastic lymphoma based on the 'tumor score.' Ann Oncol 3:711–717, 1992.
7. Isaacson P, Wright DH. Malignant lymphoma of mucosa-associated lymphoid tissue: A distinctive type of B-cell lymphoma. Cancer 52:1410–1416, 1983.
8. Warren JR, Marshall B. Unidentified curved bacilli on gastric epithelium in active chronic gastritis. Lancet 1:1273–1275, 1983.
9. Radaszkiewicz T, Dragosics B, Bauer P. Gastrointestinal malignant lymphomas of the mucosa-associated lymphoid tissue: Factors relevant to prognosis. Gastroenterology 102:1628–1638, 1992.
10. Roggero E, Zucca E, Pinotti G, Pascarella A, Capella C, Savio A, Pedrinis E, Paterlini A, Venco A, Cavalli F. Eradication of Helicobacter pylori infection in primary low-grade gastric lymphoma of mucosa-associated lymphoid tissue. Ann Intern Med 122:767–769, 1995.
11. Bayerdörffer E, Neubauer A, Rudolph B, Thiede C, Lehn N, Eidt S, Stolte M, for the MALT Lymphoma Study Group. Regression of primary gastric lymphoma of mucosa-associated lymphoid tissue type after cure of Helicobacter pylori infection. Lancet 345:1591–1594, 1995.
12. Cammarota G, Montalto M, Tursi A, Vecchio FM, Fedeli G, Gasbarrini G. Helicobacter pylori reinfection and rapid relapse of low-grade B-cell gastric lymphoma. Lancet 345:192, 1995.

13. Parsonnet J, Hansen S, Rodriguez L, Gelb AB, Warnke R, Jellum E, Orentreich N, Vogelman JH, Friedman GD. *Helicobacter pylori* infection and gastric lymphoma. N Engl J Med 330:1267–1271, 1994.

14. Isaacson PG. Gastric lymphoma and *Helicobacter pylori*. N Engl J Med 330:1310–1311, 1994.

15. Hussell T, Isaacson PG, Crabtree JE, Spencer J. The response of cells from low-grade B-cell gastric lymphomas of mucosa-associated lymphoid tissue to *Helicobacter pylori*. Lancet 342:571–574, 1993.

16. Azuma T, Konishi J, Tanaka Y, Hirai M, Ito S, Kato T, Kohli Y. Contribution of HLA-DQA gene to host's response against *Helicobacter pylori*. Lancet 343:542–543, 1994.

17. Yahanda A, Mansfield P. The role of locoregional therapy in the treatment of stage IE and IIE gastric lymphoma (abstr). Proceedings of the Society of Surgical Oncology, 47th Annual Cancer Symposium, 1994, p. 19.

18. Banks PM, Chan J, Cleary ML, Delsol G, De Wolf-Peeters C, Gatter K, Grogan TM, Harris NL, Isaacson PG, Jaffe ES, Mason D, Pileri S, Ralfkiaer E, Stein H, Warnke RA. Mantle cell lymphoma: A proposal for unification of morphologic, immunologic, and molecular data. Am J Surg Pathol 16:637–640, 1992.

19. Fisher RI, Dahlberg S, Nathwani BN, Banks PM, Miller TP, Grogan TM. A clinical analysis of two indolent lymphoma entities: Mantle cell lymphoma and marginal zone lymphoma (including the mucosa-associated lymphoid tissue and monocytoid B-cell subcategories): A Southwest Oncology Group study. Blood 85:1075–1082, 1995.

20. Stewart DA, Vose JM, Weisenburger DD, Anderson JR, Ruby EI, Bast MA, Bierman PJ, Kessinger A, Armitage JO. The role of high-dose therapy and autologous hematopoietic stem cell transplantation for mantle cell lymphoma. Ann Oncol 6:263–266, 1995.

21. Fisher RI, Gaynor ER, Dahlberg S, Oken MM, Grogan TM, Mize EM, Glick JH, Coltman CA, Miller TP. Comparison of a standard regimen (CHOP) with three intensive chemo-therapy regimens for advanced non-Hodgkin's lymphoma. N Engl J Med 328:1002–1006, 1993.

22. Velasquez WS, Cabanillas F, Salvador P, McLaughlin P, Fridrik M, Tucker S, Jagannath S, Hagemeister FB, Redman JR, Swan F, Barlogie B. Effective salvage therapy for lymphoma with cisplatin in combination with high-dose ara-C and dexamethasone (DHAP). Blood 71:117–122, 1988.

23. Philip T, Guglielmi C, Hagenbeek A, Somers R, Van Der Lelie H, Bron D, Sonneveld P, Gisselbrecht C, Cahn J-Y, Harousseau J-L, Coiffier B, Biron P, Mandelli F, Chauvin F. Autologous bone marrow transplantation as compared with salvage chemotherapy in relapses of chemotherapy-sensitive non-Hodgkin's lymphoma. N Engl J Med 333:1540–1545, 1995.

24. Vose JM. Treatment for non-Hodgkin's lymphoma in relapse. N Engl J Med 333:1565–1566, 1995.

11. Multiple endocrine neoplasia

Julie A. Miller and Jeffrey A. Norton

Introduction

The multiple endocrine neoplasia (MEN) syndromes are a family of genetic conditions characterized by a predisposition to the development of neoplasms in multiple endocrine glands. The pathologic change in affected glands is characteristically multicentric and may be expressed as hyperplasia, adenoma, or carcinoma. The MEN syndromes are inherited in an autosomal dominant manner and are classified according to the pattern of involvement (Table 1). MEN type I is characterized by parathyroid hyperplasia, pancreatic islet cell neoplasms, and adenomas of the anterior pituitary gland. Less commonly, patients with MEN-I can have adrenocortical or thyroid adenomas, lipomas, and carcinoid tumors. MEN-IIa is characterized by medullary thyroid carcinoma (MTC), adrenal pheochromocytoma, and parathyroid hyperplasia. MEN-IIb consists of medullary thyroid carcinoma, pheochromocytoma, mucosal neuromas, and a characteristic marfanoid habitus. MEN-IIb does not involve the parathyroid glands. Familial medullary thyroid carcinoma (FMTC) consists of medullary thyroid carcinoma alone without other abnormalities.

Multiple endocrine neoplasia type I

Multiple endocrine neoplasia type I (MEN-I) is an inherited endocrine disorder that includes tumors of the parathyroid gland, pancreatic islets, anterior pituitary gland, and occasionally other tissues. It is an autosomal dominant disorder.

Historical aspects

Erdheim [1] is generally credited as the first to describe associated endocrinopathies when in 1903 he reported an acromegalic patient who had a pituitary adenoma and four enlarged parathyroid glands at autopsy. Cushing and Davidoff [2] followed in 1927 by reporting a patient with a pituitary

Raphael E. Pollock (ed.), SURGICAL ONCOLOGY. Copyright © 1997. Kluwer Academic Publishers. ISBN 0-7923-9900-5. All rights reserved.

Table 1. Multiple endocrine neoplasia (MEN) syndromes and familial medullary thyroid cancer (FMTC)

Variable	MEN-I	MEN-IIa	MEN-IIb	FMTC
Mode of inheritance	Autosomal dominant	Autosomal dominant	Autosomal dominant	Autosomal dominant
Chromosome	11q 13	10	10	10
Genetic defect	Menin	RET mutation	RET mutation	RET mutation
Phenotype	No	No	Bony abnormalities Mucosal neuromas Marfanoid habitus bumpy lips	No
Medullary thyroid cancer	No	Bilateral	Bilateral	Bilateral
Course of MTC	No MTC	Virulent	Most virulent	Indolent
Pheochromocytoma	No	70% bilateral	70% bilateral	No
Parathyroid	Hyperplasia	Hyperplasia	No	No
Pancreatic islet cell tumors	Yes	No	No	No

MTC = medullary thyroid cancer.

adenoma, two parathyroid adenomas, and a pancreatic islet cell tumor. In 1945 Wermer [3] proposed that the disease was inherited in an autosomal dominant pattern after studying a kindred afflicted with tumors involving the pituitary gland, parathyroids, and pancreatic islets. A father and four of his nine children were affected. The disease was originally called multiple endocrine adenomatosis (MEA) but is currently known as MEN-I, or Wermer's syndrome.

In 1955, Zollinger and Ellison [4] reported two cases of severe recurrent peptic ulcer disease associated with pancreatic islet cell tumors. Zollinger and Ellison postulated that the islet cell tumors were ulcerogenic. McGuigan [5] in 1968 showed by immunofluorescence that gastrin was the hormone produced by the pancreatic tumors associated with the Zollinger-Ellison syndrome.

Genetics of multiple endocrine neoplasia type I

Multiple endocrine neoplasia type-I is inherited in a Mendelian autosomal dominant pattern. Oncogenesis in the MEN syndromes may require two separate mutational events. A germ-line mutation in a tumor suppressor gene confers susceptibility to neoplastic changes in the involved endocrine tissues. Elimination of the remaining normal allele through a second somatic mutational event, or 'second hit,' unmasks the inherited recessive mutation, resulting in neoplastic change. The occurrence of multiple second hits would then result in multiple clones of neoplastic cells and the multicentric involvement characteristically seen in affected tissues.

The gene responsible for MEN-I has been mapped to the long arm of chromosome 11 (11q13; see Table 1) [6]. Allelic losses of chromosome 11q13

214

have been found in parathyroid, pancreatic, and pituitary tumor tissues from both patients with MEN-I and those with sporadic tumors [7–12]. DNA sequencing from a minimal interval on 11q13 has recently identified the gene responsible for MEN-I. The MEN-I gene contains 10 exons and encodes a 2.8-kilobase transcript which translates into a predicted 610 amino acid product termed menin [12]. Menin exhibits no similarities to any previously known proteins so its function remains to be determined.

Because the exact gene has been sequenced, DNA studies can be used to determine whether an individual from an MEN-I kindred has inherited the gene. This study should save patients considerable time and expense, and it will eliminate the need for annual biochemical screening of kindred members who have not inherited the gene. In family members identified to have the MEN-I gene, biochemical screening should begin in the teenage years. Patients should be questioned and examined for kidney stones, lipomas, Cushing's syndrome, hypoglycemia, peptic ulcer disease, headaches, acromegaly, and visual field defects. Fasting serum levels of calcium, glucose, prolactin, gastrin, and pancreatic polypeptide should be obtained.

Parathyroid disease

Incidence. Primary hyperparathyroidism is the most common expression of MEN-I approaching 100% prevalence by 40 years of age [13]. All MEN-I patients have four-gland hyperplasia, in contrast to the less than 20% incidence of multiglandular involvement among sporadic cases.

Presentation. Primary hyperparathyroidism is usually the first biochemical abnormality detected in MEN-I. It tends to occur in the third decade of life, earlier than sporadic cases. Clinical features are similar to those of sporadic cases of primary hyperparathyroidism, and include asymptomatic hypercalcemia, fatigue, bone and abdominal pain, nephrolithiasis, and decreased bone density.

Diagnosis. The diagnosis is made by the detection of elevated serum levels of calcium and intact parathyroid hormone. Twenty-four hour urinary levels of calcium should also be measured and are elevated.

Treatment. Subtotal $3\frac{1}{2}$ gland parathyroidectomy has often been employed but is complicated by the recurrence of hyperparathyroidism up to 40% of the time [14] and permanent hypoparathyroidism approximately 25% of the time [15]. For these reasons, Wells and associates [16] have advocated total parathyroidectomy with autotransplantation of parathyroid tissue to the muscle of the nondominant forearm. With the autograft, the risk of permanent hypoparathyroidism is reduced, and should there be a recurrence of hyperparathyroidism, a reexploration of the forearm can be done under local anesthesia, avoiding the hazards of a neck reexploration.

Pancreaticoduodenal disease

Incidence. Pancreatic or duodenal islet cell tumors or carcinoid tumors are the second most common manifestations of MEN-I, occurring in approximately 30–80% of patients. The pathologic change is typically multicentric. Over 95% of MEN-I patients who develop pancreatic islet cell tumors will already have primary hyperparathyroidism at the time of diagnosis. The most common functional islet cell tumor in patients with MEN-I is gastrinoma, but virtually any islet cell tumor can occur in patients with MEN-I, including insulinoma, glucagonoma, vasoactive intestinal peptide (VIPoma), growth hormone releasing factor (GRFoma), somatostatinoma, pancreatic peptide (PPoma), and carcinoid tumor.

Presentation and diagnosis. Patients with MEN-I account for 20–30% of all cases of the Zollinger-Ellison syndrome (ZES). Symptoms of gastrinoma are related to gastric acid hypersecretion and include severe peptic ulcer disease, secretory diarrhea, esophagitis, and occasionally, abdominal pain. Gastrinomas in the setting of MEN-I are usually multifocal and malignant, often with regional or distant metastases at presentation. To diagnose ZES, all antisecretory medications must be discontinued. Elevated basal gastric acid output (>15 mEq/hr) and elevated fasting serum levels of gastrin (>100 pg/ml) are strongly suggestive of gastrinoma. If necessary, a secretin stimulation test can confirm the diagnosis. Secretin, 2 U/kg given intravenously, causes an increase in serum levels of gastrin >200 pg/ml over basal levels in approximately 85% of patients with ZES.

Patients with insulinomas, the second most common islet cell tumor in MEN-I patients, present with neuroglycopenic symptoms from hypoglycemia during fasting. Neuroglycopenia can cause sweating, dizziness, personality changes, drowsiness, coma, or seizures. While 80% of sporadic insulinomas are solitary, tumors are usually multicentric in the setting of MEN-I. Approximately 5–10% of insulinomas are malignant. Insulinomas are diagnosed by documenting fasting hypoglycemia (<40 mg/dl) with inappropriately elevated serum levels of insulin (>5 μU/ml) and C-peptide.

Glucagonomas are rare. They can be asymptomatic or can cause symptoms of cachexia, hypoaminoacidemia, anemia, type II diabetes mellitus, and thromboembolic disease. Patients with glucagonoma have a characteristic rash, called necrolytic migratory erythema, and an elevated plasma level of glucagon (>500 pg/ml).

Patients with VIPomas present with severe watery diarrhea (>5 l/day), dehydration, hypochloremia, hypokalemia, hypercalcemia, and elevated plasma levels of VIP.

Treatment. Because gastrinomas in the setting of MEN-I tend to be small and multicentric, they often cannot be localized by computed tomography (CT) or

216

angiography. Labeled somatostatin scintigraphy (OctreoScan) images most gastrinomas (80% sensitivity). Portal venous sampling with measurement of gastrin levels frequently localizes the source of excessive gastrin secretion to either the pancreatic head or the wall of the duodenum (gastrinoma triangle). In these patients, medical management with the H_2-antagonists (famotidine) and proton-pump inhibitors (omeprazole) is used to effectively control acid hypersecretion and its complications. Because calcium is a potent gastrin secretagogue, surgical correction of primary hyperparathyroidism in MEN-I patients greatly facilitates medical control of ZES. If a pancreatic or duodenal tumor 2–3 cm in size is identified on CT, OctreoScan, or angiogram, surgical resection of the islet cell tumor is recommended, as 50% of gastrinomas this size are malignant, with liver or nodal metastases. At the time of surgery, intraoperative ultrasound should be used to identify other pancreatic islet cell tumors that may have been missed on preoperative imaging. Further, duodenotomy is performed in MEN-1 patients with ZES because small duodenal carcinoid tumors that stain positive for gastrin have been identified in these individuals. Pancreatic body or tail islet cell tumors are removed by subtotal or distal pancreatectomy splenectomy. Pancreatic head or duodenal tumors are either enucleated or excised. Whipple pancreaticoduodenectomy has not been recommended because these tumors are indolent, even when malignant. With aggressive medical management and surgical debulking of primary and liver metastases, many patients tolerate the malignancy well and enjoy relatively long survival.

In contrast, there is no ideal medical treatment for insulinomas. Frequent feedings, calcium channel blockers, and octreotide have been used, but patients still develop hypoglycemia. Insulinomas in the setting of MEN-I are often large and solitary, but they may be multiple. These patients are usually treated with subtotal pancreatectomy to remove the islet cell tumor. Patients most often become asymptomatic and normoglycemic postoperatively. Patients with multifocal pancreatic or diffuse metastatic disease may respond to treatment with streptozotocin, diazoxide, or octreotide.

Pituitary tumors

Incidence. Adenomas of the anterior pituitary occur in 15–50% of MEN-I patients. Most of these tumors secrete prolactin, but tumors secreting adrenocorticotropic hormone (ACTH), growth hormone (GH), and thyroid stimulating hormone (TSH) may also occur.

Presentation. Pituitary neoplasms cause symptoms either by mass effects or by hormone hypersecretion. Patients may experience headaches, visual field cuts (bitemporal hemianopsia), or hypopituitarism caused by compression of the normal pituitary by the tumor. Prolactinomas cause amenorrhea/ galactorrhea in females or hypogonadism in males. Patients may present with acromegaly or hyperthyroidism from hypersecretion of GH or TSH, respectively. Patients with MEN-I and Cushing's syndrome may have ACTH hypersecretion from a pituitary adenoma (Cushing's disease), a foregut carcinoid or islet cell tumor secreting ACTH (ectopic ACTH), or even an adrenal cortical tumor secreting cortisol.

Diagnosis. Diagnosis is made based on clinical symptoms, serum hormone levels, and imaging studies. In a patient with Cushing's syndrome, a complete evaluation is necessary to determine the precise cause of the hypercortisolism. Studies include the dexamethasone suppression test, petrosal sinus sampling, and imaging studies of the pituitary, adrenals, and if ectopic ACTH is suspected, either CT or MRI of the chest and pancreas.

Treatment. Ablation of pituitary tumors may be achieved by surgery or irradiation. Prolactinomas can be treated medically with bromocriptine, a dopamine agonist and inhibitor of prolactin secretion.

Other manifestations

Other tumors in patients with MEN-I include adrenocortical adenomas in up to 40% and thyroid adenomas in up to 15% of MEN-I patients. Hypersecretion from these tumors is uncommon. Rarely, adrenocortical and thyroid carcinomas, multiple lipomas, and bronchial, thymic, gastric, or intestinal carcinoid tumors can also occur. One patient with a combination of MEN-I and MEN-IIa has been reported. He had metastatic medullary thyroid carcinoma (MTC), bilateral pheochromocytomas, and ZES caused by a pancreatic islet cell tumor within the pancreatic head.

Multiple endocrine neoplasia types IIa and IIb, and familial medullary thyroid carcinoma

Multiple endocrine neoplasia type IIa (MEN-IIa) is an inherited disease syndrome that is characterized by MTC, pheochromocytoma, and parathyroid hyperplasia. Multiple endocrine neoplasia type IIb (MEN-IIb) is an inherited disease syndrome that is characterized by medullary thyroid carcinoma, pheochromocytoma, mucosal neuromas, marfanoid habitus, intestinal ganglioneuromas, and corneal nerve hypertrophy. Parathyroid disease is not part of MEN-IIb.

Familial MTC is a disease that occurs without any other endocrine abnormality. The pattern of inheritance in all these syndromes is autosomal dominant, with a high degree of penetrance and variable expression. Each is associated with a genetic abnormality at chromosome 10. A missense mutation is seen in the RET oncogene (see Table 1).

218

Medullary thyroid cancer was first described as a distinct clinical and pathologic entity, with a high incidence of lymph node metastases, solid histologic pattern, and stromal material with the staining properties of amyloid by Hazard et al. in 1959 [17]. Two years later, in 1961, Sipple [18] noted an association of thyroid carcinoma with pheochromocytoma. In the following years, Williams noticed that the thyroid cancer associated with pheochromocytomas was MTC [19] and correctly deduced that the parafollicular cells, or C-cells, were the cell of origin in MTC [20]. These cells were later shown to secrete calcitonin.

Tashjihan et al. [21] first described a radioimmunoassay for calcitonin and demonstrated that calcitonin was elevated in patients with MTC. In 1968, Steiner et al. [22] introduced the term *MEN-II* to describe the familial occurrence of MTC, pheochromocytoma, and parathyroid hyperplasia. This syndrome is now known as MEN-IIa or Sipple's syndrome.

Williams and Pollack [23] were the first to describe patients with medullary thyroid carcinoma, pheochromocytoma, and multiple mucosal neuromas, and Chong and associates [24] suggested that this syndrome be called MEN-IIb.

Genetics of MEN-IIa, IIb, and familial medullary thyroid carcinoma

The gene for multiple Endocrine Neoplasia type IIa has been localized to the pericentromeric region of chromosome 10. More recent studies have mapped the gene for MEN-IIa and IIb to the region of chromosome 10 (10q11.2) that contains the RET protooncogene [25]. This gene encodes a transmembrane tyrosine kinase receptor and has been shown to be consistently expressed in neuroblastomas, pheochromocytomas, and MTCs [26,27]. Furthermore, the RET protooncogene is expressed in the mouse embryo in precursors of the thyroid C-cells, enteric nervous system, adrenal medulla, and parathyroid glands [28].

Germ-line mutations in the RET protooncogene have been identified in MEN-IIa, MEN-IIb, and FMTC, and somatic *ret* mutations have been found in some patients with sporadic MTC and pheochromocytomas. The tyrosine kinase receptor encoded by the RET protooncogene is believed to be involved in the proliferation, migration, and survival of a variety of neuronal lineages [28]. However, the mechanism by which *ret* mutations cause endocrine neoplasia is thus far unknown. Studies in a medullary thyroid carcinoma cell line showing one wild-type and one mutated *ret* allele in MTC cells suggest that *ret* mutations cause a dominant oncogenic conversion rather than loss of tumor suppressor function [29].

Interestingly, the autosomal dominant form of Hirschprung's disease has also been attributed to mutations in the RET protooncogene [30,31]. Although MEN-IIa has sometimes been associated with Hirschprung's disease, the *ret* mutations of MEN-II seem to confer hyperfunction of the gene, whereas those of Hirschprung's disease seem to be loss of function mutations [32].

Medullary thyroid cancer

Incidence. Medullary thyroid carcinoma accounts for 5% of all thyroid malignancies. The majority of these are sporadic cases — only 20% occur in a familial pattern, in the setting of MEN-IIa, MEN-IIb, or, less commonly, FMTC. All patients identified to carry the genetic mutations of MEN-IIa, MEN-IIb, or FMTC will develop MTC.

Presentation. Medullary thyroid carcinoma is usually the first abnormality expressed in both MEN-IIa and MEN-IIb. The MTC associated with MEN-IIb occurs earlier (sometimes before 2 years of age) than it does in patients with MEN-IIa (usually in the second or third decades) or in sporadic cases (fifth or sixth decades). While MTC is almost always unilateral in sporadic cases, it is virtually always bilateral and multicentric in the familial cases, with foci predominantly in the upper lobes. Diffuse C-cell hyperplasia is also a frequent finding.

Diagnosis. Asymptomatic members of kindreds with MEN-IIa or FMTC may be screened genetically for the RET protooncogene mutation or biochemi-

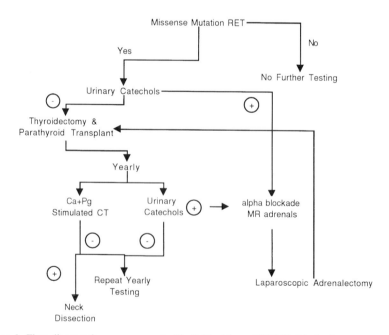

Figure 1. Flow diagram for management of individual from MEN-IIa kindred.

cally for medullary thyroid carcinoma (Fig. 1). If medullary thyroid carcinoma is present, patients will usually have elevated fasting serum levels of calcitonin. Initially, either calcium infusion or pentagastrin injection was used as a provocative agent for the early diagnosis of MTC in individuals at risk. Subsequently, it has been shown that the sequential intravenous administration of calcium followed by pentagastrin stimulated higher peak levels of plasma CT than either agent alone [33]. Kindred members with clinically occult MEN-IIa whose MTC was diagnosed by provocative testing were younger, had smaller primary tumors, had a lower incidence of lymph node metastases, and were more often cured following total thyroidectomy [34]. However, calcitonin testing is currently obsolete, as detection of missense mutations in RET in peripheral leukocytes of individuals at risk is the current preferred method of diagnosis.

Patients with MEN-IIb can be identified at birth or in early infancy by their characteristic phenotype. These individuals have a marfanoid habitus, prognathism, puffy lips, poor dentition, and multiple mucosal neuromas. Corneal nerve hypertrophy, as seen on slit-lamp examination, is also observed. Although MEN-IIb is also inherited, most of these patients have developed the disease from sporadic mutations. MEN-IIb patients usually do not have large kindreds because the MTC is more lethal. Most will have positive lymph nodes at the time of diagnosis. Individuals with MEN-IIb always have the germ-line RET mutation in the intracellular portion of the transmembrane tyrosine kinase receptor.

Treatment. Total thyroidectomy with central lymph node dissection is indicated in all patients with MEN-IIa, MEN-IIb, or FMTC, as the cancer is virtually always bilateral and multifocal. Patients with gross evidence of regional lymph node disease should receive ipsilateral neck dissection as well. Postoperatively, patients are monitored for recurrent disease with repeat baseline fasting calcitonin levels or calcitonin levels in response to calcium-pentagastrin stimulation tests. Until recently, repeat neck exploration in an attempt to resect residual disease has infrequently caused normalization of elevated plasma calcitonin levels. However, Tisell and colleagues [35] have reported 11 patients with MTC with persistently elevated plasma CT levels after total thyroidectomy and central zone lymphadenectomy. These patients underwent reoperation and meticulous superior mediastinal and bilateral lymph node dissection under magnification with the intent of removing all tumor in the neck. Stimulated postoperative plasma CT levels were normalized after reoperation in four (33%) of the patients who proved to have a few microscopic metastases.

The course of patients with MEN-IIa and MEN-IIb is essentially that of the MTC. Medullary thyroid carcinoma exhibits variable biologic aggressiveness within the different MEN syndromes and sometimes from kindred to kindred. Individuals with FMTC have the best prognosis, as the disease is indolent and surgical cure is often obtained. Prognosis is intermediate in patients with MEN-IIa, and the worst in MEN-IIb, as the cancer occurs at a younger age, is frequently spread to lymph nodes, and is much more aggressive.

In patients with MTC in the setting of MEN-IIa or MEN-IIb, it is necessary to rule out the presence of pheochromocytoma by obtaining 24-hour urine levels of vanillylmandelic acid (VMA), metanephrines, and total catecholamines. An occult pheochromocytoma could cause a fatal hypertensive crisis during surgery. If a patient with MTC is found to have a pheochromocytoma, adrenalectomy should be performed first, followed by a thyroidectomy 1–2 weeks later.

Pheochromocytoma

Incidence. Adrenal medullary pheochromocytoma occurs in approximately 50% of patients with MEN-IIa and MEN-IIb. The tumors usually appear in the second or third decade of life, concurrent with or a few years after the detection of MTC. These tumors are bilateral 60–80% of the time and usually are not malignant.

Presentation. Pheochromocytomas can cause severe frontal headaches, episodic hypertension, sweating, and palpitations. They may also be asymptomatic, detected by biochemical screening.

Diagnosis. The diagnosis of pheochromocytoma is made by detection of elevated 24-hour urinary levels of VMA, metanephrines, or total catecholamines. Imaging studies are used to identify which adrenal gland is involved with tumor. CT, MRI, and ^{131}I-MIBG scans have each been utilized by some groups. MR scan has some specificity for pheochromocytoma because the tumor appears bright on the T2-weighted image. ^{131}I-MIBG scan images pheochromocytoma based on function because MIBG is utilized in catecholamine biosynthesis. It has a 90% sensitivity. Both MR and CT can reliably detect intra-adrenal pheochromocytomas as small as 1 cm (sensitivity 80–90%).

Treatment. Patients with pheochromocytoma require preoperative alpha-adrenergic blockade with phenoxybenzamine, followed by beta-blockade if tachycardia or arrythmias develop. Beta-blockade without prior alpha-blockade is dangerous because patients are subjected to unopposed vasoconstriction. During surgery, it is necessary to remove the affected adrenal gland as identified by preoperative imaging. This procedure is now being done laparoscopically to shorten hospital stay and to improve the length of convalescence. Bilateral pheochromocytomas require bilateral adrenalectomy. Some authors recommend bilateral adrenalectomy for all individuals with pheochromocytoma in the setting of MEN-II because bilateral adrenal medullary hyperplasia is detected in 70% of these patients. Other authors advocate unilateral adrenalectomy if the contralateral gland is normal on CT, MR, or MIBG. This approach is acceptable, and such patients should be followed closely at 6-month to yearly intervals for recurrence in the remaining adrenal gland. However, recurrence usually does not occur until approximately 10 years.

Parathyroid disease

Parathyroid hyperplasia occurs in approximately 50% of patients with MEN-IIa and does not occur in patients with MEN-IIb or familial MTC. Most patients are asymptomatic, and their parathyroid disease is picked up on routine labs. When patients have symptomatic hypercalcemia, the most frequent manifestation is nephrolithiasis. Patients are treated with either a $3\frac{1}{2}$-gland or a 4-gland parathyroidectomy, with autotransplantation into the muscle of the nondominant forearm.

Gastrointestinal disease

Some individuals with MEN-IIa have Hirschsprung's disease, which has been associated with RET mutations. Patients with MEN-IIb may develop constipation, megacolon, and diverticular disease as a result of abnormal peristalsis caused by their intestinal ganglioneuromas. Constipation should be treated as symptoms arise. Medullary thyroid carcinoma can secrete a wide variety of peptide hormones that cause diarrhea. Patients who have metastatic MTC frequently develop secretory diarrhea.

References

1. Erdheim J. Zur normalen und pathologischen Histologie der Glandula thyreoidea, parathyreoidea, und hypophesis. Beitr Pathol Anat Allg Pathol 33:158, 1903.
2. Cushing H, Davidoff SM. The Pathological Findings in Four Autopsied Cases of Acromegaly with a Discussion of their Significance. Monograph 22. New York. The Rockefeller Institute for Medical Research, 1927.
3. Wermer P. Endocrine adenomatosis and peptic ulcer in a large kindred: Inherited multiple tumors and mosaic pleiotropism in man. Am J Med 35:205, 1963.
4. Zollinger RM, Ellison EH. Primary peptic ulceration of the jejunum associated with islet cell tumors of the pancreas. Ann Surg 142:709, 1955.
5. McGuigan JE. Gastric mucosal intracellular localization of gastrin by immunofluorescence. Gastroenterology 55:315, 1968.
6. Larsson C, Skogseid B, Oberg K, Nakamura V, Nordenskjold M. Multiple endocrine neoplasia type 1 gene maps to chromosome 11 and is lost in insulinoma. Nature 332:85, 1988.
7. Arnold A. Molecular mechanisms of parathyroid neoplasia. Endocrinol Metab Clin North Am 23:1, 1994.
8. Melmed S. Pituitary neoplasia. Endocrinol Metab Clin North Am 23:1, 1994.
9. Larsson C, Friedman E. Localization and identification of the multiple endocrine neoplasia type 1 disease gene. Endocrinol Metab Clin North Am 23:1, 1994.

10. Lyons J, Landis CA, Harsh G, et al. Two G-protein oncogenes in human endocrine tumors. Science. 249:655–659, 1990.

11. Landis CA, Masters SB, Spada A, Pace AM, Bourne HR, Vallar L. GTPase inhibiting mutations activate the alpha chain of Gs and stimulate adenyl cyclase in human pituitary tumors. Nature 340:692–696, 1989.

12. Chandrasekharappa SC, Guru SC, Manickam P, et al. Positional cloning of the gene for Multiple Endocrine Neoplasia-type 1. Science 276:404–407, 1997.

13. Mallette LE. Management of hyperparathyroidism in the multiple endocrine neoplasia syndromes and other familial endocrinopathies. Endocrinol Metab Clin North Am 23:1, 1994.

14. Prinz RA, Bamvros OI, Sellu D, Lynn JA. Subtotal parathyroidectomy for primary chief cell hyperplasia in the multiple endocrine neoplasia type I syndrome. Ann Surg 193:26, 1981.

15. van Heerden JA, Kent RB, Sizemore GW, Grant CS, ReMine WM. Primary hyperparathyroidism in patients with multiple endocrine neopalsia syndromes: Surgical experience. Arch Surg 118:533, 1983.

16. Wells SA, Jr., Farndon JR, Dale JK, Leight GE, Dilley WG. Long term evaluation of patients with primary parathyroid hyperplasia managed by total parathyroidectomy and heterotopic autotransplantation. Ann Surg 192:451, 1980.

17. Hazard JB, Hawk WA, Crile G, Jr. Medullary (solid) carcinoma of the thyroid: A clinico-pathologic entity. J Clin endocrinol Metab 19:152, 1959.

18. Sipple JH. The association of pheochromocytoma with carcinoma of the thyroid gland. Am J Med 31:163, 1961.

19. Williams ED. A review of 17 cases of carcinoma of the thyroid and pheochromocytoma. J Clin Pathol 18:288, 1965.

20. Williams ED. Histogenesis of medullary carcinoma of the thyroid. J Clin Pathol 19:114, 1966.

21. Tashjihan AH, Jr., Howland BG, Melvin KEW, Hill CS, Jr. Immunoassay of human calcitonin: Clinical measurement, relation to serum calcium, and studies in patients with medullary carcinoma. N Engl J Med 283:890, 1970.

22. Steiner AL, Goodman AD, Powers SR. Study of a kindred with pheochromocytoma, medullary thyroid carcinoma, hyperparathyroidism, and Cushing's disease: Multiple endocrine neoplasia type 2. Medicine 47:371, 1968.

23. Williams ED, Pollack DJ. Multiple mucosal neuromata with endocrine tumours: A syndrome allied to von Recklinghausen's disease. J Pathol Bacteriol 91:71, 1966.

24. Chong GC, Beahrs OH, Sizemore GW, Woolner LH. Medullary carcinoma of the thyroid gland. Cancer 35:695, 1975.

25. Lairmore TC, Dou S, Howe JR, et al. A 1.5 megabase yeast artificial chromosome cintig from human chromosome 10q11.2 connecting three genetic loci (RET, D10S94, and D10S102) closely linked to the MEN-2A locus. Proc Natl Acad Sci USA 90:492–496, 1993.

26. Nagao M, Ishizaka Y, Nakagawara A, et al. Expression of RET proto-oncogene in human neuroblastomas. Jpn J Cancer Res 81:309–312, 1990.

27. Santoro M, Rosati R, Grieco M, Berlingieri MT, D'Amato GL, de Franciscis V, Fusco A. The RET proto-oncogene is consistently expressed in human pheochromocytomas and medullary thyroid carcinomas. Oncogene 5:1595–1598, 1990.

28. Pachnis V, Mankoo B, Costantini F. Expression of the c-*ret* proto-oncogene during mouse embryogenesis. Development 119:1005–1017, 1993.

29. Santoro M, Carlomagno F, Romano A, et al. Activation of RET as a dominant transforming gene by germline mutations of MEN 2A and MEN 2B. Science 267:381–383, 1995.

30. Romeo G, Ranchetto P, Luo V, et al. Point mutations affecting the tyrosine kinase domain of the RET proto-oncogene in Hirschprung's disease. Nature 367:377–378, 1994.

31. Edery P, Lyonnet S, Mulligan LM, et al. Mutations of the RET proto-oncogene in Hirschprung's disease. Nature 367:378–380, 1994.

32. van Heyningen V. One gene: Four syndromes. Nature 367:319–320, 1994.

33. Wells SA, Jr., Baylin SB, Linehan WM, Farrell RE, Cox EB, Cooper CW. Provocative agents and the diagnosis of medullary carcinoma of the thyroid gland. Ann Surg 188:139, 1978.

34. Wells SA, Jr., Baylin SB, Gann DS, Farrell RE, Dilley WG, Preissig SH, Linehan WM, Cooper CW. Medullary thyroid carcinoma: Relationship of method of diagnosis to pathologic staging. Ann Surg 188:377, 1978.
35. Tisell LE, Hansson G, Jansson S, Salander H. Reoperation in the treatment of asymptomatic metastasizing medullary thyroid carcinoma. Surgery 99:60–66, 1986.

12. Advances in the diagnosis and treatment of gastrointestinal neuroendocrine tumors

Jeffrey E. Lee and Douglas B. Evans

Introduction

Gastrointestinal neuroendocrine tumors are rare neoplasms that share a common histology and biochemical features yet differ widely in their natural histories. Recent advances in our understanding of the biology of these tumors have been helpful in designing diagnostic localization strategies, selecting patients for appropriate treatment, and developing novel therapeutic approaches. Gastrointestinal neuroendocrine tumors constitute approximately 2% of all malignant gastrointestinal tumors [1]. They are classically divided into the carcinoid tumors and the pancreatic islet cell tumors. Neuroendocrine tumors have been described as being comprised of APUD (amine-precursor uptake and decarboxylation) cells [2,3].

A fundamental unifying concept is that neuroendocrine tumor cells have vesicles containing peptides that can act in an endocrine or paracrine fashion [4]. It is important to note, however, that not all neuroendocrine tumors are of neural crest origin [5]. Furthermore, a universal neuroendocrine marker has not been identified [6]. In addition to gastrointestinal neuroendocrine tumors, the neuroendocrine tumor family can be most broadly described to also include multiple endocrine neoplasia (MEN) type I–associated pituitary adenomas, MEN II–associated medullary thyroid carcinoma and pheochromocytomas, as well as paragangliomas, parathyroid adenomas, melanomas, Merkel cell tumors, and small cell lung carcinomas [4]. While neuroendocrine tumors, including those of gastrointestinal origin, are diverse in terms of their natural histories, there are some common aspects of the tumor biology of carcinoids and pancreatic islet cell tumors that have influenced recent developments in diagnostic localization and therapy.

Diagnosis

While the majority of gastrointestinal neuroendocrine tumors, with the exception of insulinomas, are malignant, benign and malignant gastrointestinal neuroendocrine tumors cannot be distinguished based on histology. Local invasion, regional metastases, or distant metastases must be present for an unequivocal diagnosis of malignancy [7].

A presumptive diagnosis of neuroendocrine tumor can often be made based on routine histopathologic examination. Immunoreactivity with neuron-specific enolase, chromogranin A, or synaptophysin can confirm the diagnosis [6]. The clinical presentation of patients with gastrointestinal neuroendocrine tumors depends on the pathologic type, hormonal status, anatomic location, and stage of the primary tumor.

Clinically nonfunctioning tumors typically include foregut (bronchopulmonary, stomach, duodenum) carcinoids, hindgut (transverse and descending colon, rectum) carcinoids, localized midgut (jejunum, ileum, appendix, ascending colon) carcinoids, and clinically nonfunctioning islet cell carcinomas [pancreatic polypeptide(PP)-omas and neurotensinomas]. In the absence of distant metastases, these tumors usually are found incidentally, as in the case of most appendiceal [8], gastric [9], and rectal carcinoids [10,11], or they may present due to mass effect or intestinal obstruction [12]. In the case of nonfunctioning tumors, symptom development may be delayed until quite late in the clinical course. The combination of normal liver function tests, an active and nearly asymptomatic patient, and a grossly enlarged liver is characteristic enough of metastatic neuroendocrine tumor to suggest the diagnosis [13]. Fine-needle aspiration biopsy can confirm the diagnosis and allow for treatment planning.

Functioning neuroendocrine tumors are classified based on their predominant hormonal syndromes, even when immunocytochemistry or serum hormone levels demonstrate a tumor to be polyhormonal. Functional carcinoid tumors produce the carcinoid syndrome, manifested by flushing, diarrhea, wheezing, and valvular heart disease. In almost all cases, and especially with midgut carcinoids, the carcinoid syndrome only occurs after the development of distant (hepatic) metastases [12,13]. The diagnosis of carcinoid syndrome is made by the demonstration of elevated urinary 5-hydroxyindoleacetic acid (5-HIAA) levels on 24-hour collection. 5-HIAA is the major metabolite of serotonin. Serotonin and its metabolites are present at elevated levels in the serum of the overwhelming majority of patients with the carcinoid syndrome; usually levels of these substances correlate with the severity of symptoms and changes in tumor mass [14,15]. Serotonin together with tachykinans, including substance P, may be responsible for flushing and wheezing in these patients [12,15]. The etiology of heart disease in patients with the carcinoid syndrome remains unclear, although the severity of heart disease correlates with urinary 5-HIAA excretion [15,16].

Functioning pancreatic endocrine tumors include the gastrinomas and insulinomas, as well as the rarer VIPomas, glucagonomas, and somatostatinomas. In each case, the diagnosis of a functioning pancreatic neuroendocrine tumor rests on the demonstration of elevation of the appropriate hormone level. For example, a diagnosis of gastrinoma is based on the findings of elevated fasting hypergastrinemia together with basal gastric acid hypersecretion and is confirmed by secretin provocative testing [17,18], while a diagnosis of insulinoma is suggested by the presence of simultaneous fasting hypoglycemia and an inappropriately elevated insulin level, and is confirmed by determining plasma proinsulin, C peptide, insulin antibodies, and sulfonylurea levels [15,18].

Preoperative localization and staging

Preoperative localization and staging has become increasingly important and effective in the evaluation of patients with gastrointestinal neuroendocrine tumors. Tumor biology influences the effectiveness of localization and staging strategies. Contrast-enhanced high resolution CT scan or angiography can demonstrate characteristic vascular primary tumors or hepatic metastases. Contrast-enhanced MRI scan can also detect both primary tumors as well as hepatic metastases [15,19]. However, neither CT nor MRI scanning is particularly sensitive at detecting characteristically small primary insulinomas or gastrinomas, with reported sensitivities ranging from 9% to 75% depending on the resolution of the specific technique used and on selection biases inherent in the population studied [20].

In experienced hands, preoperative upper endoscopy with ultrasound can localize primary gastrinomas and insulinomas [20–23]. However, the technique is better at identifying neuroendocrine tumors in the pancreatic head than the tail and is better at identifying pancreatic as opposed to duodenal gastrinomas [20–22].

The majority of gastrointestinal neuroendocrine tumors possess high-affinity receptors for somatostatin [18,20]. This has enabled successful localization of gastrointestinal neuroendocrine tumors in many patients using the radiolabled somatostatin analogue octreotide [24–27]. However, radiolabeled octreotide is less useful in patients with small tumors (e.g., primary gastrinomas and insulinomas) and in tumors that less frequently express somatostatin receptors (insulinomas) [18,20,24,26,28]. Octreotide scintigraphy may prove to be most useful as a staging modality, identifying metastatic disease in patients with gastrointestinal neuroendocrine tumors.

Selective portal venous sampling for hormone levels and intraarterial provocative injection with hepatic venous sampling have been useful in the preoperative regionalization of pancreatic islet cell tumors [29]. Venous sampling for hormones has also been used to regionalize gastrointestinal carcinoids. Recent reports on regionalizing pancreatic islet cell tumors have preferred selective intraarterial provocative injection with hepatic venous sampling over selective venous sampling because it is somewhat less technically demanding, more comfortable for the patient, safer, and appears to be at least as accurate [30–36]. Secretin is used as the provocative agent to regionalize gastrinomas; calcium is used in regionalization of insulinomas [18].

In a recent summary of the experience with this technique at the National Institutes of Health, Doppman et al. reported successful localization in 22 of 25 patients with insulinomas (sensitivity 88%) [32]. In this procedure, calcium gluconate is injected into the arteries supplying the pancreatic head (gastroduodenal and superior mesenteric) and the body and tail (splenic artery) of the pancreas. Insulin levels are measured in samples taken from the right and left hepatic veins 30, 60, and 120 seconds after calcium injection. A twofold increase in baseline insulin level taken from the right hepatic vein 30 or 60 seconds after injection is considered diagnostic of regionalization to the segment of the pancreas supplied by the selectively injected artery. Caution must be used in the interpretation of regionalization studies; tumors in the neck or proximal body of the pancreas can appear to drain via a head/uncinate pattern. In the series of patients reported by Doppman et al., all three false localizations were proximal body tumors. Two of these three patients had responses to both gastroduodenal artery and splenic injections; the third patient had a response to superior mesenteric artery injection.

Controversy exists regarding the need for extensive preoperative localization studies in the patient with insulinoma. It has been argued that following adequate preoperative evaluation to establish the diagnosis biochemically, the combination of intraoperative palpation of the pancreas along with introperative ultrasound has such a high likelihood of success that invasive localization studies, such as angiography, or regionalization studies, such as selective venous sampling or selective intraarterial provocative calcium injection and hepatic venous sampling, are unnecessary [37–41]. However, our philosophy has been to maximize the chances of a satisfactory result from initial laparotomy and to avoid the need for 'blind' pancreatectomy. Without regionalizing information, 'blind' distal pancreatectomy has a 50% chance of failure because insulinomas are distributed equally throughout the pancreas [42]. Therefore, in patients in whom symptoms of hypoglycemia are sufficiently severe or dangerous as to mandate pancreatectomy in the event a primary tumor is not identified and in whom there is doubt regarding the location of the primary tumor based on radiologic imaging, our policy has been to perform regionalization with provocative selective intraarterial calcium injection. This approach follows that advocated by others [18,32,43–45]. If the results of two noninvasive imaging studies of a patient with a biochemical diagnosis of insulinoma demonstrate a primary tumor at the same site, an invasive regionalization study is not done. However, in the face of negative or equivocal noninvasive imaging, we favor preoperative pancreatic arteriography with calcium injection. We would consider a preoperative regionalization study demonstrating a tumor in the pancreatic tail sufficient evidence alone for distal pancreatectomy in the rare event a tumor was not identified by the combination of palpation and intraoperative ultrasound in a significantly symptomatic patient.

All patients with a clinical and biochemical diagnosis of gastrinoma should undergo preoperative localization. Standard radiographic imaging often fails to identify these small tumors. Secretin-enhanced selective arteriography may demonstrate a tumor blush. While simultaneous hepatic and peripheral venous sampling for gastrin has been used to regionalize gastrinomas, preoperative regionalization of gastrinomas has thus far not been demonstrated to alter operative management and is not recommended outside of an investigational setting [18].

Intraoperative localization

As discussed earlier, ultrasonography is an established technique for the intraoperative identification of gastrointestinal neuroendocrine tumors [37,41,44]. While palpation is more sensitive than intraoperative ultrasound for the identification of duodenal carcinoids, the two techniques are equally effective for the identification of pancreatic carcinoids. Furthermore, intraoperative ultrasound is more sensitive than palpation for the identification of insulinomas; nonpalpable tumors can be identified by intraoperative ultrasonography. Both palpation and intraoperative ultrasound are more sensitive than any preoperative imaging modality for the detection of small pancreatic neuroendocrine tumors [20].

Intraoperative endoscopic transillumination, along with duodenotomy and palpation, may be helpful in the identification of primary duodenal carcinoids [20,46]. Recently, intraoperative localization of neuroendocrine pancreatic tumors using radiolabeled octreotide and a handheld gamma-detecting probe has been described [47]. In a preliminary report, eight patients with neuroendocrine tumors (four carcinoid, two gastrinoma, one glucagonoma, and one VIPoma) had successful intraoperative localization using this technique. Occult disease, not detected by standard imaging modalities or intraoperative exploration, was detected by the intraoperative gamma probe in two patients. Background interference by normal tissue binding of octreotide remains a problem, however, and its sensitivity in detecting, for example, occult primary gastrinomas remains to be established before the utility of this new technology can be determined.

Surgery

Surgical decision making in the patient with a gastrointestinal neuroendocrine tumor depends on a sound understanding of the biology and natural history of the disease. Information on the hormonal status of the tumor, its stage, and ideally the location of the primary is necessary before a decision about the appropriate surgical procedure can be made. Surgery remains the only potentially curative therapy for gastrointestinal neuroendocrine tumors.

It is appropriate to base surgery for primary carcinoids on location, size, and histology. Overall, carcinoid tumors smaller than 1 cm have a less than 2%

incidence of metastases at presentation, those between 1 and 2 cm a 10–20% incidence of metastases, and those over 2 cm a 60–90% incidence of metastases [11,48]. Appendectomy is appropriate treatment for appendiceal carcinoids less than 1 cm in size. It seems prudent to treat larger appendiceal carcinoids by right hemicolectomy [48], although some authors recommend a more conservative approach for tumors between 1 and 2 cm.

As for appendiceal carcinoids, metastases in rectal carcinoids are strongly associated with size. Within a given tumor size, the probability of metastases correlates with muscularis propria invasion [11]. Rectal carcinoids less than 1 cm can be treated with local excision [11,48]. Intermediate-size (1–2 cm) rectal carcinoids should be removed initally by local full-thickness excision; muscularis propria invasion mandates a low anterior or a posterior (Kraske) approach to resection. Sphincter preservation should be a priority; abdominoperineal resection is rarely necessary. Patients with rectal carcinoids over 2 cm have a high incidence of distant metastatic disease and a poor prognosis; radical spincter-ablating surgery in these patients should be performed very selectively.

Appropriate treatment of small intestinal carcinoids is controversial. However, since malignancy for small intestinal carcinoids is not clearly related to size, it seems prudent to perform en-bloc mesenteric lymphadenectomy when resecting these tumors [48]. Furthermore, mesenteric nodal involvement and tumor desmoplastic reaction from primary or recurrent tumor can result in symptoms of obstruction, and primary or recurrent nodal disease extending to the root of the mesentery can make complete resection of these tumors difficult and potentially hazardous. Therefore, we advocate that even small tumors without apparent nodal disease be treated with primary en-bloc mesenteric lymphadenectomy to avoid the potential for significant local problems associated with later locoregional recurrence.

Gastric carcinoids usually occur in the setting of hypergastrinemia and have a relatively benign clinical course [49]. Hypergastrinemia-associated gastric carcinoids and duodenal carcinoids smaller than 1 cm can be removed endoscopically or by local excision. The rarer sporadic gastric carcinoids and larger tumors should be treated by wide local excision or gastrectomy, depending on tumor location. An occasional patient with the carcinoid syndrome and hepatic metastases anatomically amenable to surgical resection may benefit from an aggressive approach [15,50,51].

Modern control of gastric acid hypersecretion in patients with gastrinomas has revolutionized the care of these patients. Following control of gastric acid hypersecretion, patients with sporadic gastrinoma should be staged, localized, and considered for surgical treatment. Isolated and regionally confined gastrinomas should be resected. Surgical debulking of MEN-I patients with metastatic gastrinoma remains controversial [52–60]. While only a minority of MEN-I patients will be rendered secretin-stimulation test negative by surgical resection, highly selected patients may benefit from an aggressive surgical approach.

Patients with nonfunctioning islet cell tumors should undergo resection in the absence of distant metastatic disease [61]. Criteria for resectability include a lack of encasement of the celiac axis or superior mesenteric artery (SMA) and a lack of occlusion of the superior-mesenteric-portal venous confluence. Segmental resection of the superior mesenteric-portal venous confluence can be safely performed; however, posterior or retroperitoneal extension to the origin of the celiac axis or SMA is typically the limiting factor in obtaining a locally curative resection for tumors of the pancreatic head. It is clear that margin-positive, palliative resection provides no survival benefit in patients with more common adenocarcinoma of the pancreas, and we have also avoided this approach in patients with islet cell tumors. However, direct infiltrative retroperitoneal invasion of the origin of the celiac axis and SMA is not as common with islet cell tumors as with adenocarcinoma, making more extended resections theoretically possible. In addition, large islet cell tumors of the pancreatic head may encase the common hepatic artery while sparing the SMA. Extended resection to include hepatic revascularization may warrant consideration in the subset of patients with locally advanced nonmetastatic islet cell tumors if operative mortality and morbidity can be minimized and negative margins obtained (Fig. 1). There is generally little role for palliative resection in the treatment of patients with metastatic nonfunctioning islet cell carcinoma. However, selected patients with low-volume liver metastases and a symptomatic or impending symptomatic primary tumor may derive palliative benefit from resection of the primary tumor.

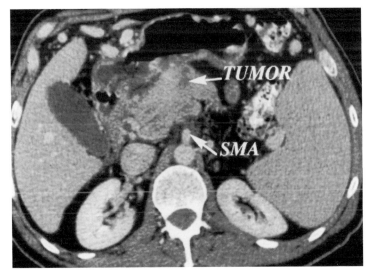

Figure 1. CT scan of a large, hypervascular islet cell tumor of the body of the pancreas that encased the hepatic artery yet maintained a normal fat plane between the tumor and the superior mesenteric artery.

Systemic therapy

Chemotherapy for gastrointestinal neuroendocrine tumors is generally reserved for patients with symptoms from hormone overproduction or mass effect, or who have rapidly progressive disease. The most effective regimens are those that contain streptozotocin [62]. For metastatic islet cell carcinomas, the combination of streptozotocin plus doxorubicin is superior to streptozotocin plus fluorouracil and results in a survival improvement [63,64]. Carcinoid tumors are generally more resistant to chemotherapy than malignant islet cell tumors [62].

Octreotide is effective at relieving symtoms and reducing hormone levels in patients with the carcinoid symdrome, and can be life saving in cases of carcinoid crisis. Control of symptoms can occur in 70–90% of patients with metastatic carcinoid tumors [65,66]. Biochemical partial responses occur in the majority of patients [66]. Radiographic partial responses may be noted in a minority of patients; some studies suggest improved survival in those undergoing octreotide therapy.

Octreotide can control symptoms in patients with pancreatic neuroendocrine tumors [67]. Octreotide is effective in relieving symptoms of diarrhea, dehydration, and hypokalemia in VIPoma patients, and in releiving peptic ulceration in gastrinoma patients, hypoglycemia in glucagonoma patients, and necrolytic skin lesions in somatostatinoma patients [65]. Unfortunately, while octreotide seems to be particularly effective in patients with VIPomas or glucagonomas, tachyphylaxis occurs rapidly and little or no effect on tumor growth is seen [68].

Interferon-α can be effective in the palliative treatment of patients with either pancreatic neuroendocrine tumors or the carcinoid syndrome [69]. Subjective symptomatic improvement is seen in the majority of treated patients. Objective tumor responses are less common. Interferon therapy is associated with significant side effects; this must be taken into account in selecting interferon as palliative therapy.

Regional therapy

Surgical or radiographic hepatic artery occlusion has been used for many years to treat patients with hepatic metastases from gastrointestinal neuroendocrine tumors [51]. Radiographic hepatic artery embolization is often combined with chemotherapy [70,71]. This combination is helpful in reducing carcinoid syndrome symptoms. However, the procedure requires careful patient selection and operator expertise to be performed safely; even in experienced hands, toxicity is significant and mortality can occur [70].

Liver transplantation has been proposed for a highly select subset of patients with hepatic metastases from neuroendocrine tumors [72,73]. Selection criteria include control of the primary tumor, absence of distant metastatic

234

disease, and hepatic progression despite chemotherapy and embolization [72]. This treatment must currently be considered highly investigational.

References

1. Oberg K. Treatment of neuroendocrine tumors. Cancer Treat Rev 20:331–355, 1994.
2. Pearse HGE. The APUD concept and hormone production. Clin Endocrinol Metab 9:211, 1980.
3. Erlandson RA. Tumors of the endocrine/neuroendocrine system: An overview. Ultrastructur Pathol 18:149–170, 1994.
4. Langley K. The neuroendocrine concept today. Ann NY Acad Sci 733:1–17, 1994.
5. Pearse HGE, Tabor TT. Embryology of the diffuse neuroendocrine system and its relationship to the common peptides. Fed Proc 38:2288, 1979.
6. Kloppel G, Heitz PU. Classification of normal and neoplastic neuroendocrine cells. Ann NY Acad Sci 733:18–23, 1994.
7. Haller DG. Endocrine tumors of the gastrointestinal tract. Curr Opin Oncol 6:72–76, 1994.
8. Moertel CG, Dockerty MB, Judd ES. Carcinoid tumors of the vermiform appendix. Cancer 21:270, 1968.
9. Davies MG, Dowd GO, McEntree GP, Hennessey TPJ. Primary gastric carcinoid tumors: A view on management. Br J Surg 77:1013, 1990.
10. Federspiel BH, Burke AP, Sokin LH, Shekitka KM, Helwig EB. Rectal and colonic carcinoids. Cancer 65:135, 1990.
11. Mani S, Modlin IM, Ballantyne G, Ahlman H, West B. Carcinoid tumors of the rectum. J Am Coll Surg 179:231–248, 1994.
12. Feldman JM. Carcinoid tumors and the carcinoid syndrome. Curr Probl Surg 26:835, 1989.
13. Moertel CG. An odyssey in the land of small tumors. J Clin Oncol 5:1502, 1987.
14. Feldman JM. Carcinoid tumors and syndrome. Semin Oncol 14:237, 1987.
15. Kvols LK. Metastatic carcinoid tumors and the malignant carcinoid syndrome. Ann NY Acad Sci 733:464–470, 1994.
16. Lundlin L, Norheim I, Landelius J, Oberg K, Theodorsson-Norheim E. Carcinoid heart disease: Relationship of circulating vasoactive substances to ultrasound-detectable cardiac abnormalities. Circulation 77:264, 1988.
17. Wolfe MM, Jensen RT. Zollinger-Ellison syndrome: Current concepts in diagnosis and management. N Engl J Med 317:1200, 1987.
18. Perry RR, Vinik, AI. Diagnosis and management of functionioning islet cell tumors. J Clin Endocrinol Metab 80:2273–2278, 1995.
19. Moore NR, Rogers CE, Britton BJ. Magnetic resonance imaging of endocrine tumours of the pancreas. Br J Radiol 68:341–347, 1995.
20. Hammond PJ, Jackson JA, Bloom SR. Localization of pancreatic endocrine tumours. Clinical Endocrinology 40:3–14, 1994.
21. Bansal R, Kochman ML, Bude R, Nostrant TT, Elta GH, Thompson NW, Scheiman JM. Localization of neuroendocrine tumors utilizing linear-array endoscopic ultrasonography. Gastrointestinal Endoscopy 42:76–79, 1995.
22. Zimmer T, Ziegler K, Liehr RM, Stolzel U, Riecken EO, Wiedenmann B. Endosonography of neuroendocrine tumors of the stomach, duodenum, and pancreas. Ann NY Acad Sci 733:425–436, 1994.
23. Zimmer T, Ziegler K, Bader M, Fett U, Hamm B, Riecken E-O, Wiedenmann. Localisation of neuroendocrine tumours of the upper gastrointestinal tract. Gut 35:471–475, 1994.
24. Krenning EP, Kwekkeboom DJ, Oei HY, de Jong RJB, Dop FJ, Reubi JC, Lamberts SWJ. Somatostatin-receptor scintigraphy in gastroenteropancreatic tumors. An overview of European results. Ann NY Acad Sci 733:416–424, 1994.

25. Jamar F, Fiasse R, Leners N, Pauwels S. Somatostatin receptor imaging with indium-111-pentetreotide in gastroenteropancreatic neuroendocrine tumors: Safety, efficacy and impact on patient management. J Nucl Med 36:542–549, 1995.

26. Vekemans MC, Urbain JL, Charkes D. Advances in radio-imaging of neuroendocrine tumors. Curr Opin Oncol 7:63–67, 1995.

27. Schirmer WJ, Melvin WS, Rush RM, O'Dorisio TM, Pozderac RV, Olsen JO, Ellison EC. Indium-111-pentetreotide scanning versus conventional imaging techniques for the localization of gastrinoma. Surgery 118:1105–1114, 1995.

28. Reubi JC, Kvols LK, Waser B, Nagorney DM, Heitz PU, Charboneau JW, Reading CC, Moertel C. Detection of somatostatin receptors in surgical and percutaneous needle biopsy samples of carcinoids and islet cell carcinomas. Cancer Res 50:5969–5977, 1990.

29. Miller DL, Doppman JL, Metz DC, Maton PN, Norton JA, Jensen RT. Zollinger-Ellison syndrome: Technique, results, and complications of portal venous sampling. Radiology 182:235–241, 1992.

30. Imamura M, Takahashi K, Adachi H, Minematsu S, Shimada Y, Naito M, Suzuki T, Tobe T, Azuma T. Usefulness of selective arterial secretin injection test for localization of gastrinoma in the Zollinger-Ellison syndrome. Ann Surg 205:230–239, 1987.

31. Fraker DL, Norton JA. Controversies in surgical therapy for APUDomas. Semin Surg Oncol 9:437–442, 1995.

32. Doppman JL, Chang R, Fraker DL, Norton JA, Alexander HR, Miller DL, Collier E, Skarulis MC, Gorden P. Localization of insulinomas to regions of the pancreas by intra-arterial stimulation with calcium. Ann Intern Med 123:269–273, 1995.

33. Doppman JL, Miller DL, Chang R, Shawker TH, Gorden P, Norton JA. Insulinomas: Localization with selective intraarterial injection of calcium. Radiology 178:237–241, 1991.

34. Thom AK, Norton JA, Doppman JL, Miller DL, Chang R, Jensen RT. Prospective study of the use of intraarterial secretin injection and portal venous sampling to localize duodenal gastrinomas. Surgery 112:1002–1009, 1992.

35. Doppman JL, Miller DL, Chang R, Maton PN, London JF, Gardner JD, Jensen RT, Norton JA. Gastrinomas: Localization by means of selective intraarterial injection of secretin. Radiology 174:25–29, 1990.

36. Doppman JL, Miller DL, Chang R, Gorden P, Eastman RC, Norton JA. Intraarterial calcium stimulation test for detection of insulinomas. World J Surg 17:349–443, 1993.

37. van Heerden JA, Grant CS, Czako PF, Service FJ, Charboneau JW. Occult functioning insulinomas: Which localizing studies are indicated? Surgery 112:1010–1015, 1992.

38. Rothmund M. Localization of endocrine pancreatic tumors. Br J Surg 81:164–166, 1994.

39. Pedrazzoli S, Pasquali C, D'Andrea AA. surgical treatment of insulinoma. Br J Surg 81:672–676, 1994.

40. Axelrod L. Insulinoma: Cost-effective care in patients with a rare disease. Ann Intern Med 123:311–312, 1995.

41. Galiber AK, Reading CC, Charboneau JW, Sheedy PF, James EM, Gorman B, Grant CS, van Heerden JA, Telander RL. Localization of pancreatic insulinoma: Comparison of pre- and intraoperative US with CT and angiography. Radiology 166:405–408, 1988.

42. Howar TJ, Stabile BE, Zinner MJ, Chang S, Bhagavan BS, Passaro E. Anatomic distribution of pancreatic endocrine tumors. Am J Surg 159:258–264, 1990.

43. Geoghegan JG, Jackson JE, Lewis MPN, Owen ERTC, Bloom SR, Lynn JA, Williamson RCN. Localization and surgical management of insulinoma. Br J Surg 81:1025–1028, 1994.

44. Doherty GM, Doppman JL, Shawker TH, Miller DL, Eastman RC, Gordon P, Norton JA. Results of a prospective strategy to diagnose, localize, and resect insulinomas. Surgery 110:989–997, 1991.

45. Norton JA, Shawker TH, Doppman JL, Miller DL, Fraker DL, Cromack DT, Gordon P, Jensen RT. Localization and surgical treatment of occult insulinomas. Ann Surg 212:615–620, 1990.

46. Frucht H, Norton JA, London JF, Vinayek R, Doppman JL, Gardner JD, Jensen RT, Maton

PN. Detection of duodenal gastrinomas by operative endoscopic transillumination. Gastroenterology 99:1622–1627, 1990.

47. Schirmer WJ, O'Dorisio TM, Schirmer TP, Mojzisik CM, Hinkle GH, Martin EW. Intraoperative localization of neuroendocrine tumors with ^{125}I-TYR(3)-octreotide and a hand-held gamma-detecting probe. Surgery 114:745–752, 1993.

48. Delcore R, Friesen SR. Gastrointestinal neuroendocrine tumors. J Am Coll Surg 178:187–211, 1994.

49. Gilligan JG, Phil M, Lawton GP, Tang LH, West AB, Modlin IM. Gastric carcinoid tumors: The biology and therapy of an enigmatic and controversial lesion. Am J Gastroenterol 90:338–353, 1995.

50. Zogakis TG, Norton JA. Palliative operations for patients with unresectable endocrine neoplasia. Endocr Surg 75:525–539, 1995.

51. Ihse I, Persson B, Tibblin S. Neuroendocrine metastases of the liver. World J Surg 29:76–82, 1995.

52. Norton JA, Jensen RT. Unresolved surgical issues in the management of patients with Zollinger Ellison syndrome. World J Surg 15:151–159, 1991.

53. Thompson NW, Bondeson AG, Bondeson L, et al. The surgical treatment of gastrinoma in MEN-1 patients. Surgery 106:1081–1086, 1989.

54. van Heerden JA, Smith SL, Miller LJ. Management of the Zollinger-Ellison syndrome in patients with multiple endocrine neoplasia type I. Surgery 100:971–977, 1986.

55. Sheppard BC, Norton JA, Doppman JL, et al. Management of islet cell tumors in patients with multiple endocrine neoplasm, a prospective study. Surgery 106:1108–1118, 1989.

56. Mignon M, Rusniewski P, Podevin P, Sabbagh L, Cadiot G, Rigaud D, Bonfils S. Current approach to the management of gastrinoma and insulinoma in adults with multiple endocrine neoplasia type 1. World J Surg 17:489–497, 1993.

57. Pipeleers-Marichal M, Somers G, Willems G, et al. Gastrinomas in the duodenums of patients with multiple endocrine neoplasia type I and the Zollinger-Ellison syndrome. N Engl J Med 322:723–727, 1990.

58. Cherner JA, Sawyers JL. Benefit of resection of metastatic gastrinoma in multiple endocrine neoplasia type-1. Gastroenterology 102:1049–1053, 1992.

59. Modlin IM, Lawton GP. Evolution of a operative strategy for diagnosis and management of duodenal gastrinomas. J Am Coll Surg 197:611–625, 1994.

60. Pasieka JL, McLeod MK, Thompson NW, Burney RE. Surgical approach to insulinomas. Arch Surg 127:442–447, 1992.

61. Evans DB, Skibber JM, Lee JE, Cleary KR, Ajani JA, Gagel RF, Sellin RV, Fenogliio CJ, Merrell RC, Hickey RC. Nonfunctioning islet cell carcinoma of the pancreas. Surgery 114:11175–11182, 1993.

62. Oberg K. Endocrine tumors of the gastrointestinal tract: Systemic treatment. Anticancer Drugs 5:503–519, 1994.

63. Moertel CG, Hanley JA, Johnsson LA. Streptozocin alone compared with streptozocin plus fluorouracil in the treatment of advanced islet cell carcinoma. N Engl J Med 303:1189–1194, 1980.

64. Moertel CG, Lefkopoulo M, Lipsitz M. Streptozocin-doxorubicin, streptozocin-fluorouracil or chlorozotocin in the treatment of advanced islet-cell carcinoma. N Engl J Med 326:519–523, 1992.

65. Lamberts SWJ, van der Lely A-J, Herder WW, Hofland LJ. Octreotide. N Engl J Med 334:246–253, 1996.

66. Kvols LK, Moertel CG, O'Connell MJ, Schutt AJ, Rubin J, Hahn RG. Treatment of the majignant carcinoid syndrome. Evaluation of a long-acting somatostatin analogue. N Engl J Med 315:663–666, 1984.

67. Kvols LK, Buck M, Moertel CG, Schutt AJ, Rubin J, O'Connell MJ, Hahn RG. Treatment of metastatic islet cell carcinoma with a somatostatin analogue (SMS 201–995). Ann Intern Med 107:162–168, 1987.

68. Wynick D, Anderson JV, Williams SJ, Bloom SR. Resistance of metastatic pancreatic endo-crine tumours after long-term treatment with the somatostatin analogue octreotide (SMS 201–995). Clin Endocrinol 30:385–565, 1989.

69. Oberg K, Eriksson B, Janson ET. The clinical use of interferons in the management of neuroendocrine gastroenteropancreatic tumors. Ann NY Acad Sci 733:471–478, 1994.

70. Ajani JA, Carrasco CH, Wallace S. Neuroendocrine tumors metastatic to the liver. Vascular occlusion therapy. Ann NY Acad Sci 733:479–487, 1994.

71. Perry LJ, Stuart K, Stokes KR, Clouse ME. Hepatic arterial chemoembolization for meta-static neuroendocrine tumors. Surgery 116:1111–1117, 1994.

72. Bechstein WO, Neuhaus P. Liver transplantation for hepatic metastases of neuroendocrine tumors. Ann NY Acad Sci 733:507–514, 1994.

73. Curtiss SI, Mor E, Schwartz ME, Sung MW, Hytiroglou P, Thung SN, Sheiner PA, Emre S, Miller CM. A rational approach to the use of hepatic transplantation in the treatment of metastatic neuroendocrine tumors. J Am Coll Surg 180:184–187, 1995.

13. Contemporary Approaches to Gastric Carcinoma

Blake Cady

Introduction

Gastric carcinoma represents a fascinating disease in terms of the history, development, philosophy, and future of the field of surgical oncology. Many facets of gastric carcinoma intrigue us: the long-term decline in incidence in the United States and other western countries [1], the rapid improvement in stage that has been seen in Japan as a result of widespread population screening [2], the evolution of sophisticated histologic analysis separating better and poorer prognostic histologic types (Lauren classification) [3], the recent significant proximal shift in the location of gastric cancers [4], the inability to find any effective systemic therapy to improve prognosis [5], and the unsubstantiated enthusiasm for a far more radical surgical approach [6,7] to gastric cancer, including radical lymph node removal, recreating a philosophical trend and surgical strategy of the 1950s long since discredited in all other human cancer surgery. This last feature has led to several randomized trials comparing the extent of regional lymph node and stomach resection in an appropriate attempt to evaluate the revived surgical philosophy and strategy [6,8–10]. The history of gastric cancer surgery and the results of these recent prospective clinical trials reaffirms and supports basic surgical oncology principles.

It may now be forgotten in the United States that as recently as 1950 gastric adenocarcinoma was the leading cancer cause of death in men [1]. It was also the second leading cause of cancer death in women in the 1930s [1]. As a result of a continuing decline in incidence and death from gastric cancer over the 60 years from 1935 to 1995, gastric cancer has fallen to the fifth leading cause of cancer death in men, and the seventh leading cancer cause of death in women in the United States [1]. This dramatic decrease in incidence and death continues to intrigue epidemiologists and supports clues about the etiology of gastric cancer. Alterations in diet and food preservation techniques during this time undoubtedly relate to the marked decline in the location of the distal 'epidemic' form of gastric cancer [11]. The subsequent marked increase in the proportion of proximal location gastric cancers indicates that there are at least two principal types of gastric cancer [4]. These enormous changes in gastric cancer incidence and location in the United States are now being mimicked in

Raphael E. Pollock (ed.), SURGICAL ONCOLOGY. Copyright © 1997. Kluwer Academic Publishers. ISBN 0-7923-9900-5. All rights reserved.

Japan with their rapid westernization of diet and modern food preservation techniques [12]. Thus, the unfolding story of gastric adenocarcinoma provides opportunities to appreciate epidemiological and biological aspects of this cancer, evolving principles of surgical treatment, outcomes related to disease presentation and surgical technique, and population control efforts for the entire field of surgical oncology.

Disease incidence

Figures 1 and 2 dramatically illustrate the enormous changes in the incidence and death rate from gastric cancer in the United States over the past 65 years. As food preservation shifted from pickling, smoking, and salting, to canning, drying, and, freezing, nitrites and other carcinogenic compounds gave way to those that preserve vitamin C and beta-carotene. Extensive research into the diet associations with gastric carcinoma indicate correlations with such food-preservation practices and with the amount of fresh fruits, vegetables, vitamins, and other substances contained in the diet [13]. *Heliobacter pylori* bacterial infection of the gastric mucosa may well be associated with these dietary and preservative variations, although it is still unclear whether *H. pylori* is causative or merely associated [11].

Correa has demonstrated the dietary practices associated with different populations that relate to their vastly different incidences of gastric adenocarcinoma [12]. His studies indicate that fresh vegetables, fruits, and other dietary components that contain vitamins and other substances significantly protect populations against the development of adenocarcinoma of the distal stomach [11,12]. The study of migrant populations illustrates clearly that changing dietary practices are related to changing incidences of gastric carcinoma [12]. Worldwide there is an inverse relationships between the incidence of gastric and colon carcinoma [14]. Populations with high gastric carcinoma rates have low colon carcinoma rates and vice-versa, again demonstrating well-described dietary relationships. Within three generations high gastric and low colon carcinoma rates of immigrant Asian populations change to match those of the United States. Most recently, studies indicate that the incidence of *H. pylori* infection of the stomach in children and young adults is associated with a later high incidence of distal gastric adenocarcinoma [11] and with the intestinal histologic type [15]. What is clear from all these data is the demonstration of opportunities to help control gastric adenocarcinoma throughout the world by appropriate diet and food-preservation practices.

Recent evidence suggests that poorly differentiated gastric adenocarcinoma (diffuse type of Lauren) has less correlation with known dietary and food-preservation practices than the better differentiated intestinal histologic type of Lauren [3,11,12]. In addition, the recent increased proportion of gastroesophageal junction adenocarcinoma of the stomach seems to bear no currently definable relationship to the dietary and food-preservation practices clearly associated with the distal endemic form of gastric adenocarcinoma [11–18]. Distal esophageal adenocarcinoma and metaphlastic changes in the distal esophageal mucosa (Barrett's esophagitis) presumably relate to gastric acid reflux secondary to lower esophageal sphincter dysfunction, but occur in the same patient population as proximal gastric and gastroesophageal junction cancer [19]. At the present time, no biologically plausible explanation for the pattern of simultaneous rapid increases gastroesophageal junction and distal esophagus adenocarcinoma has been developed [11,18]. Furthermore, no completely plausible explanation for the rising proportion of the genetically distinctive [20] poorly differentiated gastric adenocarcinoma has been elaborated either [11,17].

Clinical types and clinical presentation

Clinically, gastric carcinoma throughout the world presents in three basic patterns [21]. Superficial gastric carcinoma, presumably the predecessor to invasive and lethal gastric carcinoma, does not penetrate beyond the musclarias mucosa of the gastric wall, and while occasionally associated with immediately adjacent but limited lymph node metastases, it is highly, almost uniformly, curable [22]. While in the United States the gradually increasing incidence of superficial gastric cancer is of rather modest extent (up to 6–9% of cases) [4], in Japan, following extensive population screening programs, the rapid rise in the proportion of the superficial variety of gastric adenocarcinoma is such that over half of all cases encountered now are of this highly curable, extremely early form of disease [23]. These superficial carcinomas, while usually asymptomatic, are sometimes marked by epigastric pain symptoms and are more readily diagnosed by contemporary endoscopic, in contrast to previous radiological, diagnostic techniques, and are usually of the intestinal histologic type [21,24]. Thus the development of modern flexible fiberoptic endoscopic instruments enabled the Japanese to embark on screening programs that were feasible and cost effective, considering the high incidence and lethality of the disease in Japan, and the significant financial investment possible, and has yielded dramatic results in terms of markedly improving the stage at presentation and thus the outcome of surgical resection. This Japanese public health initiative provides a model for the benefits of a screening program with a suitably defined population at high risk, a logical screening technique, a manageable cost-effectiveness ratio, and a society wealthy enough to devote major resources to the effort.

The second clinical form of gastric adenocarcinoma is linitis plastica, which involves the gastric wall with a desmo-plastic reaction to diffuse cancer cell infiltration throughout the gastric wall, but relative sparing of the gastric mucosa. Linitis plastica has been known since early clinical descriptions of gastric cancer. In our reports, linitis plastica has made up a fixed proportion of cases over the 60-year time period despite the rapid decrease in overall incidence of the disease and the striking change in gastric location [4,21]. Thus, 15% or 16% of all gastric adenocarcinomas were clinically of the linitis plastica type from the 1930s to the 1990s. The fact that it presents as a fixed proportion of cases despite rapidly changing overall incidence and pattern leads to the speculation that it might represent a host response, rather than an innate disease characteristic. Essentially all linitis plastica clinical gastric cancers are of the diffuse histologic type, as might be expected, although the converse is not true: only a small proportion of diffuse histologic types are linitis plastica. Results of surgical therapy are so dismal that the clinical form of linitis plastica gastric cancer should be considered incurable [4,21]. Because of extension throughout the gastric wall, linitis plastica almost always requires a total gastrectomy for surgical removal. Even then, proximal and distal margins are frequently microscopically involved despite normal clinical appearance at re-section. The treatment of linitis plastica remains a challenge; its clinical behavior is similar to the uncommon diffuse colon cancers that present as a 'linitis plastica' type, and to diffuse 'inflammatory' breast cancer, which has been so lethal in the past but now seems to be yielding somewhat to multimodal therapy.

The majority of gastric adenocarcinomas consist of the third clinical type, a focal invasive presentation [21], with an otherwise normal gastric wall, of an ulcerated, polypoid, or localized growth that represents the traditional pattern of gastric adenocarcinoma. In proximal gastric cancers, metaplastic and dysplastic changes of the parietal mucosa are the usual background of precursor mucosal abnormalities. In focal invasive gastric adenocarcinomas, over half are of the poor-prognosis diffuse histology type, and the remainder are of the intestinal variety as defined by Lauren [3] or mixed forms [21]. The current proportions of intestinal and diffuse histologic types represent a striking reversal over the years from the vast majority being of the intestinal type [3]. Focal gastric adenocarcinomas lend themselves to a curative partial gastric resection with removal of accompanying lymph node metastases that are relatively limited in extent and few in number.

While in the past the great majority of focal lesions occurred in the antrum of the stomach, particularly at the parieto-antral cell boundary, increasingly they are in the gastroesophageal junction or upper stomach [18]. The trend towards a more proximal location in this country has also been seen in other parts of the world, particularly western Europe [25]. Historically, the focal type of gastric cancer led to the first successful gastric resections in the late 19th century by Billroth and others. In recent years, the focal form of gastric adenocarcinoma has presented at an earlier stage, with a smaller size and fewer nodal metastases [4]. Extensive lymph node metastases beyond the first echelon of perigastric nodes have always been associated with an extremely poor prognosis [4,26–30]. In the diffuse histologic variety, any lymph node metastases foretell a dismal prognosis [4,21], while with the intestinal histologic variety, reasonable prognostic expectations still occur with up to three [4] lymph node metastases, but even here the prognosis is poor with more than four nodal metastases, and progressively decreases with more numerous nodal metastases. Several articles point out the need to count the number of node metastases as the best prognostic indicator, rather than the lymph node station [28,29]. This fact, of course, calls into question the entire strategy of more extensive lymph node resections [31,32], fully in keeping with the implication of multiple lymph node metastases in virtually all other human cancers.

Histologic types

Underlying understanding of gastric carcinoma and any appreciation of a rational surgical approach must be the appreciation of the definition of and significant changes in the histologic types of gastric carcinoma as defined by Lauren [3] and as recorded particularly in Europe and increasingly accepted in the United States [11,12]. While in epidemic areas of gastric carcinoma throughout the world, the overwhelming majority of cases are of the intestinal histologic variety, as overall gastric cancer incidence declines, the relative proportion made up of the diffuse histologic type increases [11,12]. Whether this represents an absolute increase in the diffuse histologic variety or merely the disappearance of the diet-related, epidemic, intestinal histologic variety has not been totally clarified, but both aspects may well be components of the changing ratio of histologic types. In patients under 40 years of age [33,34], the majority of gastric carcinomas are of the diffuse histologic type and include a high proportion of the linitis plastica clinical variety.

It is clear from recent studies that the diffuse and intestinal histologic types are distinctly different varieties of gastric cancer, perhaps from inception, and are marked by defined differences in HLA phenotypes and perhaps other genetic markers [20]. If clinical superficial gastric carcinoma, almost uniformly of the intestinal histologic variety, is the usual antecedent of gastric cancer, both of the diffuse as well as the intestinal histologic types, it must be postulated that an earlier lower grade disease precedes a later clonal overgrowth of more poorly differentiated cells (diffuse histologic variety) by the time of clinical presentation [24]. While the progression of early intestinal type (superficial gastric cancer) to later diffuse histologic type has not been defined, studies do not report a significant enough proportion of early gastric carcinomas as being of diffuse histologic variety to explain the high incidence or even predominant diffuse histology at gastric resection [4,24]. Thus it might be assumed that the 'early,' superficial, intestinal histologic variety of gastric adenocarcinoma may progress down separate genetic or histologic pathways, to a more advanced invasive intestinal variety, or to a poorly differentiated histology following a clinical sequence that leads to overgrowth of the poorly differentiated histology, with the resultant clinical presentation as either linitis plastica or a focal clinical cancer.

Further studies of this sequence of histologic growth patterns would be of great interest in terms of understanding the diverse biology, genetic sequence, and alterations in multihit carcinogenesis, epidemiologic relationships, and progressive clinical growth patterns that may ensue from the presumption of a multiple-step carcinogenesis [24]. Such an intriguing area of investigation might resemble a progression from in-situ to invasive cancer currently accepted in breast carcinoma, with a definition of at least two varieties of duct carcinoma in situ, apparently separated by genetic phenotypes, into different clinical patterns and variable potential for progressive growth to clinical invasive cancers.

Surgical approaches and philosophies

The first attempts at gastric resection in the late 1800s were necessarily relatively conservative or limited in extent. The magnitude of gastric surgery, risk of surgical complications, and high operative mortality mandated a surgical approach of modest extent in our current terms. As a matter of fact, the first successful proximal gastric resection did not occur until the late 1930s [35]. In the 1940s, with the ability to transfuse blood, use antibiotics, apply knowledge of sophisticated pathophysiological responses to surgery, and manage operative trauma, the capacity to do more extensive and radical surgery rapidly increased [36]. By 1953 the first report of a super-radical gastric resection was published [37]. The failure of the increasingly radical surgical philosophy of the 1950s and 1960s to improve results led to a return to a generally more conservative surgical philosophy in this country, as emphasized by Hoerr [38]. The decline in the doctrinaire radical resectional philosophy of the 1950s and 1960s as the standard model of the surgical approach to gastric cancer (and all other cancers) was reversed in gastric cancer in the 1980s under the influence of reports of radical gastric resection and regional lymphadenectomy from Japan, which culminated in the assumption that a left upper quadrant exenteration would improve results of resection for gastric cancer [7,39].

As this chapter is published, the philosophical battleground is shifting back to a more conservative, safer approach based on the results of several randomized prospective trials that indicate no benefit from extended resections [8–10]. It is to be expected that the wave of enthusiasm for super-radical surgery in gastric cancer proposed by Japanese authors and promoted by many others will go the way of the super-radical approach to surgery in lung, esophagus, colon, and breast cancers and in melanoma and sarcoma surgery. The appreciation that the basic biological features of these cancers control disease outcome rather than variations of surgical technique will lead to a more conservative general surgical philosophy in stomach cancer, as it has in all other cancers studied. Since outcome in our common cancers is overwhelmingly related to systemic metastases, not local or regional nodal recurrence, improvements in outcome will require increasing effectiveness of adjuvant systemic therapy, not more extensive surgical procedures to remove even larger portions of primary organs or surrounding regional lymph node tissues.

244

For these reasons also, radiotherapy, yet another local therapy, cannot be expected to improve outcome generally in gastric cancer [40]. Earlier disease presentation resulting from screening and general improvement in medical care will impact on increased surgical control of gastric cancer in a far more important fashion than adjusting the details or increasing the radicalness of surgical technique. Increased recognition that lymph node metastases are 'indicators, but not governors' [41] of survival following cancer surgery will also temper erroneous assumptions that ever larger lymphatic resections will in any way improve surgical outcomes, except by their use as a prognostic indicator, as a therapy selection process, or for adjuvant systemic chemo-therapy, none of which have yet been found useful in improving gastric cancer outcome when used an adjunct to operations [5,42].

Variety of surgical procedures available for resection of the stomach

The three basic surgical resections of gastric adenocarcinoma are as follows: distal gastrectomy (of greater or lessor extent), total gastrectomy with its resultant jejunoesophageal anastomoses, and proximal gastric resection with gastroesophageal anastomosis [21]. The latter has been more widely utilized in recent years because of the increasing proportions of proximal gastric and distal esophageal adenocarcinoma [16–19]. In the past decade careful defini-tions of the extent of accompanying lymph node dissection have been promul-gated [43–45]. Thus a D1 (formerly R1) resection basically removes the first echelon of regional lymph nodes, a D2 (formerly R2) resection removes the second echelon of regional lymph node anatomy, and a D3 (formerly R3) resection removes an extensive, wide-field tertiary echelon level of lymph nodes (an anatomic, not functional, classification that may or may not be regional by definition of lymphatic flow patterns).

Thus a wide variety of surgical resection options are possible, combining variously the extent of primary organ removal and the extent of lymph node removal, from doctrinaire radical total gastrectomy with wide-field lymphatic resection or even left upper quadrant exenteration, to less than total gastrectomy with wide field but not super-radical lymphatic resection, to rela-tively conservative gastric resections with adequate but not extensive margins of normal gastric wall surrounding the primary cancer and with first-echelon lymph-node removal based on a conservative surgical philosophy. Obviously admixtures of primary stomach resection and extent of lymphatic removal are practical, both in a preplanned doctrinaire fashion and in response to the extent of the primary gastric cancer or its nodal metastases. For instance, resection of the linitis plastica clinical presentation almost always requires a total gastrectomy [4,21], but the form of lymphatic resection is irrelevant because these patients are essentially incurable, and the extent of lymph node involvement is relatively unimportant because any nodal metastases are asso-ciated with an extremely poor outcome. The conceptual and doctrinal differences that these various surgical procedures represent are being played out in the contemporary surgical scene in Europe and the United States [8,46–48]; Asian surgeons [49] and others in Europe [39,48] and the United States [44] seem wedded to the more doctrinaire radical resectional approach.

One aspect of the clinical presentation of gastric cancer in countries without screening programs that affects results is the extremely small proportion of cases even eligible for assignment in prospective trials of radical lymphatic resection. In South Africa, only 9% of cases and 15% of resections were eligible for trial assignment [50], indicating the lack of impact on overall results even potentially achievable by application of a doctrinaire radical approach because of the generally advanced nature of the disease. This fraction of patients suitable for radical lymphatic resection may be somewhat larger in more recent reports from Japan, Germany, and Holland [51].

Results of surgery

With delayed clinical presentation and advanced stage of disease, early reports of outcome following surgical resection of gastric carcinoma were dismal. As late as 1980 we reported [21,36] that the curability of gastric adenocarcinoma had not changed in decades and was about 10% overall. Many reports indicated that the proportion of cases that could undergo any kind of resection was less than 50%, and that the possibility of curative resection, that is, removal of all gross disease, made up a minority of cases and only half of resected cases. [38,52–54]. Even among patients undergoing curative resection, the portion alive disease free at 5 years was 50% or less.

As extensive harvesting of lymph nodes surrounding the stomach is practiced, the possibilities of stage shifting by the 'Will Rogers' phenomenon [55] can be demonstrated. Such seemingly improved clinical outcome occurring as a result of stage shifting, rather than resulting from technical changes in operations, has been demonstrated in other cancers. Such a phenomena is frequently not recognized when cases are compared with prior results, historical controls, or specific stages, or without complete acknowledgement of all cases encountered in the time period. The reporting of results of a specific operative procedure, of only patients resected, of those resected for cure, or of newly defined operative procedures [56] involves highly selective reporting [56] and cannot be construed as representing results overall or results of less stringently defined 'curative' resections. This emphasizes that only by randomized concurrent prospective controlled trials can the true impact of changes resulting from new therapeutic measures, such as an increased extent of surgery, be demonstrated objectively and free of the bias of stage shifting, earlier diagnosis, or selective reporting. Only with the advent of randomized prospective trials has a true understanding of the effects or lack of effects of changed treatment techniques and philosophy become appreciated in osteogenic sarcoma of children, breast cancer in women, melanoma, sarcoma of extremities, colon and rectal carcinoma, and squamous cell carcinoma of the head and neck.

Thus, it is critical that the enthusiasm for super-radical gastric cancer surgery be evaluated in similar terms. Several randomized prospective trials comparing the extensiveness of gastric and lymphatic resections in the treatment of gastric adenocarcinoma have been reported [8–10]. In each trial it has been demonstrated that the radicalness of the surgical approach has no bearing on overall outcome. This lack of improvement has applied to total gastrectomy compared with less than total gastrectomy [57], as well as to radical lymph node dissection compared with less than radical lymph node dissection accompanying gastric resection [8–10]. It is worthwhile noting that the results of these contemporary trials are still to be fleshed out by reporting of other ongoing trials [48]; however, results reported to date fail to suggest any improved outcome by more radical surgical procedures, but increase operative morbidity and mortality and lead to conclusions that are similar in all other human solid tumors: the extent of resection of the primary cancer, while related to and important in controlling local recurrence rates, has no controlling impact on survival (with a few exceptions), and the extent of lymph node dissection, while related to the regional nodal recurrence rate, staging, and perhaps selection of adjuvant systemic therapy, is not causally related to overall survival. Lymph node metastases are 'indicators, but not governors, of survival' [41]; likewise, local recurrences are indicators but seldom governors of survival [58,59]. The biologic aspects of lymph node metastases in gastric cancer have been thoroughly examined in a recent article [60].

Sophisticated staging accomplished through extensive preoperative or operative diagnostic techniques may lead to more appropriate selection of therapy in individual cases and may allow comparison from institution to institution or country to country, but does not by itself cause an improvement in overall outcome, except by eliminating advanced or incurable cases through sophisticated analysis of occult distant sites of metastatic disease or through definition of poor biological behavior of the primary cancer.

Adjuvant therapy in gastric cancer

To date no systemic adjuvant chemotherapy of gastric carcinoma has been standardized because randomized prospective trials have failed to demonstrate consistent usefulness [5,42]. Recent initial enthusiasm about a highly toxic multidrug program used as induction chemotherapy has not been substantiated by later publications [61]. Continued attempts at defining such adjuvant treatment that might be both successful and of acceptable morbidity are ongoing and obviously needed.

The used of radiotherapy as an adjuvant to surgical removal of gastric cancer has not proven successful either [40], and indeed is illogical because gastric cancer mortality is almost entirely caused by systemic metastatic spread, particularly to the liver, but also transerosally to the general peritoneal cavity, rather than by an admitted high rate of local recurrence. Since radiotherapy, a local therapy, can only contribute to improvement in local control, if at all, it would be expected that programs of increased regional radicalness by any means, radiotherapy or more extensive surgery, particularly when linked with ineffective associated systemic chemotherapy, would not be successful.

The implications of the variety of gastric cancer presentations and disease feature changes needs to be appreciated. Sharply increasing proportions of more proximal location, diffuse histology, and younger patients, coupled with the failure to find a successful systemic adjuvant therapy, would lead one to predict difficulty in achieving better overall outcome in the treatment of gastric adenocarcinoma. Contrary trends that might improve survival include earlier detection, yielding a higher proportion of the superficial clinical type, and smaller cancers with fewer lymph node metastases and decreased operative mortality. The resultant of these two countervailing trends and disease features nevertheless seem to have resulted in a slightly improved outcome overall [4]. Significant opportunities exist in gastric adenocarcinoma at present to rationalize the extent of surgical resection, thus reducing operative mortality and morbidity, and to develop epidemiological and biological knowledge about the rapidly increasing gastroesophageal junction and proximal gastric cancer in order to help control this disease. Attempts to combine various types of adjuvant systemic therapy, both immunologic and chemotherapeutic, of necessity still require investigation. Perhaps even knowledge of *H. pylori* bacteriological control may help reduce the incidence of gastric cancer.

Accompanying the rapid decline in incidence of gastric carcinoma in this country has been the proportional increase of all gastric malignancies that are gastric lymphoma [62]. While this does not bear on the issue of gastric carcinoma per se, it nevertheless should alert surgeons to the fact that a higher proportion of gastric malignancies will be discovered to be lymphomas, especially when the preoperative diagnosis is not precise. The association of gastric lymphoma with *H. pylori* infection is an intriguing story in itself [63], particularly when it is realized that the mucosa associated lymphoid tumor (MALT) variety of lymphoma has been demonstrated to be curable by antibiotic elimination of *H. pylori* infections [64]. Whether all or only a proportion of gastric lymphoma may be associated with *H. pylori* infestation is an evolving story. Along with the changing clinical presentation of gastric cancer is an improving clinical presentation of gastric lymphoma. With the increasing earliness of gastric lymphoma presentation, already of a much earlier comparative stage than gastric adenocarcinoma [65], the possibilities of treating patients without gastric resection by the use of multidrug chemotherapy has been reported [66]. Again, these changing trends in disease presentation, treatment philosophy, and outcome show that with effective chemotherapy even fairly extensive malignancy can be controlled, sometimes without resection. The issue in gastric cancer is not disease extent nor extent of surgery but lack of effective

248

chemotherapy or effective chemoradiotherapy combinations for those cases too extensive or metastatic to be cured by appropriate surgery alone.

What the future holds in the realm of gastric adenocarcinoma is difficult to predict, but clearly extensive research is needed to define the epidemiology and etiology of distal esophageal adenocarcinoma and adenocarcinoma of the gastroesophageal junction and upper stomach. As improved socioeconomic development, westernization of diet, and contemporary food-preservation practices increase, gastric cancer incidence will dramatically improve throughout the world and in immigrant populations. The genetic basis and biological development of diffuse histologic-type gastric cancer needs elaboration. The role of *H. pylori* gastric mucosal infection stands as an intriguing element of epidemiology in both gastric cancer and gastric lymphoma.

Gastric cancer, like so many other human cancers, stands on the threshold of rapid development based on new epidemiologic understanding, increasing sophistication of diagnostic studies, more carefully integrated multimodal therapy, understanding of sophisticated genetic aspects of cell growth and progression of disease, and rationalization of therapy, particularly surgery. The treatment of gastric cancer and outcomes of surgery very clearly illustrate basic surgical oncology principles. Appropriate surgical resections in gastric cancer should relate to the extent of the individual disease presentation and the individual patient, not to theoretical assumptions or doctrine unsubstantiated by appropriate clinical studies, and indeed illogical from inception. The admonition of Hoerr [38] remains true today: 'The policy of small operative procedures for small cancers and extensive operative procedures for large cancers is believed to produce results that equal those of a policy calling for extensive resections for small and favorable lesions.'

References

1. Parker SL, Tong T, Bolden S, Wingo PA. Cancer Statistics, 1996. CA Cancer J Clin 65:5–27, 1996.
2. Hisamichi S. Screening for gastric cancer. World J Surg 13:31–37, 1989.
3. Lauren PA, Nevalainen TJ. Epidemiology of intestinal and diffuse types of gastric carcinoma: A time-trend study in Finland with comparison between studies from high- and low-risk areas. Cancer 71:2926–2933, 1993.
4. Salvon-Harman JC, Cady B, Nikulasson S, Khettry U, Stone MD, Lavin P. Shifting proportions of gastric adenocarcinomas. Arch Surg 129:381–389, 1994.
5. Hermans J, Bonenkamp JJ, Boon MC, Bunt AMG, Ohyama S, Sasako M, van de Velde CJH. Adjuvant therapy after curative resection for gastric cancer: Meta-analysis of randomized trials. J Clin Oncol 11:1441–1447, 1993.
6. Bunt AMG, Hermans J, Boon MC, van de Velde CJH, Sasako M, Fleuren GJ, Bruijn JA. Evaluation of the extent of lymphadenectomy in a randomized trial of western- versus Japanses-type surgery in gastric cancer. J Clin Oncol 12:417–422, 1994.
7. Sawai K, Takahashi T, Suzuki H. New trends in surgery for gastric cancer in Japan. J Surg Oncol 56:221–226, 1994.
8. Dent DM, Madden MV, Price SK. Controlled trials and the R1/R2 controversy in the management of gastric carcinoma. Surg Oncol Clin NA 2:433–441, 1993.

9. Robertson CS, Chung SCS, Woods SDS, Griffin SM, Raimes SA, Lau JTF, Soc B, Li AKC. A prospective randomized trial comparing R1 subtotal gastrectomy with R3 total gastrectomy for antral cancer. Ann Surg 222:176–182, 1994.
10. Cuschieri A, Fayers P, Fielding J, Craven J, Bancewicz J, Joypaul V, Cook P. Surgical treatment of gastric cancer postoperative morbidity and mortality after D1 and D2 resections for Gastric cancer — Preliminar results of the MRC randomized controlled surgical trial. Lancet 1996, in press.
11. Correa P. The epidemiology of gastric cancer. World J Surg 15:228–234, 1991.
12. Correa P. Clinical implications of recent developments in gastric cancer pathology and epidemiology. Semin Oncol 12:2–10, 1985.
13. Ramon JM, Serra L, Cerdo C, Oromi J. Dietary factors and gastric cancer risk: a case-control study in Japan. Cancer 71:1731–1735, 1993.
14. Cady B, Stone MD, Wayne J. Continuing trends in the prevalence of right-sided lesions among colorectal carcinomas. Arch Surg 128:505–509, 1993.
15. Endo S, Ohkusa T, Saito Y, Fujiki K, Okayasu I, Sato C. Detection of *Heliobacter pylori* infection in early stage gastric cancer. Cancer 75:2203–2208, 1995.
16. Antonioli DA, Cady B. Changing aspects of gastric adenocarcinoma. N Engl J Med 310:1538, 1984.
17. Zheng T, Mayne ST, Holford TR, Boyle P, Liu W, Chen Y, Mador M, Flannery J. The time trend and age-period-cohort effects on incidence of adenocarcinoma of the stomach in Connecticut from 1995–1989. Cancer 72:330–340, 1993.
18. Blot WJ, Devesa SS, Kneller RW, Fraumeni JF. Rising incidence of adenocarcinoma of the esophagus and gastric cardia. JAMA 265:1287–1289, 1991.
19. Menke-Pluymers MBE, Hop WCJ, Dees J, van Blankenstein M, Tilanus HW. Risk factors for the development of an adenocarcinoma in columnar-lined (Barrett) esophagus. Cancer 72:1155–1158, 1993.
20. The M, Lee YS. HLA-DR Antigen expression in intestinal-type and diffuse-type gastric carcinoma. Cancer 69:1104–1107, 1992.
21. Cady B, Rossi RL, Silverman ML, Piccione W, Heck TA. Gastric adenocarcinoma: A disease in transition. Arch Surg 124:303–308, 1989.
22. Kim JP, Hur YS, Yang HK. Lymph node metastasis as a significant prognostic factor in early gastric cancer: Analysis of 1136 early gastric cancers. Ann Surg Oncol 2:308–313, 1995.
23. Mok YJ, Koo BW, Whang CW, Kim SM, Maruyama K, Sasako M, Kinoshita T. Cancer of the stomach: A review of two hospitals in Korea and Japan. World J Surg 17:777–782, 1993.
24. Ikeda Y, Mori M, Kamakura T, Haraguchi Y, Saku M, Sugimachi K. Increased incidence of undifferentiated type of gastric cancer with tumor progression in 912 patients with early gastric cancer and 1245 with advanced gastric cancer. Cancer 73:2459–2463, 1994.
25. Siewert JR, Kottcher K, Stein HJ, Roder JD, Busch R. Problem of proximal third gastric carcinoma. World J Surg 19:523–531, 1995.
26. Saario I, Schroder T, Lempinen M, Kivilaakso E, Nordling S. Analysis of 58 patietns surviving more than ten years after operative treatment of gastric cancer. Arch Surg 122:1052–1054, 1987.
27. Msika S, Chastang C, Houry S, Lacaine F, Huguier M. Lymph node involvement as the only prognostic factor in curative resected gastric carcinoma: A multivariate analysis. World J Surg 13:121–123, 1989.
28. Ichikura T, Tominatsu S, Okusa Y, Uefuji K, Tamakuma S. Comparison of the prognostic significance between the number of metastatic lymph nodes and nodal stage based on their location in patients with gastric cancer. J Clin Oncol 11:2194–1900, 1993.
29. Isozaki H, Okajima K, Kawashima Y, Yamada S, Nakata E, Nishimura J, Ichinona T. Prognostic value of the number of metastatic lymph nodes in gastric cancer with radical surgery. J Surg Oncol 53:247–251, 1993.
30. Jakl RJ, Miholic J, Koller R, Markis E, Wolner E. Prognostic factors in adenocarcinoma of the cardia. Am J Surg 169:316–319, 1995.

31. Lee WJ, Lee WC, Houng SJ, Shun CT, Houng RL, Lee PH, Chang KJ, Wei TC, Chen KM. Survival after resection of gastric cancer and prognostic relevance of systematic lymph node dissection: Twenty years experience in Taiwan. World J Surg 19:707–713, 1995.
32. Jatzko GR, Kisborg PH, Denk H, Klimfinger M, Stettner HM. A 10-year experience with Japanese-type radical lymph node dissection for gastric cancer outside of Japan. Cancer 76:1302–1312, 1995.
33. Tso PL, Bringaze WL, Dauterive AH, Correa P, Cohn I. Gastric carcinoma in the young. Cancer 59:1362–1365, 1987.
34. Maeta M, Yamashiro H, Oka A, Tsujitani S, Ikeguchi M, Kaibara N. Gastric cancer in the young, with special reference to 14 pregnancy-associated cases: Analysis based on 2325 consecutive cases of gastric cancer. J Surg Oncol 58:191–195, 1995.
35. Marshall SF, Adamson NE, Jr. Carcinoma of the stomach: Follow-up results in a series of 1708 patients.Surg Clin NA 39:703, 1959.
36. Cady B, Ramsden DA, Stein A, Haggitt RC. Gastric cancer: contemporary aspects. Am J Surg 133:423–429, 1977.
37. Appleby LH. The coeliac axis in the expansion of the operation for gastric carcinoma. Cancer 6:704, 1953.
38. Hoerr SO. Prognosis for carcinoma of the stomach. Surg Gynecol Obstet 137:205–209, 1973.
39. Kockerling F, Reck T, Gall FP. Extended gastrectomy: Who benefits? World J Surg 19:541–545, 1995.
40. Sindelar WF, Kinsella TJ, Tepper JE, DeLaney TF, Maher MM, Smith R, Rosenberg SA, Glatstein E. Randomized trial of intraoperative radiotherapy in carcinoma of the stomach. Am J Surg 165:178–187, 1993.
41. Cady B. Lymph node metastases indicators, but not governors of survival. Arch Surg 119:1067–1072, 1984.
42. Fuchs CS, Mayer RJ. Gastric carcinoma. N Engl J Med 333:32–41, 1995.
43. Nio Y, Tsubono M, Kawabata K, Masai Y, Hayashi H, Meyer C, Inoue K, Tobe T. Comparison of survival curves of gastric cancer patients after surgery accoding to the UICC stage classification and the general rules for gastric cancer study by the Japanese Research Society for Gastric Cancer. Ann Surg 221:47–53, 1993.
44. Shriver CD, Karpeh M, Brennan MF. Extended lymph node dissection in gastric cancer. Surg Oncol Clin NA 2:393–411, 1993.
45. Adachi Y, Oshiro T, Okuyama T, Kamakura T, Mori M, Maehara Y, Sugimachi K. A simple classification of lymph node level in gastric carcinoma. Am J Surg 169:382–385, 1995.
46. Douglass HO, Jr. R2 dissection in the treatment of gastric malignancy. Surg Oncol Clin NA 2:413–458, 1993.
47. Cady B. Comments on the appropriateness of extended resection in gastric adenocarcinoma. Surg Oncol Clin NA 2:459–466, 1993.
48. Bonenkamp JJ, van de Velde CJH, Kampschoer GHM, Hermans J, Hermanek P, Bemelmans M, Gouma DJ, Sasako M, Maruyama K. Comparison of factors influencing the prognosis of Japanese, German, and Dutch gastric cancer patients. World J Surg 17:410–415, 1993.
49. Maruyama K, Sasako M, Kinoshita T, Sano T, Katai H, Okajima K. Pancreas-preserving total gastrectomy for proximal gastric cancer. World J Surg 19:532–536, 1995.
50. Dent DM, Madden MV, Price SK. Randomized comparison of R1 and R2 gastrectomy for gastric carcinoma. Br J Surg 75:110–112, 1988.
51. Bollschweiler E, Boettcher K, Hoelscher AH, Sasako M, Kinoshita T, Maruyama K, Siewert JR. Is the prognosis for Japanese and German patients with gastric cancer really different? Cancer 71:2921–2924, 1993.
52. Dupont JB, Jr., Lee JR, Burton GR, Cohn I, Jr. Adenocarcinoma of the stomach: Review of 1497 cases. Cancer 41:941–947, 1978.
53. Adashek K, Sanger J, Longmire WP, Jr. Cancer of the stomach: Review of consecutive ten year intervals. Ann Surg 219:6–10, 1979.

54. Weed TE, Nuessle W, Ochsner A. Carcinoma of the stomach: Why are we failing to improve survival? Ann Surg 193:407–413, 1981.
55. Feinstein AR, Sosin DM, Wells CK. The Will Rogers phenomenon: stage migration and new diagnostic techniques as a source of misleading statistics for survival in cancer. N Engl J Med 312:1604–1608, 1985.
56. Mendes de Almeida JC, Bettencourt A, Santos Costa C, Mendes de Almeida JM. Curative surgery for gastric cancer: Study of 166 consecutive patients. World J Surg 21:889–895, 1994.
57. Gouzi JL, Huguier M, Fagniez PL, Launois B, Flamant Y, Lacaine F, Paquet JC, Hay JM. Total versus subtotal gastrectomy for adenocarcinoma of the gastric antrum. Ann Surg 209:162–166, 1989.
58. Fisher B, Anderson S, Fisher ER, et al. Significance of ipsilateral breast tumor recurrence after lumpectomy. Lancet 338:327–331, 1991.
59. Balch CM, Urist MM, Karakousis CP, Smith TJ, Temple WJ, Drzewiecki K, Jewell WR, Bartolucci AA, Mihm MC, Jr., Barnhill R, Wanebo HJ. Efficacy of 2-cm surgical margins for intermediate-thickness melanomas (1 to 4 mm): Results of a multi-institutional randomized surgical trial. Ann Surg 221:262–269, 1993.
60. Hundahl SA. Gastric cancer nodal metastases: Biological significance and therapeutic considerations. Surg Oncol Clin NA 5:1–16, 1996.
61. Lerner A, Gonin R, Steele GD, Jr., et al. Etoposide, doxorubicin, and cisplatin chemotherapy for advanced gastric adenocarcinoma. J Clin Oncol 10:536–540, 1992.
62. Severson RK, Davis S. Increasing incidence of primary gastric lymphoma. Cancer 66:1283–1287, 1990.
63. Parsonnet J, Hansen S, Rodriguez L, Gelb AB, Warnke RA, Jellum E, Orentreich N, Vogelmen JH, Friedman GD. *Helicobacter pylori* infection and gastric lymphoma. N Engl J Med 330:1267–1270, 1994.
64. Nakamura S, Akazawa K, Yao T, Tsuneyoshi M. Primary gastric lymphoma: A clinicopathologic study of 233 cases with special reference to evaluation with the MIB-1 index. Cancer 76:1313–1324, 1995.
65. Lim FE, Hartman AS, Tan ECG, Cady B, Meissner WA. Factors in the prognosis of gastric lymphoma. Cancer 39:1715–1720, 1977.
66. Frazee RC, Robert J. Gastric lymphoma treatment, medical versus surgical. Surg Clin NA 72:1283–1287, 1992.

14. New strategies in locally advanced breast cancer

S. Eva Singletary, Kapil Dhingra, and Di-Hua Yu

Introduction

A combined modality approach, with the integration of systemic chemotherapy and/or hormonal therapy with surgery and irradiation, is considered
the standard of care in the treatment of locally advanced breast cancer. Since
the mid-1970s, patients with primary breast cancers larger than 5 cm in diameter (T3, stage IIB), with skin or chest wall involvement (T4, stage IIIB), or
with matted or fixed axillary lymph nodes (N2, stage IIIA), have been treated
at The University of Texas M.D. Anderson Cancer Center with a doxorubicin-
based combination chemotherapy for three to four cycles prior to local
therapy, which is followed by completion of systemic therapy and irradiation
[1]. Because the histological response of tumor shrinkage within the surgical
specimen is a more reliable prognostic indicator than clinical response [2,3],
patients with residual tumor greater than 1 cm^3 in size are crossed over to a
different chemotherapy regimen after surgery. Currently, a promising alternative is the drug paclitaxel (Taxol), which has been shown to be effective even
in tumors that are anthracycline resistant [4,5]. However, it is still unclear
whether this approach will significantly improve overall survival rates.

Although studies such as the National Surgical Adjuvant Breast Protocol
B-18 have not yet confirmed a survival advantage for patients who receive
induction chemotherapy, the use of chemotherapy in patients with intact
tumors prior to surgical intervention may identify patients who have a poorer
prognostic outlook (i.e., patients with four or more positive axillary lymph
nodes after induction chemotherapy) and therefore qualify for dose-intensive
chemotherapy programs or other investigational protocols.

Quality-of-life issues are also important. Experience has shown that induction chemotherapy is well tolerated by patients and that patients who receive
induction chemotherapy can undergo surgical procedures without increased
rates of infection or delayed wound healing [6]. Tumor downstaging may allow
the options of breast-preservation surgery or, if mastectomy is needed, immediate reconstruction. The concern that the surgeon may miss a 'window of
opportunity' to resect operable disease has been allayed by the discovery that
tumor progression rarely occurs during induction chemotherapy. In the few

Raphael E. Pollock (ed.), SURGICAL ONCOLOGY. Copyright © 1997. Kluwer Academic Publishers.
ISBN 0-7923-9900-5. All rights reserved.

patients with tumor progression during chemotherapy, the dismal survival rate reflects a disease process beyond that treatable by the surgical knife.

This chapter addresses the current status of breast-preservation surgery after tumor downstaging, the role of axillary node dissection, the feasibility of immediate reconstruction in selected patients with locally advanced breast cancer, and recent innovative strategies in systemic therapy and basic science research.

Breast-preservation surgery after tumor downstaging

The question of whether breast-preservation surgery should be performed for locally advanced disease was raised because of observations of tumor downstaging after induction chemotherapy in mastectomy specimens that had no evidence of residual tumor or residual tumor less than $1 \, cm^3$. If the primary role of surgery is local control, particularly in patients at high risk of occult micrometastases, the extent of surgery that is necessary after achieving tumor reduction with systemic therapy is unclear.

In a retrospective review at the M.D. Anderson Cancer Center [7] of 143 patients with stages from IIB through selected stage IV (positive supraclavicular lymph nodes) who responded with at least 50% tumor shrinkage to induction combination chemotherapy based on doxorubicin and then underwent complete mastectomy, the most common factors associated with multiple quadrant tumor involvement were persistent skin edema of the breast (65%), residual tumor size larger than 4 cm (56%), extensive intramammary lymphatic invasion (20%), and known mammographic evidence of multicentric disease (16%). According to the eligibility criteria for breast preservation (Table 1), 33 (23%) of these 143 patients could have had a segmental mastectomy (wide local excision) and axillary node dissection rather than a modified radical mastectomy. None of these 33 patients were found to have tumor in other quadrants of the breast in the mastectomy specimens, and at a median follow-up of 34 months none had experienced a chest wall recurrence. In contrast, of 110 patients who were considered not good candidates for breast-preservation surgery, 55 (50%) had tumor in other quadrants: 22 (40%) involving two quadrants, 9 (16%) involving three quadrants, and 24 (44%) involving the entire breast.

In a subsequent prospective M.D. Anderson clinical trial (1989–1990) of 203 evaluable patients with stage IIA (primary tumors greater than 2 cm but not exceeding 5 cm), stage IIB, stage IIIA-B, or selected stage IV (positive supraclavicular lymph nodes) breast cancers who completed four cycles of induction chemotherapy (5-fluorouracil, doxorubicin, and cyclophosphamide), breast preservation was elected and performed in 51 (25%) using the previously established criteria (see Table 1). The rate of breast preservation for patients with dermal lymphatic involvement (stage IIIB) was only 6%

Table 1. Criteria for breast-conservation surgery after induction chemotherapy for locally advanced breast cancer

---

Resolution of skin edema (dermal lymphatic involvement)
Residual tumor size <5 cm
Absence of extensive intramammary lymphatic invasion
Absence of extensive suspicious microcalcifications
No known evidence of multicentricity
Patient's desire for breast preservation

---

because of the usual persistence of central skin edema. With a median follow-up of greater than 43 months (range, 29–61 months), only four patients had relapses in the breast, and two of these patients remained disease free after mastectomy.

Other investigators have also described the feasibility of breast preservation after tumor downstaging with induction chemotherapy. Schwartz et al. [8] reported that 39% of stage II and stage III patients who received induction chemotherapy to maximum clinical response underwent breast-preservation surgery. Only one patient in this series developed recurrent disease in the breast; the median follow-up was 29 months. Since 1990, these investigators have performed breast-preservation surgery in approximately three fourths of their patients who have responded to preoperative chemotherapy.

Induction chemotherapy is now being used in patients with smaller primary tumors (2–5 cm). In a pilot study by Bonadonna et al. [9] of 227 women with primary tumors at least 3 cm in diameter without skin or chest wall involvement, patients whose tumors were downstaged by preoperative chemotherapy to less than 3 cm at surgery underwent quadrantectomy (minimum margin of 2 cm) and irradiation (5 fractions for a total dose of 60 Gray in 6 weeks). One of five different drug regimens was used for three to four cycles preoperatively, and additional postoperative chemotherapy (two to three cycles) was given to patients with positive nodes and to those with negative nodes but estrogen receptor-negative tumors. A clinical response of 50% or greater tumor shrinkage by palpation prior to surgery was observed in 78% of patients. Breast preservation was possible in 91% of patients with an initial tumor size of 3–5 cm (n = 183) and in 73% of patients with an initial tumor size larger than 5 cm (n = 37). At a median follow-up of 30 months from completion of preoperative chemotherapy, the local recurrence rate was 2% and the overall survival rate was 93%.

Role of axillary node dissection

Because breast-preservation surgery is often possible on an outpatient basis, under local anesthesia with intravenous sedation, the next question to resolve

255

is whether axillary node dissection can be omitted. As these patients receive systemic therapy based on the initial size of the primary tumor, the staging information obtained from an axillary node dissection after induction chemotherapy would be helpful only in selecting patients who have a poor prognosis and may desire to participate in dose-intensive chemotherapy trials or other investigational studies [10]. Unfortunately, we still do not know if high-dose chemotherapy significantly prolongs survival in the subset of patients with tumors that are resistant to standard chemotherapy.

In the National Surgical Adjuvant Breast Project (NSABP) B-04 trial, which compared radical mastectomy to total mastectomy with or without irradiation [11], the survival rates for patients receiving radical mastectomy and those receiving total mastectomy were equivalent. However, another issue in the role of axillary node dissection is the need for local control of the axilla. Of those patients treated with total mastectomy alone in NSABP B-04, 20% developed regional disease and required a delayed axillary node dissection; fewer than 2% presented with an inoperable axilla. Although up to 33% of patients treated with total mastectomy alone in this protocol did have some axillary lymph nodes removed with the specimen, in keeping with the philosophy of ensuring complete removal of the breast, including the tail of Spence, recent studies [12,13] in which axilla were observed rather than dissected have reported the same range of axillary relapse rates (15–20%). If the assumption was made that occult microscopic nodal disease always led to clinical manifestation of disease, one would have anticipated a relapse rate as high as 50%.

Whether modern-day chemotherapy can substitute for surgical control of the axilla is still unknown. Some investigators have demonstrated a lower rate of locoregional recurrence after mastectomy with adjuvant chemotherapy than after mastectomy and radiotherapy alone [14]. However, the optimal local control of regional recurrence for locally advanced disease was provided by using both systemic therapy and irradiation. The addition of radiation has been shown to decrease the rate of recurrence in the nondissected clinically negative axilla to less than 3% [15,16]. Like the psychological trauma of locoregional recurrence after breast-preservation surgery, this aspect of the benefit-risk ratio of irradiation of the axilla should be considered regardless of whether survival is affected. At M.D. Anderson, patients with T2-3, N0-1 breast cancers who received four cycles of paclitaxel versus 5-fluorouracil, doxorubicin, and cyclophosphamide (FAC) preoperatively and were downstaged to become potential breast-preservation candidates with a clinically negative axilla are randomized to receive either irradiation of the axilla or a standard level I-II axillary node dissection (removal of lymph nodes lateral and posterior to the pectoralis minor muscle). After surgery, systemic therapy (four cycles of FAC) is completed. The breast and nodal basin are consolidated with irradiation, which includes the lower axilla if not dissected, and, in selected patients, the supraclavicular fossa (Fig. 1).

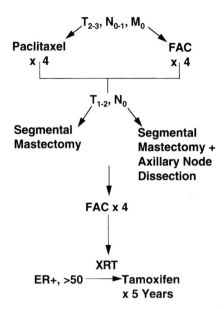

Figure 1. Flow diagram of the M.D. Anderson Cancer Center protocol for treatment of patients with T2-3, N0-1 carcinoma of the breast. FAC = 5-fluorouracil, doxorubicin, cyclophosphamide; XRT = radiation therapy; ER$^+$ = estrogen receptor positive.

Feasibility of immediate breast reconstruction

For patients with locally advanced breast cancer who are not candidates for breast preservation or who elect to have standard mastectomy, controversy exists about whether breast reconstructive surgery should be delayed until completion of both adjuvant chemotherapy and irradiation. One fear, that reconstruction would mask the detection of a locoregional recurrence, led many surgeons to advocate a 2-year waiting period for reconstruction following mastectomy, because the majority of recurrent disease would by then have become manifest.

However, the rate of regional recurrences after mastectomy with immediate reconstruction is the same as after mastectomy without reconstruction. With a median follow-up of 5.4 years, Slavin et al. [17] reported a 11.7% regional recurrence rate in their series of 120 patients who underwent immediate flap reconstruction after a standard mastectomy for stage II or stage III breast cancer. In 545 patients who underwent immediate reconstruction for all stages of breast cancer at M.D. Anderson, the overall incidence of regional recurrence was 2.6%. Of 95 patients who were more than 4 years in follow-up from surgery, the recurrence rate was 4.2%. This incidence is similar to that previously described by Buzdar et al. [14] at M.D. Anderson for patients who underwent mastectomy without reconstruction followed by adjuvant doxorubicin-based chemotherapy. When a regional recurrence develops, it is

257

usually located in the skin or subcutaneous tissue of the mastectomy flap and is detected by physical examination. Routine postmastectomy mammograms of the reconstructed breast mound are not useful and can create confusion if fat necrosis is present [18,19].

Another area of concern was whether immediate reconstruction would hamper the completion of both adjuvant chemotherapy, and, if indicated, irradiation. The experience at M.D. Anderson indicates that immediate reconstruction has not interfered with the resumption of chemotherapy. The risk of complications from immediate reconstruction is very low, especially with the use of a myocutaneous flap [20,21]. Subsequent irradiation of a breast mound reconstructed from autogenous tissue for patients at high risk of regional recurrence or for the treatment of the recurrence has not impaired the flap's blood supply or affected the cosmetic result if there is no pre-existing fat necrosis (Fig. 2). In 19 patients in a series from M.D. Anderson [22] who received postoperative radiotherapy after reconstruction with a transrectus abdominis myocutaneous flap (TRAM) for either known local recurrence (n = 4) or as adjuvant therapy for high risk of recurrence (n = 15), the cosmetic result was dependent on the initial outcome of the reconstruction. If fat necrosis was present, irradiation accentuated the fibrosis and volume loss.

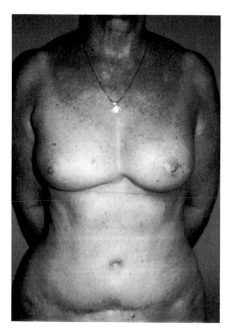

Figure 2. Excellent cosmetic result after postoperative irradiation of the left reconstructed breast mound and nodal basins following a skin-sparing modified radical mastectomy and immediate TRAM reconstruction. Nipple reconstruction was performed later using local skin flaps for the nipple projection with the areola simulated by tattooing. TRAM = transrectus abdominis musculocutaneous flap.

The use of tissue expansion for implant reconstruction before or after irradiation has been disappointing, with a high complication rate as well as patient discomfort and dissatisfaction [23]. The M.D. Anderson series of patients who received submuscular implants revealed that the rates of capsular contrasture (Baker III or greater), pain, implant exposure, and implant removal were significantly high (p = 0.028) in 13 patients with implants within an irradiated field than in 230 patients with implants who received no irradiation [24]. Results were slightly improved when comparing 19 patients with implants placed beneath autogenous reconstruction in an irradiated area to 36 patients with implants and autogenous reconstruction without irradiation (p = 0.717). The optimal result is most likely achieved by avoiding implants and using only autogenous tissue for reconstruction in patients who will receive adjuvant radiotherapy.

Thus, in selected patients with a good response to induction chemotherapy (i.e., tumor shrinkage) who desire immediate breast reconstruction, or when debulking surgical procedures are required, the preference is to use an autogenous tissue flap rather than implants to create a breast mound. If for palliation, it is also preferred to provide skin coverage of the operative defect with a tissue flap and avoid the need for skin grafts [25]. This use of a myocutaneous flap for breast reconstruction before or after irradiation has not interfered with the resumption of chemotherapy or the detection of locoregional recurrence.

Strategies to improve systemic therapy of locally advanced breast cancer

Systemic chemotherapy has been used as the initial treatment for locally advanced breast cancer for over 20 years. Several clinical trials have demonstrated the ability to achieve a partial response (>50% tumor shrinkage) in 50–95% of patients, including a 5–25% clinical complete remission rate by using anthracycline-containing combinations [26–33]. As a consequence of the high frequency of objective responses, downstaging of locally advanced breast cancer can be achieved in approximately 70% of patients [1]. However, a pathological complete remission occurs in only one half to two thirds of patients who achieve a clinical complete remission [1,2]. An important observation in these trials has been the correlation of clinicopathologic response with long-term disease-free survival. Seventy-five percent of patients who achieve a complete remission can be expected to be disease free after a 5-year follow-up, in contrast with patients with a partial or minor response in whom 5-year disease-free survival rates are 30% and 14%, respectively [1,34].

However, despite an aggressive multimodality treatment approach, only 30% of patients can be expected to be long-term survivors [1]. The extent of primary tumor shrinkage is not sufficient to permit breast preservation in many patients [7,8]. Therefore, it is essential to develop new strategies for better local as well as systemic disease control.

Strategies in clinical research

The four types of treatment strategies that have the potential to improve upon current systemic treatments for locally advanced breast cancer include: (1) dose-intensive chemotherapy, (2) non–cross-resistant chemotherapeutic regimens, (3) improved selection and individualization of chemotherapy regimens, and (4) novel targeted therapies.

Dose-intensive chemotherapy

Delivery of high-dose chemotherapy (above conventional maximal tolerated dose) is limited by both myeloid and nonmyeloid toxic effects. Therefore, early attempts at dose escalation generally did not succeed in delivering significantly higher doses of chemotherapy [35]. Hematopoietic growth factors, that is, granulocyte colony-stimulating factor (G-CSF) and granulocyte-macrophage colony-stimulating factor (GM-CSF), allow moderate (25–30%) increases in delivered dose intensity [36–38]. While this degree of increase may appear relatively small, the dose-response curve for breast cancer appears to be quite steep in this range of dose. Therefore, such an increase in dose intensity may translate into a significantly greater antitumor effect [39–41]. Early results from several clinical studies, which show increased response rates with growth factor–supported dose-intensive therapy, have provided direct support for this expectation [36,38]. Unfortunately, the interpretation of many of these trials is confounded by inclusion of both patients with locally advanced breast cancer as well as those with metastatic breast cancer. These two groups of patients differ considerably in extent of disease, tolerance of chemotherapy, extent of prior chemotherapy, and chemosensitivity. Prospective trials to evaluate the clinical therapeutic impact of growth factor–supported, dose-intensive outpatient chemotherapy regimens are in progress [39–41].

At M.D. Anderson, a prospective, randomized trial was initiated in 1991 to compare standard FAC (5-FU, $500\,mg/m^2$, days 1 and 3; Adriamycin (doxorubicin), $50\,mg/m^2$ by infusion over 48 hours; and cyclophosphamide, $500\,mg/m^2$, day 1) with escalated-dose FAC (5-FU, $600\,mg/m^2$, days 1 and 3; doxorubicin, $60\,mg/m^2$ by infusion over 48 hours; cyclophosphamide, $1000\,mg/m^2$, day 1) + G-CSF (Amgen, Inc.). Four cycles of induction chemotherapy were given to patients with locally advanced breast cancer in an attempt to downstage the disease. Preliminary results from the first 97 patients [42] showed that high-dose FAC + G-CSF resulted in a statistically significant higher response rate (76% vs. 98%; $p = 0.002$) and degree of downstaging of disease (53% vs. 77%; $p = 0.02$). However, this was achieved at the expense of a significantly higher requirement for platelet and packed red blood cell transfusion and a higher incidence of neutropenic fever despite G-CSF administration. Thus, these results show the need for improved support for trilineage hematopoiesis to ameliorate the toxicity and to further increase the antitumor efficacy. The next generation of trials in this area should evaluate the roles of thrombopoietin and stem-cell growth factor in enhancing the effectiveness of this regimen.

The use of hematopoietic stem cells, obtained from either peripheral blood or bone marrow, can permit the administration of higher doses of chemotherapy than can be delivered in conjunction with only myeloid growth factors. Because of its significant morbidity, early trials of high-dose chemotherapy followed by autologous stem-cell rescue were confined to patients with metastatic breast cancer. Recent trials have begun to investigate high-dose chemotherapy potential clinical usefulness for patients with high-risk primary breast cancer (e.g., those with ≥ 10 positive lymph nodes or with locally advanced breast cancer and ≥ 4 positive lymph nodes after neoadjuvant chemotherapy) [43,44]. Aggressive utilization of outpatient resources has reduced the need for hospitalization and, therefore, the cost of such programs. Further improvements in this area can be expected from optimization of high-dose chemotherapy regimens and availability of trilineage hematopoietic growth factors.

Non–cross-resistant chemotherapy programs

Anthracycline-containing regimens have been the mainstay for neoadjuvant chemotherapy of locally advanced breast cancer [26,28–33]. The use of potentially non–cross-resistant regimens is a conceptually attractive proposition to improve the response and survival rates. Until recently, this strategy was limited by the number of potentially effective drugs. The addition of methotrexate and Vinca alkaloids to anthracycline-containing adjuvant therapy programs did not substantially alter the outcome. The discovery of several new, effective chemotherapeutic agents, for example, taxanes (paclitaxel and docetaxel) and vinorelbine, has sparked renewed interest in this area. Whether these drugs can be beneficial to patients receiving anthracycline-containing combinations will be determined by the results of clinical trials now in progress (see Fig. 1).

Prediction of therapeutic responsiveness

The clinical response to an induction chemotherapy regimen may range from no response to a complete remission. If the chemosensitivity of a breast tumor could be predicted before or soon after initiation of chemotherapy, it would facilitate the selection of an optimal treatment regimen for that particular tumor. A number of cellular proteins involved in mediating drug resistance have been identified, including MDR1 (multidrug resistance or P-glycoprotein), MRP (multidrug resistance–associated protein), glutathione S-transferase, and dihydrofolate reductase [45]. In primary breast cancer, P-glycoprotein expression is generally infrequent [46,47], but in patients with locally advanced breast cancer, it is detectable at a high frequency and appears to be associated with a poor response to chemotherapy [48,49]. Most of the other drug resistance–associated proteins are not detectable at a sufficiently high frequency, have not been studied in adequate detail, or are not reliable enough in predicting in vivo drug resistance. Several investigators have considered the use of in vitro chemosensitivity-directed therapy. Older in vitro assays did not meet widespread clinical acceptance because they required prolonged cultures and could not be performed in all cases. They could predict chemoresistance accurately, but they were poor predictors of chemosensitivity. The newer assays that do not involve extended culture of breast tumor cells and preserve cellular spatial relationships hold promise in this regard [50]. Even if these assays predict chemoresistance only, they may allow exclusion of ineffective chemotherapy drugs from the treatment combination and allow dose escalation of potentially effective drugs, especially in conjunction with hematopoietic growth factors.

Prediction of chemosensitivity based on the in-vivo effects of chemotherapeutic drugs on the tumor is a relatively new area of investigation. Changes in flow cytometric DNA profiles and nuclear morphometric features in sequential fine-needle aspirates obtained from breast tumors before and after administration of chemotherapy have been shown to correlate with subsequent objective tumor regression in some pilot studies but not in others [51,52]. More detailed studies are needed to investigate the optimal time for the performance of flow cytometry following chemotherapy. Furthermore, these studies need to be performed in conjunction with an assessment of cell cycle checkpoints (e.g., *p53*), which are important determinants of chemosensitivity in breast tumor cells [53].

While flow cytometry measures alterations in DNA content and cell cycle characteristics, positron emission tomography allows an assessment of metabolic alterations in breast tumors following chemotherapy. In pilot studies, decreased radiotracer uptake was detected 1–2 weeks after the first course of chemotherapy in the majority of patients who eventually demonstrated a major clinical response [54,55]. The utility of magnetic resonance imaging has also been investigated in a similar fashion in preliminary studies. More detailed prospective studies are needed to determine if these relatively expensive modalities can be utilized with sufficient accuracy and cost effectiveness so as to justify their routine use during neoadjuvant chemotherapy.

Newer targets for therapy

Rapid advances in our understanding of molecular genetic and biochemical changes underlying mammary carcinogenesis have led to the identification of several specific targets for novel therapeutic approaches [56]. These include genetic alterations, such as amplified/activated oncogenes and inactivated/deleted tumor suppressor genes, as well as transcriptional/post-transcriptional abnormalities of cellular proteins [57]. The potential approaches to target these molecules include monoclonal antibodies, either alone or conjugated to chemical toxins/prodrugs/radioisotopes, active specific immunotherapy (i.e., vaccines), and gene therapy (i.e., transfection of genetic material) to either suppress an oncogene or to replace the product of an inactivated tumor suppressor gene [57–62]. An advantage of these approaches is that they target critical lesions that are relevant to tumor biology. More importantly, they are tumor specific, in contrast to most chemotherapeutic agents, which kill proliferating normal as well as tumor cells. All of these approaches are in early stages of development. Critical issues of delivery to the target site and antitumor efficacy are being addressed in a number of phase I/II trials. Over the next few years, the more effective approaches will probably begin to be tested in primary locally advanced breast cancer.

An interesting observation in these trials has been the synergistic interaction of these novel targeted therapies with conventional chemotherapeutic agents. For example, antibodies against c-erbB-2 and epidermal growth factor receptor (EGFR) oncogene products (both are cell-surface tyrosine kinase receptors) can synergize with cisplatin, doxorubicin and cyclophosphamide to kill breast cancer cells [63,64]. This concept is now being tested in the adjuvant setting by using a combination of doxorubicin, cyclophosphamide, and an antibody against the c-erbB-2 protein.

Strategies in basic science research

The c-erbB-2 gene (also known as HER-2, neu, or NGL) encodes a transmembane protein of 185 kDa, p185, which has extensive sequence homology to EGFR [65,66]. Similar to EGFR, p185 is a transmembrane glycoprotein with intrinsic tyrosine kinase activity [67–69]. Amplification or overexpression of the c-erbB-2 gene has been found in 20–30% of the tumors of breast cancer patients [70]. Patients whose breast cancers overexpress c-erbB-2 have a significantly lower survival rate and a shorter time to relapse than patients whose tumors do not overexpress the gene. Moreover, high levels of expression of p185 in the tumor have been positively correlated with lymph node metastasis in breast cancers [70–73]. We have demonstrated that expression of the mutation-activated rat neu oncogene is sufficient to induce higher metastatic potential in 3T3 cells [74] and that overexpression of p185 enhances the metastatic potential of human lung cancer cells [75]. Recent investigations focusing on c-erbB-2 expression and breast cancer response to therapy indicate that c-erbB-2 may have value in predicting response to certain treatments.

C-erbB-2 expression and breast cancer response to chemotherapy

Nonresponsiveness of some breast cancer cells to chemotherapy and the appearance of resistant cell populations upon relapse pose major obstacles to the ultimate success of the cancer therapy. Standard combination chemotherapeu-

263

tic regimens, consisting of either cyclophosphamide/methorexate/5-fluorouracil (CMF) or cyclophosphamide/doxorubicin/5-fluorouracil (CAF), are associated with response rates in previously untreated patients of 35–80% and in previously treated patients of 10–40% [76]. One clinical study has demonstrated that breast tumors that overexpress c-erbB-2/neu were less responsive to CMF-containing adjuvant chemotherapy regimens than those tumors that express a normal amount of the gene product [77]. It has also been reported that patients with node-positive early breast tumors that overexpress c-erbB-2 may benefit from higher doses of chemotherapy [78].

In another investigation, the influence of the pattern of c-erbB-2–encoded p185 immunostaining (membranous or cytoplasmic) on outcome in node-positive patients who did or did not receive adjuvant therapy was examined. This investigation revealed that the difference in survival rates between cases with positive and negative staining was only significant among patients receiving adjuvant chemotherapy or hormone therapy [79]. However, other investigators found no survival correlation with c-erbB-2 or p53 protein expression when examined by immunohistochemistry in a limited series of 81 patients with primary breast carcinomas treated with an adjuvant chemotherapy with a median follow-up of 5 years [80].

C-erbB-2 expression and breast cancer response to endocrine therapy

Growth of human breast cells is closely regulated by steroid hormone as well as peptide hormone receptors. Members of both receptor classes are important prognostic factors in human breast cancer. Clinical data indicate that overexpression of the c-erbB-2 gene is associated with an estrogen receptor–negative phenotype. For example, in a nonrandomized study of 871 primary invasive breast tumors, c-erbB-2 activation was significantly correlated with shorter disease-free and overall survival in the subgroup of patients receiving adjuvant tamoxifen therapy but not in the untreated group. Further subcategorization demonstrated the relationship to poor prognosis to be confined to lymph node–positive and steroid receptor–positive tumors [81]. This observation suggests that steroid receptor–positive and c-erbB-2–positive breast tumors are resistant to tamoxifen therapy. Another recent study demonstrated that estrogen receptor–positive breast cancer patients with elevated serum p185 levels are less likely to respond to hormone treatment than patients with nondetectable or low levels of p185 [82]. In an effort to clarify the potential of oncogene amplifications as markers for the prediction of relapse-free survival and response to first-line endocrine therapy and subsequent chemotherapy in patients with recurrent breast cancer, Berns et al. found that c-erbB-2/neu amplification was associated with a less favorable response to endocrine therapy; the objective response rate was only 17% and the progression-free survival rate only 4% at 12 months in patients who developed metastatic disease and who had received first-line hormonal therapy (n = 114)

[83]. These data demonstrate a link between the hormone receptor and growth factor receptor pathways and suggest that one mechanism for development of endocrine resistance in human breast cancers may involve overexpression of the c-erbB-2/neu receptor.

Evidence from laboratory investigations

In addition to the reported clinical correlations between overexpression of c-erbB-2 and resistance to chemotherapy and hormone therapy, experimental data from several laboratory studies have provided more direct evidence that c-erbB-2 overexpression can confer drug resistance in cancer cells.

Tsai et al. assessed the differences in c-erbB-2/neu messenger RNA expression and in-vitro drug sensitivity [as IC_{50} values determined by the tetrazolium-based methylthiotetrazole (MTT) assay] to doxorubicin, carmustine, cisplatin, melphalan, mitomycin, and etoposide in a panel of 20 non–small-cell lung carcinoma cell lines (NSCLC) cell lines established from untreated patients [84]. They found a statistically significant correlation between the IC_{50} values for all six drugs and the degree of HER-2/neu gene expression in all 20 cell lines (r = 0.67–0.86; p < 0.005). These findings indicate that overexpression of c-erbB-2/neu is a marker for intrinsic multidrug resistance in NSCLC cell lines. Recently, it has been further demonstrated that NSCLC cell line H460 transfected with c-erbB-2 cDNA manifested enhanced expression of p185, which led to intrinsic chemoresistance to doxorubicin, cisplatin, mitomycin, and etoposide [85].

Several studies have demonstrated that anti-p185 antibodies are synergistic with chemotherapeutic drugs (such as cisplatin) in inhibiting breast and ovarian cancer cell growth in vitro [86–88]. In an earlier study, Hancock et al. used a monoclonal antibody (TAb 250) specific to an extracellular epitope of the c-erbB-2 protein (gp185). TAb 250 inhibited the in-vitro proliferation of human breast tumor cell lines that overexpress c-erbB-2 in a dose-dependent manner [86]. Treatment of cells with combinations of cis-diammedichloroplatinum (CDDP) and TAb 250 resulted in a significantly enhanced cytotoxic effect in cell lines exhibiting high levels of p185, but not in a cell line exhibiting no detectable level of p185. This synergistic cytotoxicity was apparent at antibody concentrations that showed no inhibitory effect alone. Athymic mice bearing subcutaneous xenografts of human tumor cells expressing high levels of p185 showed a greatly enhanced inhibition of tumor growth when treated with TAb 250 and CDDP than with the antibody or CDDP alone. However, TAb 250 did not enhance the growth-inhibitory effect of CDDP on tumor xenografts that were not expressing p185.

Benz et al. assessed the chemo-endocrine sensitivity of estrogen receptor–positive MCF-7 breast cancer cells transfected with full-length c-erbB-2/HER-2 cDNA [89]. These p185-overexpressing transfectants had acquired two- to fourfold resistance to cisplatin and were no longer sensitive to the antiestrogen tamoxifen. In addition, the MCF/HER2 tumors in nude mice exhibited hormone-dependent, tamoxifen-resistant growth, which supports the possibility that p185 overexpression in human breast cancers is linked to resistance to therapy.

To further examine the relationship between overexpression of the c-erbB-2/*neu*–encoded p185 protein and increased drug resistance in human breast cancer cells, Yu et al. tested a panel of established human breast cancer cell lines that express p185 at different levels for their sensitivity to the chemotherapy agents paclitaxel and docetaxel [90]. Higher levels of expression of p185 in these cell lines correlated with increased resistance to paclitaxel and docetaxel. N29 monoclonal antibodies that can specifically downregulate p185 were able to sensitize the p185-overexpressing breast cancer cells to paclitaxel. To further investigate whether p185 overexpression can indeed lead to increased paclitaxel resistance, human c-erbB-2/*neu* cDNA was inserted into the very low p185-expressing MDA-MB-435 human breast cancer cells, and paclitaxel sensitivities were examined among the parental MDA-MB-435 cells and stable transfectants with increased expression of p185. The p185-overexpressing MDA-MB-435 transfectants were more resistant to paclitaxel than the parental cells. The increased resistance to paclitaxel and docetaxel was found only in c-erbB-2/*neu*–transformed cells. These data indicate that overexpression of p185 can lead to intrinsic paclitaxel resistance.

Conclusions

The goals of surgery in locally advanced breast cancer are to obtain adequate locoregional control with minimal disfigurement and to enable accurate staging to determine prognosis and assist in clinical decision making. Close cooperation and clear communication between members of the multidisciplinary breast cancer team are necessary to determine whether the patient is a candidate for breast preservation, or immediate reconstruction if mastectomy is performed. Translational research that brings new treatment concepts from the laboratory to the clinical arena is essential for progress to continue in the management of locally advanced breast cancer.

References

1. Hortobagyi GN, Ames FC, Buzdar AU, Kau SW, McNeese MD, Paulus D, Hug V, Holmes FA, Romsdahl MM, Fraschini G, McBride CM, Martin RG, Montague E. Management of stage III primary breast cancer with primary cheomotherapy, surgery, and radiation therapy. Cancer 62:2507–2516, 1988.
2. Feldman LD, Hortobagyi GN, Buzdar AU, Ames FC, Blumenschein GR. Pathological assessment of response to induction chemotherapy in breast cancer. Cancer Res 46:2578–2581, 1986.

3. McCready DR, Hortobagyi GN, Kau SW, Smith TL, Buzdar AU, Balch CM. The prognostic significance of lymph node metastases after preoperative chemotherapy for locally advanced breast cancer. Arch Surg 124:21–25, 1989.
4. Holmes FA, Walters RS, Theriault RL, Forman AD, Newton LK, Raber MN, Buzdar AU, Frye DK, Hortobagyi GN. Phase II trial of Taxol, an active drug in the treatment of metastatic breast cancer. J Natl Cancer Inst 83:1797–1805, 1991.
5. Pazdur R, Kudelka AP, Kavanagh JJ, Cohen PR, Raber MN. The taxoids: Paclitaxel (Taxol) and docetaxel (Taxotere). Cancer Treat Rev 19:351–386, 1993.
6. Broadwater JR, Edwards MJ, Kuglen C, Hortobagyi GN, Ames FC, Balch CM. Mastectomy following preoperative chemotherapy. Ann Surg 213:126–129, 1991.
7. Singletary SE, McNeese MD, Hortobagyi GN. Feasibility of breast conservation surgery after induction chemotherapy for locally advanced carcinoma. Cancer 69:2849–2852, 1992.
8. Schwartz GF, Birchansky CA, Komarnicky LT, Mansfield CM, Cantor RI, Biermann WA, Fellin FM, McFarlane J. Induction chemotherapy followed by breast conservation for locally advanced carcinoma of the breast. Cancer 73:362–369, 1994.
9. Bonadonna G, Veronesi U, Brambilla C, Ferrari L, Passoni P, Coopmands de Yoldi GF, Luini A, Greco M, Valagussa P. Primary chemotherapy for resectable breast cancer. Recent Results Cancer Res 127:113–117, 1993.
10. Lin PP, Allison DC, Wainstock J, Miller KD, Dooley WC, Friedman N, Baker RR. Impact of axillary lymph node dissection on the therapy of breast cancer patients. J Clin Oncol 11:1536–1544, 1993.
11. Fisher B, Redmond C, Fisher ER, Bauer M, Wolmark N, Wickerham L, Deutsch M, Montague E, Margolese R, Foster R. Ten-year results of a randomized clinical trial comparing radical mastectomy and total mastectomy with or without radiation. N Engl J Med 312:674–681, 1985.
12. Cady B. The need to reexamine axillary lymph node dissection in invasive breast cancer. Cancer 73:505–508, 1994.
13. Lythgoe JP, Palmer MK. Manchester regional breast study — 5 and 10 year results. Br J Surg 69:693–696, 1982.
14. Buzdar AU, McNeese MD, Hortobagyi GN, Smith TL, Kau S, Fraschini G, Hug V, Ellerbrock N, Holmes FA, Ames F, Singletary SE. Is chemotherapy effective in reducing the local failure rate in patients with operable breast cancer? Cancer 65:394–399, 1990.
15. Haffty BG, McKhann C, Beinfield M, Fischer D, Fischer JJ. Breast conservation therapy without axillary dissection. Arch Surg 128:1315–1319, 1993.
16. Taylor ME, Perez CA, Garcia DM, Myerson R, Philpott G, Levy J, Simpson JR, Tucker G, Rush C. Regional nodal management and patterns of failure following conservative surgery and radiation therapy for stage I and II breast cancer. Int J Radiat Oncol Biol Phys 26:593–599, 1993.
17. Slavin SA, Love SM, Goldwyn RM. Recurrent breast cancer following immediate reconstruction with myocutaneous flaps. Plast Reconstr Surg 93:1191–1204, 1994.
18. Holmes FA, Singletary SE, Kroll S, Holbert JM, Paulus DD, Libshitz HI, Sniege N. Fat necrosis in an autogeneously reconstructed breast mimicking recurrent carcinoma at mammography. Breast Dis 1:211–218, 1988.
19. Lee CH, Poplack SP, Stahl RS. Mammographic appearance of the transverse rectus abdominis musculocutaneous (TRAM) flap. Breast Dis 7:99–107, 1994.
20. Kroll SS, Ames FC, Singletary SE, Schusterman MA. The oncologic risks of skin preservation at mastectomy when combined with immediate reconstruction of the breast. Surg Gynecol Obstet 172:17–20, 1991.
21. Schusterman MA, Kroll SS, Miller MJ, Reece GP, Baldwin BJ, Robb GL, Altmyer CS, Ames FC, Singletary SE, Ross MI, Balch CM. The free TRAM flap for breast reconstruction: One center's experience with 211 consecutive cases. Ann Plast Surg 32:234–241, 1994.
22. Hunt K, Baldwin B, Singletary E, Ames F, Strom E, McNeese M, Kroll S. Postoperative radiotherapy does not interfere with TRAM flap viability or cosmetic results in patients with

high risk breast cancer. Proceedings of the 48th Cancer Symposium of the Society of Surgical Oncology, abstract 30, 1995, p 43.

23. Halpern J, McNeese MD, Kroll SS, Ellerbroek N. Irradiation of prosthetically augmented breasts: A retrospective study on toxicity and cosmetic results. Int J Radiat Oncol Biol Phys 18:189–191, 1990.
24. Evans GRD, Schusterman MA, Kroll SS, Miller MJ, Reece GP, Robb GL, Ainslie N. Reconstruction and the radiated breast: Is there a role for implant? Proceedings of the 48th Cancer Symposium of the Society of Surgical Oncology, abstract 106, 1995, p 62.
25. Singletary SE. Surgical management of locally advanced breast cancer. Semin Radiat Oncol 4:254–259, 1994.
26. Touboul E, Lefranc J-P, Blondon J, Ozsahin M, Mauban S, Schwartz LH, Schlienger M, Laugier A, Guerin RA. Multidisciplinary treatment approach to locally advanced noninflammatory breast cancer using chemotherapy and radiotherapy with or without surgery. Radiother Oncol 25:167–175, 1992.
27. Hortobagyi GN, Blumenschein GR, Spanos W, Montague E, Buzdar A, Yap H, Schell F. Multimodal treatment of locoregionally advanced breast cancer. Cancer 51:763–786, 1983.
28. DeLena M, Zucali R, Viganotti G, Valagussa P, Bonadonna G. Combined chemotherapy-radiotherapy approach in locally advanced (T3b-T4) breast cancer. Cancer Chemother Pharmacol 1:53–59, 1978.
29. DeLena M, Varini M, Zucali R, Rovini D, Viganotti G, Valagussa P, Veronesi U, Bonadonna G. Multimodal treatment for locally advanced breast cancer. Results of chemotherapy-radiotherapy versus chemotherapy-surgery. Cancer Clin Trials 4:229–236, 1981.
30. Rubens RD, Sexton S, Tong D, Winter PJ, Knight RK, Hayward JL. Combined chemotherapy and radiotherapy for locally advanced breast cancer. Eur J Cancer 16:351–356, 1980.
31. Hobar PC, Jones RC, Schouten J, Leitch AM, Hendler F. Multimodality treatment of locally advanced breast carcinoma. Arch Surg 123:951–955, 1988.
32. Conte PF, Alama A, Bertelli G, Canavese G, Carnino F, Catturich A, DiMarco E, Gardin G, Jacomuzzi A, Monzeglio C, Mossetti C, Nicolin A, Pronzato P, Rosso R. Chemotherapy with estrogenic recruitment and surgery in locally advanced breast cancer: Clinical and cytokinetic results. Int J Cancer 40:490–494, 1987.
33. Perloff M, Lesnick GJ, Korzun A, Chu F, Holland JF, Thirlwell MP, Ellison RR, Carey RW, Leone L, Weinberg V, Rice MA, Wood WC. Combination chemotherapy with mastectomy or radiotherapy for stage III breast carcinoma: A cancer and leukemia group B study. J Clin Oncol 6:261–269, 1988.
34. Jacquillat C, Baillet F, Weil M, Auclerc G, Housset M, Auclerc MF, Sellami M, Jindani A, Thill L, Soubrane C, Khayat D. Results of a conservative treatment combining induction (neoadjuvant) and consolidation chemotherapy, hormonotherapy, and external and interstitial irradiation in 98 patients with locally advanced breast cancer (IIIA–IIIB). Cancer 61:1977–1982, 1987.
35. Hortobagyi GN, Buzdar AU, Bodey GP, Kau S, Rodriguez V, Legha SS, Yap H-Y, Blumenschein GR. High-dose induction chemotherapy of metastatic breast cancer in protected environment: A prospective randomized study. J Clin Oncol 5:178–184, 1987.
36. Ardizzoni A, Venturini M, Sertoli MR, Giannessi PG, Brema F, Danova M, Testore F, Mariani GL, Pennucci MC, Queirolo P, Silvestro S, Bruzzi P, Lionetto R, Latini F, Rosso R. Granulocyte-macrophage colony-stimulating factor (GM-CSF) allows acceleration and dose intensity increase of CEF chemotherapy: A randomised study in patients with advanced breast cancer. Br J Cancer 69:358–391, 1994.
37. Mamounas EP, Anderson S, Wickerham DL, Clark R, Stoller R, Hamm JT, Stewart JA, Bear HD, Glass AG, Bornstein R, Fisher B. The efficacy of recombinant human granulocyte colony-stimulating factor and recombinant human granulocyte macrophage colony-stimulating factor in permitting the administration of higher doses of cyclophosphamide in a doxorubicin-cyclophosphamide combination. Am J Clin Oncol 17:374–381, 1994.
38. Van Hoef MEHM, Baumann I, Lange C, Luft T, de Wyneter EA, Ranson M, Morgenstern

GR, Yvers A, Dexter TM, Testa NG, Howell A. Dose-escalating induction chemotherapy supported by lenograstim preceding high-dose consolidation chemotherapy for advanced breast cancer. Ann Oncol 3:217–224, 1994.

39. Hryniuk WM. Average relative dose intensity and the impact on design of clinical trials. Semin Oncol 14:65–74, 1987.

40. Focan C, Andrien JM, Closon MT, Dicato M, Driesschaert P, Focan-Henrard D, Lemaire M, Lobelle JP, Longree L, Ries F. Dose-response relationship of epirubicin-based first-line chemotherapy for advanced breast cancer: A prospective randomized trial. J Clin Oncol 11:1253–1263, 1993.

41. Wood WC, Budman DR, Korzun AH, Cooper MR, Younger J, Hart RD, Moore A, Ellerton JA, Norton L, Ferree CR, Ballow AC, Frei E III, Henderson IC. Dose and dose intensity of adjuvant chemotherapy for stage II, node-positive breast carcinoma. N Engl J Med 330:1253–1259, 1994.

42. Dhingra K, Singletary E, Strom E, Sahin A, Esparza L, Valero V, Booser D, Walters R, Hortobagyi G. Randomized trial of G-CSF (Filgrastim)-supported dose-intense neoadjuvant chemotherapy in locally advanced breast cancer (abstr). Proc Am Soc Clin Oncol 14:94, 1995.

43. Peters WP, Ross M, Vredenburgh JJ, Meisenberg B, Marks LB, Winer E, Kurtzberg J, Bast RC, Jones R, Shpall E, Wu K, Rosner G, Gilbert C, Mathias B, Coniglio D, Petros W, Henderson IC, Norton L, Weiss RB, Budman D, Hurd D. High-sose chemotherapy and autologous bone marrow support as consolidation after standard-dose adjuvant therapy for high-risk primary breast cancer. J Clin Oncol 11:1132–1143, 1993.

44. Fay J, Jones S, Lynch J, Herzig N, Christiansen L, Pineiro L, Collins R Jr, Freeman B, Herzig G. The treatment of primary breast cancer with intensive thiotepa, cyclophosphamide and hematopoietic stem cell transplantation — a phase II trial of the North American Marrow Transplant group (abstr). Proc Am Soc Clin Oncol 14:117, 1995.

45. Biedler JL. Drug resistance: Genotype versus phenotype — thirty-second G.H.A. Clowes Memorial Award lecture. Cancer Res 54:666–678, 1994.

46. Schneider J, Bak M, Efferth TH, Kaufmann M, Mattern J, Volm M. P-glycoprotein expression in treated and untreated human breast cancer. Br J Cancer 60:815–818, 1989.

47. Hennequin E, Delvincourt C, Pourny C, Jardillier J-C. Expression of mdr1 gene in human breast primary tumors and metastases. Breast Cancer Res Treat 26:267–274, 1993.

48. Ro J, Sahin A, Ro JY, Fritsche H, Hortobagyi G, Blick M. Immunohistochemical analysis of P-glycoprotein expression correlated with chemotherapy resistance in locally advanced breast cancer. Hum Pathol 21:787–791, 1990.

49. Verrele P, Meissonnier F, Fonck Y, Feillel V, Dionet C, Kwiatkowski F, Plagne R, Chassagne J. Clinical relevance of immunohistochemical detection of multidrug resistance P-glycoprotein in breast carcinoma. J Natl Cancer Inst 83:111–116, 1991.

50. Blackman KE, Fingert HJ, Fuller AF, Meitner PA. The fluorescent cytoprint assay in gynecological malignancies and breast cancer. Methodology and results. Contrib Gynecol Obstet 19:53–63, 1994.

51. Brifford M, Spyratos F, Hacene K, Tubiana-Hulin M, Pallud C, Giles F, Rouesse J. Evaluation of breast carcinoma chemosensitivity by flow cytometric DNA analysis and computer assisted image analysis. Cytometry 13:250–258, 1991.

52. O'Reilly SM, Camplejohn RS, Rubens RD, Richards MA. DNA flow cytometry and response to preoperative chemotherapy for primary breast cancer. Eur J Cancer 28:681–683, 1992.

53. Faille A, De Cremoux P, Extra JM, Linares G, Espie M, Bourstyn E, De Rocquancourt A, Giacchetti S, Marty M, Calvo F. p53 mutations and overexpression in locally advanced breast cancers. Br J Cancer 69:1145–1150, 1994.

54. Jansson T, Westlin JE, Ahlström H, Lilja A, Långström B, Bergh J. Positron emission tomography studies in patients with locally advanced and/or metastatic breast cancer: A method for early therapy evaluation. J Clin Oncol 13:1470–1477, 1995.

55. Nieweg OE, Wong W-H, Singletary SE, Hortobagyi GN, Kim EE. Positron emission

tomography of glucose metabolism in breast cancer: Potential for tumor detection, staging, and evaluation of chemotherapy. Ann NY Acad Sci 698:423–428, 1993.

56. Dhingra K, Hittelman WN, Hortobagyi GN. Genetic changes in breast cancer — consequences for therapy? Gene 159:59–63, 1995.

57. Callahan R, Salomon DS. Oncogenes, tumour suppressor genes and growth factors in breast cancer: Novel targets for diagnosis, prognosis and therapy. Cancer Surv 18:35–56, 1993.

58. Powis G, Kozikowski A. Growth factor and oncogene signalling pathways as targets for rational anticancer drug development. Clin Biochem 24:385–397, 1991.

59. Bundgaard H. Prodrugs as a means to improve the delivery of peptide drugs. Adv Drug Deliv Rev 8:1–38, 1992.

60. Kay MA, Ponder KP, Woo SLC. Human gene therapy: Present and future. Breast Cancer Res Treat 21:83–93, 1992.

61. Zhang Y, Yu D, Xia W, Hung M-C. HER-2/neu-targeting cancer therapy via adenovirus-mediated E1A delivery in an animal model. Oncogene 10:1947–1954, 1995.

62. Cox LA, Chen G, Lee EY-HP. Tumor suppressor genes and their roles in breast cancer. Breast Cancer Res Treat 32:19–38, 1994.

63. Baselga J, Norton L, Masui H, Pandiella A, Coplan K, Miller WH, Jr., Mendelsohn J. Antitumor effects of doxorubicin in combination with anti-epidermal growth factor receptor monoclonal antibody. J Natl Cancer Inst 85:1327–1333, 1993.

64. Hancock MC, Langton BC, Chan T, Toy P, Monahan JJ, Mischak RP, Shawver LK. A monoclonal antibody against the c-erbB-2 protein enhances the cytotoxicity of cis-diamminedichloroplatinum against human breast and overian tumor cell lines. Cancer Res 51:4575–4580, 1991.

65. Yamamoto T, Ikawa S, Akiyama T, Semba K, Nomura N, Miyajima N, Saito T, Toyoshima K. Similarity of protein encoded by the human c-erbB-2 gene to epidermal growth factor. Nature 319:230–234, 1986.

66. Bargmann CI, Hung M-C, Weinberg RA. The neu oncogene encodes an epidermal growth factor receptor-related protein. Nature 319:226–230, 1986.

67. Akiyama T, Sudo C, Ogawara H, Toyoshima K, Yamamoto T. The product of the human c-erbB-2 gene: A 185-kilodalton glycoprotein with tyrosine kinase activity. Science 232:1644–1646, 1986.

68. Coussens L, Yang-Feng TL, Liao Y-C, Chen E, Gray A, McGrath J, Seeburg PH, Libermann TA, Schlessinger J, Francke U, Levinson A, Ullrich A. Tyrosine kinase receptor with extensive homology to EGF receptor shares chromosomal location with neu oncogene. Science 230:1132–1139, 1985.

69. Stern DF, Heffernan PA, Weinberg RA. p185, a product of the neu proto-oncogene, is a receptor-like protein associated with tyrosine kinase activity. Mol Cell Biol 6:1729–1740, 1986.

70. Slamon DJ, Godolphin W, Jones LA, Holt JA, Wong SG, Keith DE, Levin WJ, Stuart SG, Udove J, Ullrich A, McGuire WL. Studies of the HER-2/neu proto-oncogene in human breast and ovarian cancer. Science 244:707–712, 1989.

71. Tauchi K, Hori S, Itoh H, Osamura RY, Tokuda Y, Tajima T. Immunohistochemical studies on oncogene products (c-erbB-2, EGFR, c-myc) and estrogen receptor in benign and malignant breast lesions. With special reference to their prognostic significance in carcinoma. Virchows Arch A Pathol Anat Histopathol 416:65–73, 1989.

72. Lacroix H, Iglehart JD, Skinner MA, Kraus MH. Overexpression of c-erbB-2 or EGF-receptor proteins present in early stage mammary carcinoma is detected simultaneously in matched priamry tumors and regional metastasis. Oncogene 4:145–151, 1989.

73. Slamon DJ, Clark GM, Wong SG, Levin WJ, Ullrich A, McGuire WL. Human breast cancer: Correlation of relapse and survival with amplification of the HER-2/neu oncogene. Science 235:177–182, 1987.

74. Yu D, Hung MC. Expression of activated rat neu oncogene is sufficient to induce experimental metastasis in 3T3 cells. Oncogene 6:1991–1996, 1991.

75. Yu D, Wang S-S, Dulski KM, Tsai C-M, Nicolson GL, Hung M-C. C-erbB-2/neu

overexpression enhanced metastatic potential in human lung cancer cells. Cancer Res 54:3260–3266, 1994.

76. Hayes DF, Henderson IC, Shapiro CL. Treatment of metastatic breast cancer: Present and future prospects. Semin Oncol 22:5–21, 1995.

77. Gusterson BA, Gelber RD, Goldhirsch A, Price KN, Save-Soderborgh J, Anbazhagan R, Styles J, Rudenstam C-M, Golouh R, Reed R, Martinez-Tello F, Tiltman A, Torhorst J, Grigolato P, Bettelheim R, Neville AM, Burki K, Castiglione M, Collins J, Lindtner J, Senn H-J, Ludwig IBCSG. Prognostic importance of c-erbB-2 expression in breast cancer. J Clin Oncol 10:1049–1056, 1992.

78. Muss HB, Thor AD, Berry DA, Kute T, Liu ET, Koerner F, Cirrincione CT, Budman DR, Wood WC, Barcos M, Henderson IC. C-erbB-2 expression and response to adjuvant therapy in women with node-positive early breast cancer. N Engl J Med 330:1260–1266, 1994.

79. Tetu B, Brisson J. Prognostic significance of HER-2/neu oncoprotein expression in node-positive breast cancer. The influence of the pattern of immunostaining and adjuvant therapy. Cancer 73:2359–2365, 1994.

80. Jacquemier J, Penault-Llorc F, Viens P, Houvenaeghel G, Hassoun J, Torrente M, Adelaide J, Birnbaum D. Breast caner response to adjuvant chemotherapy in correlation with erbB2 and p53 expression. Anticancer Res 14:2773–2778, 1994.

81. Borg A, Baldetorp B, Ferno M, Killander D, Olsson H, Ryden S, Sigurdsson H. ERBB2 amplification is associated with tamoxifen resistance in steroid-receptor positive breast cancer. Cancer Lett 81:137–144, 1994.

82. Leitzel K, Teramoto Y, Konrad K, Chinchilli VM, Volas G, Grossberg H, Harvey H, Demers L, Lipton A. Elevated serum c-erbB-2 antigen levels and decreased response to hormone therapy of breast cancer. J Clin Oncol 13:1129–1135, 1995.

83. Berns EM, Foekens JA, van Staveren IL, van Putten WLJ, de Koning HY, Portengen H, Klijn JG. Oncogene amplification and prognosis in breast cancer: Relationship with systemic treatment. Gene 159:11–18, 1995.

84. Tsai C-M, Chang K-T, Perng R-P, Mitsudomi T, Chen M-H, Kadoyama C, Gazdar AF. Correlation of intrinsic chemoresistance of non-small-cell lung cancer cell lines with HER-2/neu gene expression but not with ras gene mutation. J Natl Cancer Inst 85:897–901, 1993.

85. Tsai C-M, Yu D, Chang K-T, Wu L-H, Perng PR-P, Ibrahim NK, Hung M-C. Enhanced chemoresistance by elevation of p185[neu] levels in HER-2/neu transfected human lung cancer cells. J Natl Cancer Inst 87:682–684, 1995.

86. Hancock MC, Langton BC, Chan T, Toy P, Monahan JJ, Mischak RP, Shawver LK. A monoclonal antibody against the c-erbB-2 protein enhances the cytotoxicity of cis-diamminedichloroplatinum against human breast and ovarian tumor cell lines. Cancer Res 51:4575–4580, 1991.

87. Pietras RJ, Fendly BM, Chazin VR, Pegram MD, Howell SB, Slamon DJ. Antibody to HER-2/neu receptor blocks DNA repair after cisplatin in human breast cancer and ovarian cancer cells. Oncogene 9:1829–1838, 1994.

88. Arteaga CL, Winnier AR, Poirier MC, Lopez-Larraza DM, Shawver LK, Hurd SD, Stewart SJ. p185c-erbB-2 signaling enhances cisplatin-induced cytotoxicity in human breast carcinoma cells: Association between an oncogenic receptor tyrosine kinase and drug-induced DNA repair. Cancer Res 54:3758–3765, 1994.

89. Benz CC, Scott GK, Sarup JC, Johnson RM, Tripathy D, Coronado E, Shepard HM, Osborne CK. Estrogen-dependent, tamoxifen-resistant tumorigenic growth of MCF-7 cells transfected with HER2/neu. Breast Cancer Res Treat 24:85–95, 1993.

90. Yu D, Liu B, Wang S-S, Sun D, Ibrahim N, Price JE, Sneige N, Hortobagyi GH, Hung M-C. Overexpression of c-cerbB-2/neu in breast cancer cells confers increased resistance to Taxol and Taxotere via mdr-1-independent mechanisms. Oncogene (1996) 13, 1359–1365.

15. Biliary tract cancer

Steven A. Curley

Introduction

Cholangiocarcinomas are malignant tumors that arise from the epithelium of the intrahepatic or extrahepatic bile ducts. Cholangiocarcinomas are rare compared with hepatocellular carcinoma, comprising less than 10% of primary malignancies of the liver [1]. The autopsy incidence of cholangiocarcinoma is low also, being reported in 0.089–0.46% of necropsies [1]. Cholangiocarcinomas are diagnosed most frequently in the fifth and sixth decades of life [2]. There is only a slight male preponderance of cases of cholangiocarcinoma.

Clinical presentation

The clinical features of cholangiocarcinoma are nonspecific and depend on the location of the tumor. Tumors at the liver hilum may cause obstructive jaundice early in the course of the disease, while the primary tumor is still small. Cholangiocarcinomas that arise in peripheral bile ducts within the hepatic parenchyma usually reach a large size before becoming clinically evident. Patients with these large peripheral hepatic tumors usually present with hepatomegaly and an upper abdominal mass, abdominal and back pain, and weight loss [2]. Jaundice and ascites are late and usually preterminal sequelae in patients with large intrahepatic cholangiocarcinomas. Jaundice associated with a large hepatic cholangiocarcinoma is caused by a combination of extension of the tumor to the bifurcation of the left and right hepatic ducts and by compression of contralateral bile ducts by the expanding tumor.

Serum alkaline phosphatase levels are elevated in greater than 90% of patients with cholangiocarcinoma [2]. Serum bilirubin also is elevated in the majority of cholangiocarcinoma patients, particularly in those with a tumor arising in the central portion of the liver or the extrahepatic hilar bile ducts [3]. In contrast to hepatocellular carcinoma, serum alpha fetoprotein (AFP) levels are abnormal in less than 5% of cholangiocarcinoma patients [2]. There is an increase in serum carcinoembryonic antigen (CEA) levels in

Raphael E. Pollock (ed.), SURGICAL ONCOLOGY. Copyright © 1997. Kluwer Academic Publishers. ISBN 0-7923-9900-5. All rights reserved.

40–60% of cholangiocarcinoma patients [2,4]. Another tumor marker, CA 19-9, is elevated in over 80% of patients with cholangiocarcinoma [4]. Mild anemia occurs occasionally, but other serum laboratory studies are usually normal. However, clinically significant hypercalcemia in the absence of bone metastases has been described in several patients with large hepatic cholangiocarcinomas [5]. In one case, the hypercalcemia was shown to be caused by release of parathyroid hormone–related protein by the cholangiocarcinoma [6].

Causative factors

There are distinct differences between the factors associated with cholangiocarcinoma compared with those associated with hepatocellular carcinoma. Cholangiocarcinoma does not appear to be associated with hepatitis B or C virus infection, cirrhosis, or mycotoxin exposure [1]. Only 10–20% of cholangiocarcinomas occur in cirrhotic patients, compared with the 70–90% of hepatocellular carcinomas arising in cirrhotic livers [2,7,8]. Frequently the cirrhosis associated with cholangiocarcinomas is a subacute secondary biliary type that results from the neoplastic obstruction of the bile ducts, indicating that some cases of cirrhosis in cholangiocarcinoma patients are the result of the tumor rather than their cause.

Cholangiocarcinoma is more prevalent in Southeast Asia than in other parts of the world. The higher incidence in this geographic region is related to parasitic infection with the liver flukes *Clonorchis sinensis* and *Opisthorchis viverrini* [9,10]. Infestation by other biliary parasites, such as *Fasciola hepatica* and *Schistosomiasis japonica*, does not appear to have similar carcinogenic effects [11]. Liver flukes induce hyperplasia and adenomatous proliferation of human biliary epithelium and are associated with hepatolithiasis [12]. The association of chronic injury and cellular proliferation associated with liver fluke infestation suggests a direct etiologic role in the subsequent development of cholangiocarcinoma, but this relationship is not established unequivocally. It is interesting to note that in a Syrian Golden hamster model, administration of dimethylnitrosamine alone does not cause neoplasia, but this agent given to animals with liver fluke infection leads to the development of cholangiocarcinomas [13,14].

Several disorders that can produce chronic inflammation of the bile ducts have been associated with an increased risk of developing cholangiocarcinoma. These include polycystic liver disease, choledochal cysts, congenital dilatation of the intrahepatic bile ducts (Caroli's syndrome), sclerosing cholangitis (frequently in association with inflammatory bowel disease), hepatolithiasis, and cholelithiasis [15–22]. Hepatolithiasis is not a common disorder, and only 5–7% of patients with documented hepatic stones develop cholangiocarcinoma [23,24]. Patients who underwent diagnostic radiographs with intravenous injection of thorotrast are at high risk of developing hepatocellular carcinoma, angiosarcoma, and cholangiocarcinoma [25,26]. Cholangiocarcinoma is the most frequent hepatic neoplasm reported in patients who have received thorotrast. Because cholangiocarcinoma is a relatively rare neoplasm, it has been difficult to prove the pathogenesis of cholangiocarcinoma related to any of these factors, but it is clear that chronic inflammation of the biliary tree by any cause is associated with an increased risk of developing cholangiocarcinoma. In patients with sclerosing cholangitis, whether associated with ulcerative colitis or not, radiologic distinction between sclerosing cholangitis and cholangiocarcinoma is often impossible. A recent study showed that the serum tumor marker CA19-9 had an 89% sensitivity and 86% specificity in diagnosing cholangiocarcinoma in patients with sclerosing cholangitis [27]. Combining serum CA19-9 levels with serum CEA levels may further increase the diagnostic accuracy to detect cholangiocarcinoma in patients with sclerosing cholangitis [28].

It has been suggested that hepatocellular carcinoma and cholangiocarcinoma arise from a common hepatic progenitor or 'stem' cell in response to chronic injury and subsequent cellular proliferation [29]. Evidence supporting this theory occurs in patients who present with combined hepatocellular carcinoma and cholangiocarcinoma [30,31]. Approximately 3% of patients with hepatocellular carcinoma have histologic evidence within or adjacent to the cancer of coexistent cholangiocarcinoma [32]. Evaluation of a variety of cell surface markers in the cholangiocarcinoma and hepatocellular carcinoma cells of patients with combined tumors indicates a high degree of homology in the expression of cell surface molecules between the two malignant cell types [30,31]. Furthermore, the only consistent genetic alterations that have been detected in cholangiocarcinomas are loss of heterozygosity in regions of chromosomes 5 and 17 that are also lost in hepatocellular carcinoma [33]. These findings suggest a common origin from a pluripotential cell type in patients with combined hepatocellular carcinoma and cholangiocarcinoma, but definitive proof has not yet been elucidated.

Pathology

Cholangiocarcinomas appear grossly as firm, gray-white tumors. Cholangiocarcinomas originating in the periphery of the hepatic parenchyma usually are solitary and large, but satellite nodules occasionally are present [1,34]. Gross tumor invasion of large portal or hepatic veins occurs much less frequently than in hepatocellular carcinoma. Metastases to regional lymph nodes, the lungs, and the peritoneal cavity are more common in cholangiocarcinoma than in hepatocellular carcinoma. When the tumor causes longstanding biliary obstruction, the liver may show secondary biliary cirrhosis.

Microscopically, cholangiocarcinoma is characterized by low cuboidal cells that resemble normal biliary epithelium (Fig. 1). In more poorly differentiated tumors, solid cords of cells without lumens may be present.

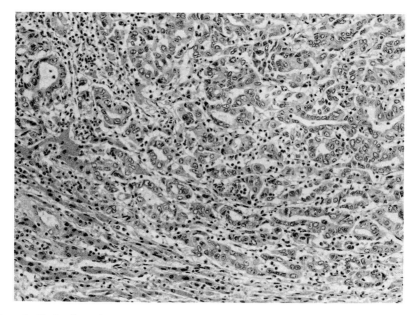

Figure 1. Cholangiocarcinoma of the liver. Large cuboidal cells with prominent nucleoli in diffuse sheets and forming glandular structures. Intracellular and intraluminal mucin can be demonstrated and distinguishes this tumor from hepatocellular carcinoma. Compressed hepatic parenchyma is seen at lower left. Magnification ×187.

Cholangiocarcinomas are mucin-secreting adenocarcinomas, and intracellular and intraluminal mucin often can be demonstrated. The presence of mucin is useful in differentiating cholangiocarcinoma from hepatocellular carcinoma. The absence of bile production by cholangiocarcinoma also is useful in distinguishing this tumor from a hepatocellular carcinoma. Immunohistochemical staining that is positive for epithelial membrane antigen and tissue polypeptide antigen may be useful in confirming a diagnosis of cholangiocarcinoma [35,36]. Varying degrees of pleomorphism, atypia, mitotic activity, hyperchromatic nuclei, and prominent nucleoli are noted from area to area in the same tumor. Cholangiocarcinomas are usually locally invasive with spread along nerves or in subepithelial layers of the bile ducts.

Treatment of intrahepatic cholangiocarcinoma

The majority of patients with intrahepatic cholangiocarcinoma present with large tumors and usually have evidence of regional lymph node, pulmonary, and/or bone metastases at the time of diagnosis. In patients who present with jaundice from large intrahepatic cholangiocarcinomas, death usually ensues within a year of diagnosis. Rarely, small peripheral cholangiocarcinomas that

276

are detected before they metastasize or cause jaundice may be resected with resultant long-term survival [7,37–39]. A study of 19 patients who underwent resection of intrahepatic cholangiocarcinoma demonstrated that patient with no porta hepatis lymph node metastases had a 13-year survival of 64% compared with 0% for patients with nodal metastases [40]. A larger cohort of 32 patients who underwent resection of intrahepatic cholangiocarcinomas confirmed the negative prognostic impact of regional lymph node metastases and large size (>5 cm diameter) of the primary tumor [41].

Orthotopic liver transplantation has been described in patients with intrahepatic cholangiocarcinoma [41–44]. The 1-year survival in series prior to 1990 was 29.4%, with only two of the patients undergoing liver transplantation alive 5 years following the transplant [42]. Almost 90% of the patients who survived at least 90 days after the liver transplant died from recurrent cholangiocarcinoma, frequently at extrahepatic sites. Recent small series of patients describe 5-year post-transplantation survival rates up to 53% [43,44]. The improved survival is based on careful selection of cholangiocarcinoma patients for liver transplantation, specifically by not transplanting patients with lymph node metastases or invasion of major intrahepatic or extrahepatic blood vessels.

Hilar bile duct cholangiocarcinoma

In 1890, Fardel first described a primary malignancy of the extrahepatic biliary tract [45]. A report in 1957 described three patients with small adenocarcinomas involving the confluence of the left and right hepatic ducts [46]. Such primary cholangiocarcinomas arising at the bifurcation of the extrahepatic biliary tree are known commonly as Klatskin's tumors, following his report in 1965 of a larger series of patients with these lesions [47].

Cholangiocarcinomas arising in the hilar bile ducts are relatively rare lesions. Extrahepatic biliary cancer has an incidence of 0.01–0.46% in autopsy series [48]. Of the 17,000 projected new cases of hepatobiliary cancers that occur annually in the United States, approximately 3000 are Klatskin's tumors [49].

Diagnosis

The usual clinical presentation of patients with hilar cholangiocarcinoma is painless jaundice. Patients also may report concomitant onset of fatigue, pruritus, fever, vague abdominal pain, and anorexia. The serum liver function tests in patients with hilar cholangiocarcinoma commonly demonstrate obstructive jaundice, with alkaline phosphatase and total bilirubin levels elevated in greater than 95% and 85% of patients, respectively [50].

The diagnosis of pancreatic cancer is considered frequently in patients presenting with painless jaundice. For this reason, a computed tomography

(CT) scan of the abdomen may be the first radiologic study obtained. Patients with painless jaundice due to pancreatic cancer may or may not have a mass in the head of the pancreas on a CT scan. They will, however, have dilation of the extrahepatic biliary tree and gallbladder. In contrast, a diagnosis of hilar cholangiocarcinoma should be suspected in the patient with painless jaundice whose CT scan demonstrates dilated intrahepatic bile ducts with a normal gallbladder and extrahepatic biliary tree. High-resolution, thin-section CT scans can provide information on the location of an obstructing tumor and on the extent of involvement of the liver and porta hepatis structures by the tumor (Figs. 2–4).

Ultrasound is the simplest noninvasive study for the jaundiced patient. Like the CT scan, ultrasound can demonstrate a nondilated gallbladder and common bile duct associated with dilated intrahepatic ducts [51]. Additionally, as gray-scale ultrasonography has improved, the diagnosis of cholangiocarcinoma is supported by finding a hilar bile duct mass in 65–90% of patients [52,53]. Ultrasound and CT scan also are useful in determining preoperatively the presence of intrahepatic tumor due to direct extension or metastases, portal vein invasion by tumor, and enlarged periportal lymph nodes, suggesting nodal metastases [53,54].

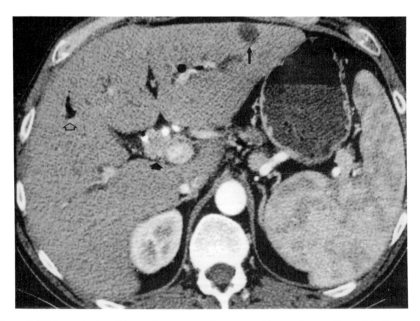

Figure 2. High-resolution, thin-section computed tomographic scan in a patient with obstructive jaundice. The scan demonstrates a tumor (solid arrow) at the hepatic hilum lying anterior and lateral to the portal vein. Dilated intrahepatic bile ducts (open arrow) and a liver metastasis (long arrow) are seen. Biopsy of the hilar tumor confirmed the diagnosis of cholangiocarcinoma.

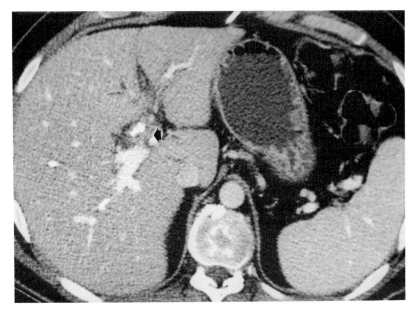

Figure 3. High-resolution, thin-section computed tomographic scan in another patient with obstructive jaundice. The scan demonstrates a tumor at the confluence of the left and right hepatic bile ducts compressing the portal vein (solid arrow). Biopsy of the hilar tumor confirmed the diagnosis of cholangiocarcinoma.

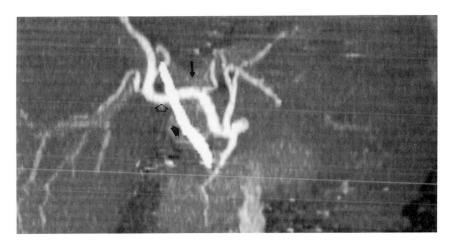

Figure 4. Vascular reconstruction of the hepatic arteries and portal vein from a bolus contrast injection spiral computed tomogram in a patient with hilar cholangiocarcinoma. There is no evidence of vascular invasion on this image, which was confirmed at the time of resection. A biliary stent (solid arrow) is seen overlying the right hepatic artery (open arrow). The portal vein is also evident (long arrow).

279

Cholangiography definitively demonstrates a lesion obstructing the left and right hepatic duct at the hilar confluence (Fig. 5), and percutaneous transhepatic cholangiography (PTC) and endoscopic retrograde cholangiopancreatography (ERCP) are both useful in assessing patients with extrahepatic biliary obstruction. A prospective, randomized comparison of PTC and ERCP in jaundiced patients concluded that both techniques had similar diagnostic accuracies [55]. PTC was 100% accurate at demonstrating obstruction at the confluence of the left and right hepatic ducts, while ERCP had an accuracy of 92% in demonstrating these lesions. ERCP has the additional benefit of providing a pancreatogram. A normal pancreatogram helps to exclude a small carcinoma of the head of the pancreas as a cause of biliary obstruction. Some

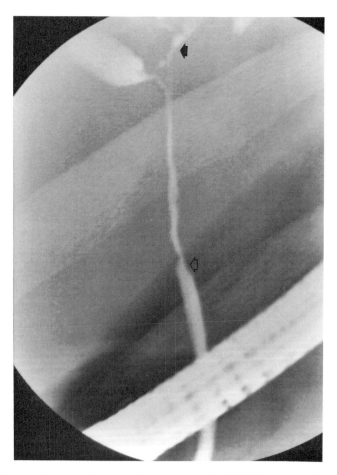

Figure 5. Endoscopic retrograde cholangiopancreatography (ERCP) showing a long stricture of the extrahepatic bile duct extending from the confluence of the left and right hepatic ducts (solid arrow) to the top of the duodenum (open arrow). Brushings obtained at the time of ERCP confirmed a diagnosis of cholangiocarcinoma.

investigators have recommended combined PTC and ERCP to establish the extent of the lesion in the bile ducts; however, such concomitant studies are helpful only in selected patients with complete obstruction of the biliary tree [56]. Cytologic specimens can be obtained at the time of PTC and ERCP. The presence of malignant cells in bile or bile duct brushings is confirmed in approximately 50% of patients undergoing PTC or ERCP [52].

Drainage of the obstructed biliary tree with partial or complete relief of jaundice and associated symptoms can be achieved with PTC. Improvements in catheter technology led to the development of endoprostheses that can be placed across the malignant obstruction into the duodenum to allow internal drainage [57]. It must be emphasized that providing symptomatic relief for patients by decompressing the biliary tract should not be the primary reason to place these catheters. Prospective, randomized studies have failed to demonstrate a benefit in terms of a decrease in hospital morbidity or mortality by preoperative decompression of biliary obstruction [58,59]. However, the catheters are useful in identifying and dissecting the hepatic duct bifurcation at the time of operation and aid in the reconstruction of the biliary tract following extirpation of the tumor [60,61]. Although ERCP can be employed to place an internal stent across a malignant hilar obstruction, the success rate with this procedure is much lower than with PTC [62].

The final radiologic study to consider is celiac and superior mesenteric arteriography with late-phase portography. Arteriography in patients with hilar cholangiocarcinoma is important because extensive encasement of the hepatic arteries or portal vein precludes curative resection. Combining the findings on cholangiography with vascular involvement by tumor on arteriography has been found to have a greater than 80% accuracy in predicting unresectability [63]. However, occasionally a patient will have compression or displacement of vascular structures rather than true malignant invasion or encasement. A high-resolution, thin-section CT scan with intravenous bolus contrast administration can demonstrate hepatic artery and portal vein involvement by a hilar tumor and obviate the need for more invasive angiographic studies. We obtain an arteriogram in less than 10% of our patients with hilar cholangiocarcinoma.

The role of laparoscopy as part of the diagnostic and staging evaluation of patients with hilar cholangiocarcinoma is being evaluated at our institution. Several patients with seemingly resectable tumors have avoided an exploratory laparotomy when peritoneal tumor implants were found with laparoscopy. Additionally, patients at high risk of developing peritoneal carcinomatosis may be identified by positive cytologic specimens obtained from laparoscopic washings.

Prognostic factors

In contrast to reports from two or three decades ago, most patients with hilar cholangiocarcinoma are now diagnosed premortem. The most important factor affecting prognosis is respectability of the tumor. Patients who undergo resection with curative intent have 3-year survival rates as high as 50% and 5-year survival rates between 10% and 44% [64,65]. Significant determinants of improved prognosis in patients undergoing curative resection include well-differentiated tumors, absence of lymph node metastases, absence of direct tumor extension into the liver, papillary histology (vs. nodular or sclerotic), serum bilirubin at presentation of less than 9 mg/dl, and a near-normal or normal performance status [65]. Palliative resection, surgical bypass procedures, and various types of intubation and drainage procedures are associated with 3-year survival rates of 0–4% [66]. Hilar cholangiocarcinomas have a poorer prognosis than do carcinomas arising in the middle or distal thirds of the extrahepatic bile duct, which is related directly to presentation of tumor at a more locally advanced stage with liver involvement by tumor and resultant lower rates of resection.

Pathologic features of the bile duct cancer are predictors of outcome. Prognosis is affected adversely if the tumor infiltrates through the serosa of the bile duct, invades directly into the liver, demonstrates vascular invasion, or has metastasized to regional lymph nodes [67]. Histologic type and grade also are important factors. Patients with the relatively unusual papillary bile duct adenocarcinoma have the most favorable prognosis, with 3-year survival rates up to 75% [66,67]. Patients with the more common nodular or sclerotic types of hilar cholangiocarcinoma have 3-year survival rates of less than 30%. Patients with well or moderately differentiated carcinomas have a 3-year survival rate of 21%, whereas no patient with a poorly differentiated carcinoma survived longer than 2 years [67].

Treatment

Resection. Resection of a hilar cholangiocarcinoma affords the patient the best chance for significant survival; however, 5-year survival rates after resection of hilar cancers are 40% in the most hopeful reports and 10% or less in other accounts. Almost all patients who die after a seemingly curative resection of the extrahepatic bile ducts do so as a result of recurrent tumor.

The patterns of failure after curative extrahepatic bile duct resection for hilar cholangiocarcinoma have been described in a few series of patients (Table 1) [68]. Locoregional tumor recurrence developed in a high percentage of patients, with failure in the liver (62%), tumor bed (42%), and regional lymph nodes (20%). The caudate lobe is the most frequent site of liver recurrence. Regional lymph nodes include porta hepatis, retroduodenal, and perigastric node groups along the gastrohepatic ligament. Distant metastasis develops in the majority of patients who exhibit a locoregional recurrence but was the site of first failure in only 24%.

Detailed anatomic studies have offered an explanation for the high incidence of liver and local recurrence following resection of a hilar cholangiocarcinoma. In a series of 25 patients undergoing surgery for hilar

Site	Frequency (%)
Liver	62
Tumor bed	42
Regional lymph nodes	20
Peritoneum	16
Lungs	71
Bone	31
Skin and subcutaneous tissue	7

cholangiocarcinoma, direct invasion of hepatic parenchyma at the hilum was noted in 12 patients (46.2%), with 11 patients (42.3%) also having carcinoma extending into the bile ducts draining the caudate lobe or directly invading the caudate lobe parenchyma [69]. A study of 106 adult human cadavers showed that 97.2% had bile ducts draining the caudate lobe that entered directly into the main left hepatic duct, right hepatic duct, or both [70]. These caudate lobe bile ducts frequently enter the main left or right hepatic ducts within 1 cm of the proper hepatic duct. Thus, a carcinoma arising at the confluence of the right and left hepatic ducts need not be of a large size to extend into the bile ducts draining the caudate lobe.

Because cholangiocarcinoma is known to spread along the wall of the bile ducts and because the caudate lobe and hepatic hilum are frequent sites of tumor recurrence following extrahepatic duct resection, a number of authors now recommend more aggressive resections to include the caudate lobe and hepatic hilar parenchyma [70–76]. The improved equipment and understanding of techniques requisite for a safe liver resection allow performance of aggressive extended resections with little or no increase in operative morbidity and mortality. The median survival associated with a more radical surgical approach has varied from 10 to 37 months, with 5-year survival rates of 20–44% and 10-year survival rates as high as 14% [70–76]. These studies clearly show that liver resection is worthwhile only if completely tumor-negative resection margins can be attained, because there were no 5-year survivors with positive resection margins. Very extensive operations that include major hepatectomy, resection of the extrahepatic bile ducts, and en-bloc pancreaticoduodenectomy have been used in patients with hilar cholangiocarcinoma [77]. Given the operative mortality rate of at least 30% and a 100% rate of complications combined with rare survival for more than 2 years, such ultraradical procedures are of dubious value.

A multimodality approach to reduce locoregional recurrence rates and improve survival after resection has been reported [78]. Of 53 patients who underwent resection of a hilar cholangiocarcinoma, 38 received postoperative external-beam radiotherapy to the resection bed at a dose of 50–60 Gy. In addition, 27 of these 38 patients received brachytherapy with iridium-192 seeds temporarily loaded into their transhepatic biliary stents in the area of the hepaticojejunostomies. These 27 patients received 20 Gy of internal radiation after completion of external-beam radiotherapy. There was no significant difference in the 1-, 2-, and 3-year survivals for patients who underwent resection with or without radiotherapy, but there were no survivors past 3 years in the group without radiotherapy. The 5- and 10-year survival rates in the group receiving radiotherapy were 11% and 5%, respectively. Stented hepaticojejunostomies allow access to the remaining biliary tree following resection of hilar cholangiocarcinomas and can be used for diagnostic and therapeutic purposes [79].

Liver transplantation. Total hepatectomy with immediate orthotopic liver transplantation has been described in 78 patients with hilar cholangio-carcinoma [43,44,80–92]. The 90-day mortality from hemorrhage, sepsis, and graft rejection was 23.1%. Of the 60 patients who survived more than 3 months following transplantation, the median survival was 11 months. In this same group of 60 patients, the 5-year survival rate was 5.0%. In patients who died more than 3 months after transplantation, death was due to tumor recurrence in 85.4%. Due to these poor results, most transplant centers no longer perform liver transplants in patients with hilar cholangiocarcinoma. Liver transplantation for hilar cholangiocarcinoma should only be considered as part of a prospective protocol evaluating multimodality treatment.

Palliation. In general, curative surgical resection is possible in less than 30% of patients with hilar cholangiocarcinoma [78,93]. In patients deemed unresectable based on the findings of diagnostic studies, laparotomy can be avoided by placing percutaneous external drains or endoscopically placed endoprostheses [94,95]. Conventional 10- or 12-French polyethylene endo-prostheses have a high rate of occlusion and cholangitis. Self-expanding metal stents placed endoscopically appear to provide improved long-term palliation because of lower rates of occlusion and cholangitis [96]. When unresectability is determined at the time of laparotomy, a decision must be made on a surgical bypass versus an operative intubation to provide drainage of the obstructed biliary tree. It is clear that techniques for surgical bypass, operative intubation, and percutaneous external drainage are equivalent in partial or complete relief of jaundice in 70–100% of patients [64]. Seemingly, the only potential advantage to the patient who undergoes surgical bypass instead of operative intubation is the absence of an external drainage catheter in the former group.

The advantage of not having an external biliary drainage catheter or an internal endoscopically placed biliary endoprosthesis should not be underesti-mated because it is known that the incidence of cholangitis and occlusion or displacement of the catheter or endoprosthesis ranges from 28% to almost 100% [94–99]. The assessments of quality of life in patients with hilar cholangiocarcinoma who undergo surgical bypass, operative intubation, or percutaneous drainage have not demonstrated a distinct advantage for one type of palliative treatment [64,100]. However, some studies suggest that the duration of well-being is longest in patients undergoing surgical bypass procedures [100–103]. There is no significant difference in survival related to the type of palliative procedure employed to relieve biliary obstruction; the median survival in patients undergoing palliative drainage is 8 months or less. However, effective palliation of biliary obstruction in patients with unresectable hilar cholangiocarcinomas is important because 50% will survive for at least 1 year, 20% will live for 2 years, and 10% will live 3 years or longer [104].

Chemotherapy. Given the high percentage of unresectable hilar cholangiocarcinomas, various chemotherapeutic regimens and radiotherapeutic regimens have been used in the hope of providing improved palliation and prolongation of survival. Adjuvant radiotherapy also has been employed following resection of tumors to reduce locoregional recurrence and potentially to improve survival [78]. Unfortunately, reports describing chemotherapy or radiotherapy for hilar cholangiocarcinoma rarely describe the treatment results in more than 10–20 patients.

A 1988 review of systemic chemotherapy for bile duct cancer noted that 97 patients had been treated with nine different treatment programs [105]. Mitomycin C, doxorubicin, and 5-fluorouracil are the agents that have shown the greatest activity against cholangiocarcinoma. The collective partial response rate in the 97 patients was 29%, with no complete responses. The median survival of these patients receiving systemic chemotherapy ranged between 6 and 11 months. No reports since 1988 have indicated a better response rate with systemic chemotherapy. With no significant increase in survival and considering the quality-of-life issues related to chemotherapeutic toxicity, systemic chemotherapy has not demonstrated a distinct advantage in patients with hilar cholangiocarcinoma.

Regional chemotherapy by hepatic artery infusion has some potential advantages over systemic chemotherapy. The proximal bile duct receives its arterial blood supply from the hepatic artery so that an increased concentration of drug can be delivered directly to the region of the tumor, including the liver. By using drugs such as 5-fluorouracil and floxuridine, systemic exposure to drug is limited because of the high rate of hepatic extraction of these agents. There are reports of 46 hilar cholangocarcinoma patients who have been treated by hepatic artery chemotherapy infusion [105,106]. The partial response rate for the entire group of patients was 43%, but there were no complete responses and no significant prolongation of survival. Hepatic artery infusion chemotherapy may have a role in palliation of patients with hilar cholangiocarcinoma, but currently available drugs do not provide improved survival.

Radiotherapy. Radiotherapy for bile duct cancer is yet more confusing due to the various types, doses, routes of administration, and association with resected and unresected tumors, all in small numbers of patients. Internal radiation with iridium-192 wires or seeds may have a palliative role in improving the patency of obstructed bile ducts; however, the number and frequency of episodes of cholangitis were not reduced, so the overall benefit is uncertain [107]. Internal radiation has been associated with prolongation of survival to an average of 16 months, and occasionally patients with unresectable disease survived more than 5 years [108–110]. Although the use of external-beam radiotherapy alone to treat patients with unresectable hilar cholangiocarcinoma has not provided significant differences in overall patient survival, rare long-term survivals have been reported [111]. Intraoperative radiotherapy also has been evaluated in association with resectable and unresectable tumors [112,113]. Again, there is a suggestion of a slight prolongation of survival in patients with unresectable tumors, but the most interesting use of intraoperative radiotherapy may be as an immediate surgical adjuvant in the resected high-risk tumor bed.

At the University of Texas M.D. Anderson Cancer Center, we have employed a treatment technique of four-field irradiation directed to the porta hepatis to a dose of 45 Gy. Patients receive 5-FU by continuous intravenous infusion during the 5-week course of external-beam irradiation. Further radiotherapy is administered by a reduced treatment field using an arc rotation to deliver an additional dose of 15–20 Gy to the primary target volume [114]. We have used this treatment plan for patients who have had a surgical biliary bypass procedure and do not have transcutaneous biliary drainage catheters. This radiation technique envelopes the target and a small portion of the duodenum with a high dose. However, in patients with existing external biliary drainage tubes, a combination of external beam plus endoluminal boost irradiation is an attractive treatment program. The favored treatment sequence is to start with external-beam irradiation to obtain tumor regression, which provides a better dose distribution from the endoluminal boost irradiation to treat any residual tumor. We currently use high-dose rate iridium-192 (^{192}Ir) implants in a fractionated treatment schedule of 4 Gy daily for 5 consecutive days. The fractionated high-dose rate treatment, along with the favorable dose distribution obtained with endoluminal therapy, may decrease late-occurring duodenitis. For patients in whom there are technical or medical limitations for fractionated therapy, a single 20 Gy boost with the high-dose technique can be used.

The use of endoluminal ^{192}Ir alone for palliative treatment of patients with unresectable hilar bile duct cancers has been reported [115]. Endoluminal doses ranged from 15 Gy to 35 Gy when combined with external-beam irradiation (usually 45–50 Gy), or when endoluminal doses of up to 60 Gy were used alone. The dose reference point may vary from 0.5 cm to 1.0 cm from the central catheter. The total nominal doses of external-beam plus endoluminal boost irradiation are between 60 Gy and 70 Gy to the tumor, and although this range exceeds the liver and small intestine tolerance, the highest doses are confined to a small volume of tissue. The median survival for patients treated by this endoluminal method, with or without external-beam irradiation, is 15–18 months. Several patients survived for more than 4 years after treatment; however, the majority of patients failed locally.

Complications with the endoluminal boost have been related mainly to cholangitis, which occurs to some degree in nearly all patients. Septic cholangitis and death occur in less than 15% of the patients because antibiotic therapy is usually effective. Prophylactic antibiotics are not recommended because flora colonizing the catheter tract became drug resistant. A better approach to reduce sepsis is to remove the drainage catheter after therapy whenever there is cholangiographic evidence of bile duct patency following treatment.

Another specialized technique that has been used for boost treatments of biliary tract cancers is electron beam intraoperative radiotherapy (EB-IORT) [116]. This technique improves the dose distribution by concentrating treatment directly on the target volume, while the uninvolved liver, adjacent duodenum, and stomach are excluded from the treatment field during surgery. Nine patients with advanced proximal biliary cancers were treated with EB-IORT in one report [117]. Patients were considered for IORT if they had residual gross or microscopic disease confined to the region of the porta hepatis, or if there was adjacent hepatic parenchymal involvement by tumor. The field size was 7–10 cm in diameter, and the IORT dose was 10–22 Gy. In five patients, additional external-beam irradiation was given. An analysis of the patients treated with EB-IORT was made with concurrent groups who were treated without radiation or with external-beam irradiation with or without ^{192}Ir endoluminal boost irradiation. There was a significant improvement in median survival for the patients receiving high-dose irradiation, regardless of boost technique, compared with those who were not irradiated (13 vs. 4.6 months, respectively). Duodenitis occurred in most of the patients who received any form of irradiation, and portal vein thrombosis was observed in one patient who was treated with EB-IORT.

Gallbladder carcinoma

Adenocarcinoma of the gallbladder is the fifth most common gastrointestinal malignancy. When compared with the worldwide incidence of hepatocellular carcinoma, gallbladder carcinoma accounts for less than 10% of the annual cases of primary hepatobiliary cancer. However, in western countries like the United States, with a low incidence of hepatocellular carcinoma, gallbladder carcinoma is relatively more prevalent, with an estimated 4000 cases diagnosed in 1993 compared with 10,000 cases of hepatocellular carcinoma in the same year [118]. Autopsy and biliary tract operation data from 112,713 patients revealed an average incidence of gallbladder carcinoma ranging from 0.55% to 1.91% [119]. Over the past three decades there appears to be a slight increase in the incidence of gallbladder carcinoma in western countries, but this may be ascribed to more thorough reporting mechanisms rather than a true increase in incidence [119]. Gallbladder carcinoma is a disease that is diagnosed most frequently in the sixth and seventh decades of life. Unlike hepatocellular carcinoma (HCC) and cholangiocarcinoma, gallbladder carcinoma has a higher incidence in females than males, with a ratio of approximately 3:1 [119]. The preponderance of this cancer in females is even greater in patients less than 40 years old, with a female-to-male ratio of 20:1 [120].

Gallbladder carcinoma is more prevalent in Southwest American Indians. The incidence of this disease is six times higher than that in non-Indian populations, and gallbladder carcinoma has been found in 6% of Southwest American Indians undergoing biliary tract surgery [121]. Gallbladder carcinoma is the second most common gastrointestinal malignancy in this population, and the youngest reported case of gallbladder carcinoma occurred in an 11-year-old Navajo girl [122].

Causative factors

There are no apparent associations between gallbladder carcinoma and hepatitis B or C virus infection, cirrhosis, or mycotoxin exposure. Similarly, chemical hepatocarcinogens have not been demonstrated clearly to increase the risk to develop gallbladder carcinoma. However, there are suggestions that workers exposed to carcinogenic substances, such as methylcholanthrene and nitrosamines, have a higher incidence and earlier onset of gallbladder carcinoma when compared with control populations [123]. Experimental studies indicate that animals exposed to hepatocarcinogens alone rarely form gallbladder carcinoma, but when the animals are also fed a gallstone-inducing diet, over 50% developed gallbladder carcinoma [124]. There is a significant association between gallstones and gallbladder carcinoma, with gallstones present in 74–92% of patients with gallbladder carcinoma [125]. The risk of developing gallbladder carcinoma increases directly with increasing gallstone size [126]. Patients with gallstones 2.0–2.9 cm in diameter have a 2.4 times higher relative risk to develop gallbladder carcinoma, whereas patients with gallstones greater than 3.0 cm in diameter have a 10.1 times higher risk of developing gallbladder carcinoma. Patients with longstanding chronic cholecystitis can develop calcification of the gallbladder wall, also known as porcelain gallbladder. It is possible that chronic inflammation and/or infection of the gallbladder increases the risk of developing gallbladder carcinoma because 22% of patients with calcified gallbladders have gallbladder carcinoma [127,128]. Furthermore, pathogenic bacteria are cultured from the gallbladders of patients with gallbladder cancer at a significantly greater frequency than patients with simple cholelithiasis [129]. Cholelithiasis and cholecystitis are more common in females, which may in part explain the higher incidence of gallbladder carcinoma in females [130].

Gallstones or other factors that cause chronic inflammation of the gallbladder mucosa may induce a series of premalignant changes. If not treated with a

288

cholecystectomy, patients with these premalignant lesions may progress to invasive gallbladder carcinoma. Epithelial dysphasia, atypical hyperplasia, and carcinoma in situ have been identified in the gallbladder mucosa of 83%, 13.5%, and 3.5%, respectively, of patients undergoing cholecystectomy for cholelithiasis or cholecystitis [131]. Areas of mucosal dysplasia can be observed in over 90% of patient with invasive gallbladder carcinoma [132]. There also is evidence that adenomatous polyps arising from the gallbladder mucosa are premalignant lesions because a review of 1605 cholecytectomies produced 11 benign adenomas, 7 adenomas with areas of malignant transformation, and 79 invasive gallbladder carcinomas [133]. Regions of residual adenomas were found in 20% of the cases of invasive gallbladder carcinoma. There appears to be an increased expression of epithelial growth factors and protooncogenes, particularly *ras*, in the progression from chronic cholecystitis to dysplasia and then to invasive carcinoma [134].

Pathology

The gross appearance of gallbladder carcinoma varies depending on the stage of the disease and extent of spread. Early stage lesions that have not infiltrated through all layers of the gallbladder wall may be indistinguishable from chronic cholecystitis. On opening the gallbladder in these early stage patients, gallstones usually are present, and there may be subtle mucosal abnormalities, such as plaquelike lesions or small ulcerations. Occasionally, a sessile or pedunculated tumor is present and suggests the diagnosis of a gallbladder carcinoma [135]. More advanced gallbladder carcinomas are grossly evident by infiltration into the liver or contiguous organs, such as the duodenum or stomach [135]. These tumors are white to grey on cut section and very firm. When associated with a calcified gallbladder, these carcinomas are extremely hard, difficult to section, and have a gritty consistency.

Microscopically, over 90% of gallbladder carcinomas are adenocarcinomas, with the remaining cases being adenosquamous carcinomas, anaplastic carcinomas, and rarely carcinoid tumors or embryonal rhabdomyosarcoma [125]. Carcinoma in situ is an early lesion, with the malignant cellular characteristics involving only the mucosal layer of the gallbladder wall (Fig. 6). Gallbladder adenocarcinomas generally have a predominant papillary or tubular arrangement of cells [135]. Papillary adenocarcinoma is characterized by an extended storma covered by columnar cells. The tubular formations of tubular adenocarcinoma may be lined by tall columnar cells or by cuboidal epithelium. Mucin production and signet-ring cells can be identified frequently in gallbladder adenocarcinomas [135]. More poorly differentiated carcinomas have solid sheets or nests of small, scattered cells infiltrating into the stroma and destroying the normal gallbladder wall architecture. The hallmark of each of these types of invasive carcinoma is infiltration into the muscle and adventitial layers of the gallbladder wall (Fig. 7). Vascular, lymphatic, and perineural invasion by the carcinoma can be demonstrated frequently.

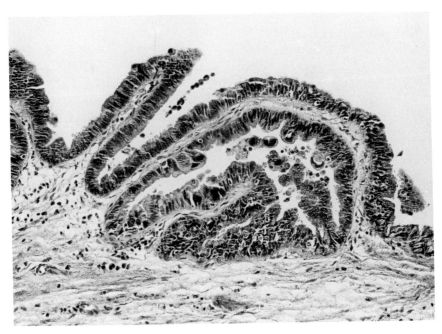

Figure 6. Carcinoma in situ of the gallbladder. The normal tall villous configuration of the mucosa is replaced by blunt, irregular villopapillary epithelium composed of increased numbers of cells with large nuclei. Nuclear polarity is absent and mitotic figures are present. Magnification ×187.

Advanced local and regional disease usually is present at the time of diagnosis of gallbladder carcinoma. Only 10% of patients with this disease have cancer confined to the gallbladder wall [125]. Direct extension of the carcinoma into the gallbladder fossa of the liver is present in 69–83% of patients [136,137]. Direct invasion of the liver usually indicates the presence of other regional disease because less than 12% of patients with liver involvement have no other sites of regional disease. Direct invasion of the extrahepatic biliary tract occurs in 57% of cases; the duodenum, stomach, or transverse colon are involved in 40%; and the pancreas is involved in 23% [119]. The hepatic artery or portal vein is encased by tumor in 15% of patients. Regional lymph node metastases in the cystic, choledochal, or pancreaticoduodenal lymphatic drainage basins are present in 42–70% of patients [136]. Somewhat more distant lymph node metastases occur along the aorta or inferior vena cava in approximately 25% of cases. Importantly, lymph node metastases can occur in the absence of liver or other contiguous organ involvement by the gallbladder carcinoma.

The pattern of lymph node metastases from gallbladder carcinoma is predictable based on anatomical studies that have identified three pathways of lymphatic drainage of the gallbladder [138]. The main pathway is the

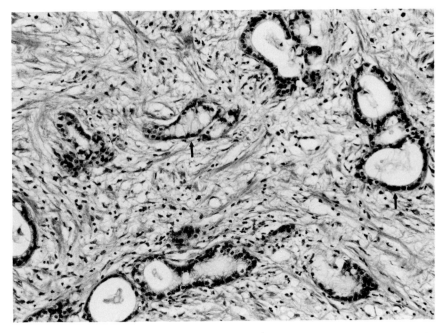

Figure 7. Poorly differentiated, invasive carcinoma of the gallbladder. Cells are mucin producing and some residual glands are present (long arrows). Magnification ×187.

cholecystoretro-pancreatic pathway, with lymphatic vessels on the anterior and posterior surface of the gallbladder that converge at a large retroportal lymph node. This principal retroportal lymph node communicates with the choledochal and pancreaticoduodenal lymph nodes. The cholecysto-celiac pathway consists of lymphatics from the anterior and posterior wall of the gallbladder that run to the left through the hepatoduodenal ligament to reach the celiac lymph nodes. The cholecysto-mesenteric pathway is lymphatic channels that run to the left in front of the portal vein and then communicate with groups of pancreaticoduodenal lymph nodes or aortico-caval lymph nodes lying near the left renal vein. The final pattern of spread of gallbladder carcinoma is related to vascular invasion. Noncontiguous liver, pulmonary, and bone metastases have been found in 66%, 24%, and 12% of gallbladder carcinoma patients, respectively [136].

The staging systems used for gallbladder carcinoma are based on the pathologic characteristics of local invasion by the tumor and lymph node metastases. Before the American Joint Cancer Committee (AJCC) developed a tumor-node-metastasis (TNM) staging schema for gallbladder carcinoma, the Nevin staging system was used frequently [139]. Studies of gallbladder carcinoma performed in Japan generally apply the staging system of the Japanese Society of Biliary Surgery [140]. Most recent studies stage patients ac-

Table 2. Comparison of the three commonly used staging systems for gallbladder carcinoma

Stage	Nevin	J.S.B.S.	A.J.C.C. TNM
I	Cancer confined to the mucosa	Cancer confined to subserosal layers	$T_{1a}N_0M_0$ $T_{1b}N_0M_0$ $T_2N_0M_0$
II	Cancer involves the mucosa and muscularis	Direct invasion of the liver and/or bile duct, porta hepatis lymph node metastases	$T_1N_1M_0$ $T_2N_1M_0$
III	Cancer extends through the serosa (all three layers of the gallbladder wall involved)	More extensive liver invasion by cancer, more extensive regional lymph node metastases (gastrohepatic, retropancreatic)	T_3AnyNM_0
IV	Tumor through all three layers of the gallbladder wall with cystic lymph node metastasis	Liver, peritoneal, and/or distant organ metastases	T_4AnyNM_0 $AnyTAnyNM_1$
V	Tumor invades the liver by direct extension and/or metastasis to any distant organ	No stage V	No stage V

J.S.B.S. = Japanese Society of Biliary Surgery; A.J.C.C. = American Joint Cancer Commission.

T = Primary tumor; T_x = primary tumor cannot be assessed; T_1 = tumor invades mucosa or muscle layer; T_{1a} = tumor invades mucosa; T_{1b} = tumor invades muscle; T_2 = tumor invades perimuscular connective tissue, no extension beyond serosa or into liver; T_3 = tumor invades beyond serosa or into one adjacent organ or both (extension <2 cm into liver); T_4 = tumor extends >2 cm into liver and/or into two or more adjacent organs (stomach, duodenum, colon, pancreas, omentum, extrahepatic bile ducts).

N = Regional lymph nodes; N_x = regional lymph nodes cannot be assessed; N_0 = no regional lymph node metastasis; N_1 = regional lymph node metastasis; N_{1a} = metastasis in cystic duct, pericholedochal, and/or gastrohepatic lymph nodes; N_{1b} = metastasis in peripancreatic, periduodenal, periportal, celiac, and/or superior mesenteric artery lymph nodes.

M = Distant metastasis; M_x = presence of distant metastasis cannot be assessed; M_0 = no distant metastasis; M_1 = distant metastasis.

cording to the TNM criteria. Carcinoma in situ corresponds to a $T_{1a}N_0M_0$ tumor in the AJCC staging system. The characteristics of these three staging systems are outlined in Table 2.

Diagnosis

The most common symptoms and signs in patients with gallbladder carcinoma are nonspecific. Right upper quadrant abdominal pain, which may or may not be exacerbated by eating a fatty meal, is the predominant presenting complaint in 75–97% of patients [119,125,141]. Right upper quadrant abdominal tenderness is present in a slightly smaller percentage of patients. These symptoms and signs usually are ascribed to cholelithiasis or cholecystitis. Nausea, vomiting, and anorexia are present in 40–64% of patients; clinically evident jaundice is present in 45%; and weight loss of greater than 10% of normal body weight is noted in 37–77%.

Although 45% of patients obviously are jaundiced at presentation, 70% of patients present with a serum bilirubin elevated at least two times greater than normal [141]. Serum alkaline phosphatase levels are elevated in two thirds of patients with gallbladder carcinoma. Alanine aminotransferase and aspartate aminotransferase levels are elevated in one third of patients and are consistent with advanced hepatic invasion and metastases. Serum carcinoembingonic antigen (CEA) levels generally are obtained only in patients diagnosed preoperatively with advanced stages of disease. In these patients with TNM stage III or IV disease, the serum CEA level is elevated in over 80% of patients [141]. The incidence of elevated serum CEA levels in early stage disease is not known.

Before ultrasonography and CT became widely available, the preoperative diagnosis rate for gallbladder carcinoma was only 8.6–16.3% [119,142]. Ultrasonography is the primary imaging study for symptomatic patients with presumed cholelithiasis or choledocholithiasis. A high-resolution ultrasound is able to detect early and locally advanced gallbladder carcinoma [143]. Early tumors as small as 5 mm can be recognized as a polypoid mass projecting into the gallbladder lumen or as a focal thickening of the gallbladder wall [144]. In patients with locally advanced gallbladder carcinoma, ultrasound can demonstrate extrahepatic and intrahepatic bile duct obstruction, regional lymphadenopathy, direct hepatic extension of tumor, and hepatic metastases. Preoperative ultrasonography may suggest the correct diagnosis in up to 75% of patients with gallbladder carcinoma [144–146]. Blood flow studies with color Doppler ultrasonography are also useful because gallbladder cancers have high velocity arterial flow in 90% of cases, while benign lesions have minimal flow [147]. CT scans are performed less frequently in patients with presumed benign biliary tract disease. However, if gallbladder carcinoma is suspected, CT findings can predict correctly the diagnosis in 88–95% of patients [148–150]. The CT characteristics of gallbladder carcinoma include diffuse or focal gallbladder wall thickness of greater than 0.5 mm in 95% of patients, gallbladder wall contrast enhancement in 95%, an intraluminal mass in 90%, direct liver invasion by tumor in 85%, regional lymphadenopathy in 65%, concomitant cholelithiasis in 52%, dilated intrahepatic or extrahepatic bile ducts in 50%, noncontiguous liver metastases in 12%, invasion of contiguous gastrointestinal tract organs in 8%, and intraluminal gallbladder gas in 4% [150]. CT also can demonstrate calcification of the gallbladder wall (Fig. 8).

Treatment

Resection. The curative resection rates for gallbladder carcinoma range from 10% to 30% [151–153]. The majority of patients are not candidates for curative resection because of extensive locoregional disease, noncontiguous liver metastases, and/or distant metastases. While it is clear that long-term survival can be achieved in some patients with resectable lesions, the extent of resection remains a controversial issue.

A large majority of surgeons consider simple cholecystectomy to be adequate treatment for gallbladder carcinoma confined to the mucosa ($T_{1a}N_0M_0$). The 5-year survival rate for patients undergoing simple cholecystectomy for

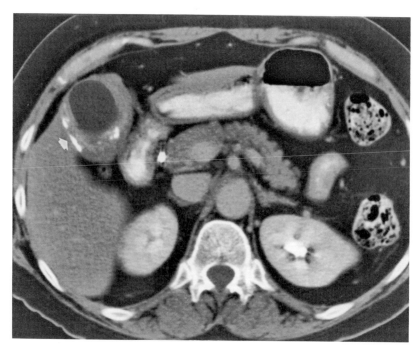

Figure 8. A high-resolution computed tomogram in a patient with gallbladder carcinoma. The marked thickening and calcification of the gallbladder wall is readily apparent (arrow).

disease confined to the mucosa ranges from 57% to 100% [154–157]. There is not universal agreement on simple cholecystectomy as the sole treatment for patients with $T_{1a}N_0M_0$ tumors; some authors recommend that extended cholecystectomy (cholecystectomy, wedge resection of the gallbladder fossa including a 3–5 cm margin of normal liver, and a cystic, pericholedochal, gastrohepatic, pancreaticoduodenal, and para-aortic lymphadenectomy) be performed to treat patients with these very early stage lesions [158,159]. These authors recommend that all gallbladders be opened at the time of cholecystectomy for frozen section evaluation of any suspicious areas in the mucosa. If an unsuspected gallbladder carcinoma is diagnosed by frozen section biopsy or if a $T_{1a}N_0M_0$ gallbladder carcinoma is diagnosed on final pathology, these authors advocate that an extended cholecystectomy be performed. The bias for this aggressive surgical treatment of $T_{1a}N_0M_0$ gallbladder carcinoma is based on the small number of cases of regional lymph node recurrences in patients treated with simple cholecystectomy alone. No rationale is provided for the liver resection because the small number of patients who did fail after simple cholecystectomy developed metastases in pericholedochal or cystic lymph nodes and not in the liver. Furthermore, the incidence of subsequent lymph node metastases in $T_{1a}N_0M_0$ patients was less than 10% in the small groups of 32 and 36 patients, respectively [158,159]. The incidence of lymph node metastases in 201 patients with gallbladder carcinoma confined to the mucosa was only 2.5% in a study of patients who underwent cholecystectomy and regional lymphadenectomy [155]. The mortality rate for extended resection ranges from 2% to 5%, and major postoperative morbidity occurs in 13–40% [154–156,160]. Therefore, the morbidity and mortality associated with extended cholecystectomy is excessive compared with the potential survival benefit that would occur in less than 5% of patients with $T_{1a}N_0M_0$ lesions.

There is a rationale for performing extended cholecystectomy in patients with T_{1b} tumors or AJCC TNM stage II and III gallbladder carcinomas (Fig. 9). In 165 patients with T_{1b} gallbladder carcinomas, there was a 15.6% incidence of regional lymph node metastasis [155]. Of 867 patients with a T_2 primary lesion, 56.1% had regional lymph node metastases [155]. The 453 patients with T_3 tumors had a 74.4% incidence of regional lymph node metastases [155]. The 5-year survival rate following extended cholecystectomy for AJCC stage II and III gallbladder carcinoma ranges from 7.5% to 37% [154–156,158,160,161]. AJCC stage II or III gallbladder carcinoma patients treated with simple cholecystectomy alone had a 0% 5-year survival rate compared with a 29% 5-year survival rate in those patients treated with extended cholecystectomy [160]. T_{1b} patients are classified as stage I in the AJCC system but, arguably, with a 15.6% incidence of regional lymph node metastases, long-term survival benefit may occur in a significant number of these patients who undergo an extended cholecystectomy (see Fig. 9).

All authors do not perform an en-bloc resection of the extrahepatic bile duct as part of an extended cholecystectomy. Because gallbladder carcinoma

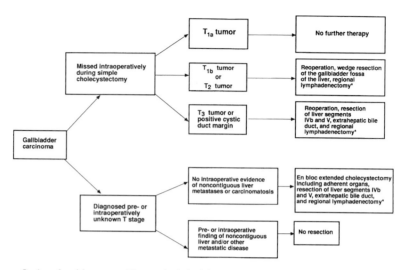

Figure 9. An algorithm to guide surgical decision making in treating gallbladder carcinoma. Regional lymphadenectomy includes complete dissection of the cystic, pericholedochal, pancreaticoduodenal, gastrohepatic, and para-aortic lymph nodes.

is found to invade the extrahepatic bile duct in 57% of cases, with almost all cases occurring in patients with T_3 or T_4 tumors, an en-bloc resection of the proper hepatic and common bile duct with Roux-en-Y hepaticojejunostomy should be included in an extended cholecystectomy of transmurally invasive tumors. This includes those cases in whom a clinically unsuspected gallbladder carcinoma is diagnosed pathologically following a simple cholecystectomy with a positive margin at the cystic duct.

Extremely radical operations have been proposed for patients with extensive $T_3N_1M_0$ or $T_4N_{0-1}M_0$ tumors. This includes hepatopancreaticoduodenectomy and abdominal organ cluster transplantation for locally advanced gallbladder carcinoma [155,162,163]. The operative mortality rate for these radical procedures is at least 15% with a greater than 90% incidence of major morbidity. Resection of the portal vein and/or hepatic artery with vascular reconstruction frequently is necessary to resect completely all gross malignant disease. The largest report of patients undergoing hepatopancreaticoduodenectomy for gallbladder carcinoma is 150 cases from Japan, with a 5-year survival rate of 14% [155]. The patients who did not die from intraoperative or postoperative complications all succumbed to recurrent and/or metastatic carcinoma.

It is estimated that 70,000 laparoscopic cholecystectomies are performed each year in the United States [164]. On average, gallbladder carcinoma is diagnosed in 2% of patients undergoing cholecystectomy for presumed benign biliary tract disease [119]. Thus, approximately 1400 patients annually who undergo laparoscopic cholecystectomy could suffer inadvertent dissemination of gallbladder carcinoma [164–169]. The spillage of tumor cells at the time of laparoscopic cholecystectomy has caused seeding of peritoneal surfaces and laparoscopy tracts in several patients. This dissemination of tumor cells is an unfortunate occurrence because it may preclude a potentially curative open resection and limit the patient's long-term survival. Because of the large number of cholecystectomies being performed laparoscopically and the small but measurable risk of dissemination of tumor cells, it has been recommended that (1) unless the surgeon feels capable of performing a definitive extended cholecystectomy for gallbladder carcinoma, cases in whom gallbladder carcinoma is suspected preoperatively by clinical or radiologic criteria should be referred without laparoscopy, laparotomy, or percutaneous biopsy; and (2) if gallbladder carcinoma is suspected on visual inspection during an attempted laparoscopic cholecystectomy, either an open definitive operation should be performed or the operation should be terminated without biopsy and the patient referred for appropriate surgical therapy [165].

Palliation. The majority of patients with gallbladder carcinoma are diagnosed at an advanced, unresectable stage of disease. As in patients with hilar bile duct cancer, relief of symptomatic jaundice is a consideration. Patients with unresectable gallbladder carcinoma frequently have extensive involvement of the extrahepatic bile duct and may have bulky porta hepatis lymphadenopathy, which makes endoscopic placement of an internal stent difficult. When unresectable gallbladder carcinoma is diagnosed at the time of laparotomy, a surgical biliary bypass, such as an intrahepatic cholangioenteric anastomosis, can be performed and results in significant symptomatic relief in greater than 90% of patients [64]. When the diagnosis is made based on radiographic and percutaneous biopsy findings, jaundice can be relieved by placement of percutaneous transhepatic biliary catheters.

In contrast to patients with hilar bile duct carcinoma in which gastroduodenal obstruction is a relatively rare event, between 30% and 50% of patients with advanced gallbladder carcinoma will develop a clinically significant element of gastroduodenal obstruction [170]. This can be treated surgically with a bypass procedure, such as gastrojejunostomy, or by placement of a decompressing gastrostomy tube and feeding jejunostomy tube. A percutaneous endoscopic gastrostomy tube also can be used to decompress the obstructed stomach in patients with advanced disease and limited expected survival.

Chemotherapy. Studies that describe the results of chemotherapeutic treatment for unresectable or metastatic gallbladder carcinoma suffer from small numbers of patients and inclusion of patients with hilar bile duct carcinoma. A study of 53 patients with gallbladder carcinoma who received systemic chemotherapy with 5-fluorouracil (5-FU) or 5-FU plus other chemotherapeutic agents showed objective antitumor responses in 12% or less of the patients in each treatment arm [171]. Fluoropyrimidines combined with doxorubicin administered systemically have produced objective response rates of 30–40% [172,173]. Complete remission is rare and transient following such systemic chemotherapy regimens, and the median survival is 11 months or less. The toxicities associated with these treatments are not insignificant, and the survival benefit is only a few months greater than that of patients who received no treatment.

Hepatic arterial infusion chemotherapy also has been described in small numbers of patients with locally advancd gallbladder carcinoma. Partial response rates of 55–60% and complete response rates of 9% have been reported [174–176]. However, the median duration of response was only 3 months, and all patients developed progressive disease. There have been no patients who survived more than 4 years after beginning hepatic arterial chemotherapy. The median survival of 12–14 months with hepatic arterial infusion chemotherapy is not a major improvement over the median survival in patients treated with intravenous chemotherapy. There may be less frequent and less severe systemic toxicity with hepatic arterial infusion chemotherapy, but the magnitude of this benefit is slight and does not justify routine use of this approach to treat unresectable gallbladder carcinoma. Currently, there are not particularly compelling cytotoxic chemotherapeutic agents to treat locally unresectable or metastatic primary hepatobiliary malignancies.

Radiation therapy. Analysis of the patterns of failure after resection of gallbladder carcinoma revealed that local recurrence was the site of first, and in a significant number of cases the only site, of failure in over one half of the patients [119,177]. External-beam radiation therapy to a total dose of 45 Gy can produce radiographic evidence of tumor reduction in 20–70% of these tumors and provide temporary relief of jaundice in up to 80% of patients [625–627]. In general, external-beam radiation therapy is a palliative treatment. The median survival for locally advanced gallbladder carcinoma patients treated with radiation therapy is approximately 10 months [177–180]. Occasional long-term survivors are reported following treatment with higher doses of radiation therapy or with administration of radiation-sensitizing chemotherapeutic agents such as 5-FU during external-beam radiation therapy [177]. However, extrahepatic bile duct stricture has been reported in several of the long-term survivors treated with high doses of radiation therapy [181].

Intraoperative radiation therapy with a dose of 20–30 Gy has been delivered to treat unresectable gallbladder carcinoma [182,183]. Recanalization of obstructed extrahepatic bile ducts occurs in the majority of patients treated with this technique. Intraoperative radiation therapy has not been associated with increased operative or postoperative morbidity in patients with unresectable tumors. The median survival of patients treated with intraoperative radiation therapy is less than 12 months, and this treatment modality appears to palliate biliary tract obstruction without significantly improving survival.

Multidisciplinary approaches

The majority of patients who undergo an extended cholecystectomy or more radical resection for AJCC stage II, III, or IV gallbladder carcinoma develop tumor recurrence and die as a result of their disease. Nonrandomized studies and case reports have suggested that overall survival can be improved by administering adjuvant radiation therapy and/or chemotherapy after resection of stage II, III, or IV tumors [184,185]. Unfortunately, the number of patients who have received postsurgical adjuvant treatment is small, and a variety of treatment regimens have been used. In a nonrandomized study, nine patients with stage IV gallbladder carcinoma were treated with complete surgical resection alone, while 17 patients were treated with complete resection combined with 20–30 Gy of intraoperative radiation therapy [186]. Ten of these 17 patients also received 36.4 Gy of postoperative external-beam radiation therapy. The surgical procedures performed in both groups of patients included extended cholecystectomy and a variety of more radical procedures, including hepatopancreaticoduodenectomy. There were no 3-year survivors in the 9 patients treated with resection alone, but there was a 10.1% 3-year survival in the 17 patients treated with resection and radiation therapy. Unfortunately, there are no randomized trials of patients with stage II and III gallbladder carcinoma treated with a coherent program of adjuvant therapy. Such trials will be necessary to demonstrate an improvement in survival in patients who receive adjuvant therapies after a curative resection for gallbladder carcinoma.

References

1. Anthony PP. Tumours and tumour-like lesions of the liver and biliary tract. In MacSween RNM, Anthony PP, Scheuer PJ (eds). Pathology of the Liver, 2nd ed. Edinburgh: Churchill Livingstone, 1987, p 574.
2. Moto R, Kawarada Y. Diagnosis and treatment of cholangiocarcinoma and cystic adenocarcinoma of the liver. In Okuda K, Ishak KG (eds). Neoplasms of the Liver. Tokyo: Springer-Verlag, 1987, p 381.
3. Pitt H, Dooley W, Yeo C, Cameron J. Malignancies of the biliary tract. Curr Probl Surg 32:1, 1995.
4. Jalanko H, Kuusela P, Roberts P, et al. Comparison of a new tumor marker, CA 19-9T, with α-fetoprotein and carcinoembryonic antigen in patients with upper gastrointestinal disease. J Clin Pathol 37:218, 1984.
5. Oldenburg WA, Van Heerden PA, Sizemore GW, et al. Hypercalcemia and primary hepatic tumors. Arch Surg 117:1363, 1982.
6. Davis JM, Sadasivan R, Dwyer T, et al. Case report: Cholangiocarcinoma and hypercalcemia. Am J Med Sci 307:350, 1994.
7. The Liver Cancer Study Group of Japan. Primary liver cancer in Japan. Cancer 54:1747, 1984.
8. Chearanai O, Pleggvanit U, Domrongsak D, et al. Primary liver cancer, angiographic study of 127 cases. J Med Assoc Thailand 67:482, 1984.
9. Schwartz DA. Cholangiocarcinoma associated with liver fluke infection: A preventable source of morbidity in Asian immigrants. Am J Gastroenterol 81:76, 1986.

10. Kurathong S, Lerdverasirikul P, Wonkpaitoon V, et al. *Opisthorchis viverrini* infection and cholagiocarcinoma. A prospective, case-controlled study. Gastoenterology 89:151, 1985.
11. Nakashima T, Okuda K, Kojiro M, et al. Primary liver cancer coincident with *Schistosomiasis japonica*. A study of 23 necropsies. Cancer 36:1483, 1975.
12. Nakanuma Y, Terada T, Tanka Y. Are hepatolithiasis and cholangiocarcinoma aetiologically related? A morphological study of 12 cases of hepatoliathiasis associated with cholangiocarcinoma. Virchows Arch A Pathol Anat Histopathol 406:43, 1985.
13. Thamavit W, Phamarapravati N, Sahaphong S, et al. Effects of dimethylnitrosamine on induction of cholangiocarcinoma in *Opisthorchis viverrini*-infected Syrian golden hamsters. Cancer Res 38:4634, 1978.
14. Prempracha N, Tengchaisri T, Chawengkirttikul R, et al. Identification and potential use of a soluble tumor antigen for the detection of liver-fluke-associated cholangiocarcinoma induced in a hamster model. Int J Cancer 57:691, 1994.
15. Landais P, Drunfeld JP, Droz D, et al. Cholangiocellular carcinoma in polycystic kidney and liver disease. Arch Intern Med 144:2274, 1984.
16. Voyles CR, Smadja C, Shands W, Blumgart LH. Carcinoma in choledochal cysts. Age-related incidence. Arch Surg 118:986, 1983.
17. Imaura M, Miyashita T, Tani T, et al. Cholangiocellular carcinoma associated with multiple liver cysts. Am J Gastroenterol 79:790, 1984.
18. Dayton MT, Longmire WP, Tompkins RK. Caroli's disease: A premalignant condition. Am J Surg 145:41, 1983.
19. Wee A, Ludwig L, Coffey RJ, et al. Hepatobiliary carcinoma ssociated with primary sclerosing cholangitis and chronic ulcerative colitis. Hum Pathol 16:719, 1985.
20. Chen PH, Lo HW, Wang CS, et al. Cholangiocarcinoma in hepatolithiasis. J Clin Gastroenterol 6:539, 1984.
21. Koga A, Ichimiya H, Yamaguchi, et al. Hepatolithiasis associated with cholangiocarcinoma, possible etiologic significance. Cancer 55:2826, 1985.
22. Yoshimoto H, Ikeda S, Tanaka M, Matsumoto S. Intrahepatic cholangiocarcinoma associated with hepatolithiasis. Gastrointest Endosc 31:260, 1985.
23. Chen MF, Jan YY, Wang CS, et al. A reappraisal of cholangiocarcinoma in patient with hepatolithiasis. Cancer 71:2461, 1993.
24. Chijiiwa K, Ichimiya H, Kuroki S, et al. Later development of cholangiocarcinoma after the treatment of hepatolithiasis. Surgery 177:279, 1993.
25. Ito Y, Kojiro J, Nakashima T, Mori T. Pathomorphologic characteristics of 102 cases of thorotrast-related hepatocellular carcinoma, cholangiocarcinoma and hepatic angiosarcoma. Cancer 62:1153, 1988.
26. Rubel LR, Ishak KG. Thorotrast-associated cholangiocarcinoma. An epidemiologic and clinicopathologic study. Cancer 50:1408, 1982.
27. Nichols JC, Gores GJ, LaRusso NF, et al. Diagnostic role of serum CA 19-9 for cholangiocarcinoma in patients with primary sclerosing cholangitis. Mayo Clin Proc 68:874, 1993.
28. Ramage JK, Donaghy A, Farrant JM, et al. Serum tumor markers for the diagnosis of cholangiocarcinoma in primary sclerosing cholangitis. Gastroenterology 108:865, 1995.
29. Sell S, Dunsford HA. Evidence for the stem cell origin of hepatocellular carcinoma and cholangiocarcinoma. Am J Pathol 134:1347, 1989.
30. Okada Y, Jinno K, Moriwaki S, et al. Expression of ABH and Lewis blood group antigens in combined hepatocellular-cholangiocarcinoma. Possible evidence for the hepatocellular origin of combined hepatocellular-cholangiocarcinoma. Cancer 60:345, 1985.
31. Goodman ZD, Ishak KG, Longloss JM, et al. Combined hepatocellular-cholangiocarcinoma. A histologic and immunohistochemical study. Cancer 55:124, 1985.
32. Aoki K, Takayasu K, Kawano T, et al. Combined hepatocellular carcinoma and cholangiocarcinoma: Clinical features and computed tomographic findings. Hepatology 18:1090, 1993.

33. Ding SF, Delhanty JDA, Dowles JS, et al. Loss of constitutional heterozygosity on chromosomes 5 and 17 in cholangiocarcinoma. Br J Cancer 67:1007, 1993.
34. Weinbren K, Matum SS. Pathological aspects of cholangiocarcinoma. J Pathol 139:217, 1983.
35. Bonetti F, Chilosi M, Posa R, et al. Epithelial membrane antigen expression in cholangiocarcinoma. A useful immunohistochemical tool for differential diagnosis with hepatocarcinoma. Virchows Arch A Pathol Anat Histopathol 401:307, 1983.
36. Pastolero GC, Wakabayashi T, Oka T, Mori S. Tissue polypeptide antigen: A marker antigen differentiating cholangiolar tumors from other hepatic tumors. Am J Clin Pathol 87:168, 1987.
37. Sixth report. Liver Cancer Study Group of Japan. Primary liver cancer in Japan. Cancer 60:1400, 1987.
38. Okuda K and The Liver Cancer Study Group of Japan: Primary Liver cancers in Japan. Cancer 45:2663, 1980.
39. Liguory C, Canard JM. Tumours of the biliary system. Clin Gastroenterol 12:269, 1983.
40. Chou FF, Sheen-Chen SM, Chen CL, et al. Prognostic factors of resectable intrahepatic cholangiocarcinoma. J Surg Oncol 59:40, 1995.
41. Pichlmayr R, Lamesch P, Weimann A, Tusch G, Ringe B. Surgical treatment of cholangiocellular carcinoma. World J Surg 19:83, 1995.
42. Curley SA, Levin B, Rich TA. Liver and bile ducts. In Abeloff MD, Armitage JO, Lichter AS, Niederhuber JE (eds). Clinical Oncology. London: Churchill Livingston, 1995, p 1305.
43. Sansalone CV, Colella G, Caccamo L, et al. Orthotopic liver transplantation for primary biliary tumors: Milan multicenter experience. Transplant Proc 26:3561, 1994.
44. Goldstein RM, Stone M, Tillery GW, et al. Is liver transplantation indicated for cholangiocarcinoma? Am J Surg 166:768, 1993.
45. Fardel D. Malignant neoplasms of the extrahepatic biliary ducts. Ann Surg 76:205, 1922.
46. Altemeier WA, Gall EA, Zinninger MM, et al. Sclerosing carcinoma of the major intrahepatic bile ducts. Arch Surg 75:450, 1957.
47. Klatskin G. Adenocarcinoma of the hepatic duct at its bifurcation within the porta hepatis. Am J Med 38:241, 1965.
48. Sako K, Seitzinger GL, Garside E. Carcinoma of the extrahepatic bile ducts: Review of the literature and report of six cases. Surgery 41:416, 1957.
49. Longmire WP, Jr. Tumors of the extrahepatic biliary radicles. Curr Prob Cancer 1:1, 1976.
50. Faintuck J, Levin B. Diagnosis of bile duct cancer. In Wanebo HJ (ed). Hepatic and Biliary Cancer. New York: Marcel Dekker, 1982, p 299.
51. Wheeler PG, Dawson JL, Nunnerly H, et al. Newer techniques in the diagnosis and treatment of proximal bile duct carcinoma — an analysis of 41 consecutive patients. Q J Med 50:247, 1981.
52. Okuda K, Ohto M, Tsuchiya Y. The role of ultrasound, percutaneous transhepatic cholangiography, computed tomographic scanning, and magnetic resonance imaging in the preoperative assessment of bile duct cancer. World J Surg 12:18, 1988.
53. Garber ST, Donald JJ, Lees WR. Cholangiocarcinoma: Ultrasound features and correlation of tumor position with survival. Abdom Imaging 18:69, 1993.
54. Neumaier CE, Bertolotto M, Perrone R, Martinoli C, et al. Staging of hilar cholangiocarcinoma with ultrasound. J Clin Ultrasound 23:173, 1995.
55. Elias E, Hamlyn AN, Jain S, et al. A randomized trial of percutaneous transhepatic cholangiography with the Chiba needle versus ERCP for bile duct visualization in jaundice. Gastroenterology 71:439, 1976.
56. Tanaka M, Ogawa Y, Matsumoto S, et al. The role of endoscopic retrograde cholangiopancreatography in preoperative assessment of bile duct cancer. World J Surg 12:27, 1988.
57. Yamakawa T, Esguerra R, Kaneko H, et al. Percutaneous transhepatic endoprosthesis in malignant obstruction of the bile duct. World J Surg 12:78, 1988.

58. Pitt HA, Gomes AS, Lois JF, et al. Does preoperative percutaneous biliary drainage reduce operative risk or increase hospital cost? Ann Surg 201:545, 1985.
59. McPherson GAD, Benjamin IS, Hodjson HJF, et al. Pre-operative percutaneous transhepatic biliary drainage: The results of a controlled trial. Br J Surg 71:371, 1984.
60. Cameron JL, Broe P, Zuidema GD. Proximal bile duct tumors: Surgical management with silastic transhepatic biliary stents. Ann Surg 196:412, 1982.
61. Crist DW, Kadir S, Cameron JL. The value of preoperatively placed percutaneous biliary catheters in reconstruction of the proximal part of the biliary tree. Surg Gynecol Obstet 165:421, 1987.
62. Soehendra N, Grimm H. Endoscopic retrograde drainage for bile duct cancer. World J Surg 12:85, 1988.
63. Voyles CR, Bowley NJ, Allison DJ, et al. Carcinoma of the proximal extrahepatic biliary tree, radiologic assessment and therapeutic alternatives. Ann Surg 197:188, 1983.
64. Bismuth H, Castaing D, Traynor O. Resection or palliation: Priority of surgery in the treatment of hilar cancer. World J Surg 12:39, 1988.
65. Nagorney DM, Donohue JH, Farnell MB, et al. Outcomes after curative resections of cholangiocarcinoma. Arch Surg 128:871, 1993.
66. Tompkins RK, Thomas D, Wile A, et al. Prognostic factors in bile duct carcinoma. Ann Surg 194:447, 1981.
67. Ouchi K, Suzuki M, Hashimoto L, et al. Histologic findings and prognostic factors in carcinoma of the upper bile duct. Am J Surg 157:552, 1989.
68. Mittal B, Deutsch M, Iwatsuki S. Primary cancers of the extrahepatic biliary passages. Int J Radiat Oncol Biol Phys 11:849, 1985.
69. Mizumoto R, Kawarada Y, Suzuki H. Surgical treatment of hilar carcinoma of the bile duct. Surg Gynecol Obstet 162:153, 1986.
70. Mizumoto R, Suzuki H. Surgical anatomy of the hepatic hilum with special reference to the caudate lobe. World J Surg 12:2, 1988.
71. Bengmark S, Ekberg H, Evander A, et al. Major liver resection for hilar cholangiocarcinoma. Ann Surg 207:120, 1988.
72. Iwasaki Y, Okamura T, Ozaki A, et al. Surgical treatment for carcinoma at the confluence of the major hepatic ducts. Surg Gynecol Obstet 162:457, 1986.
73. White TT. Skeletization resection and central hepatic resection in the treatment of bile duct cancer. World J Surg 12:48, 1988.
74. Pinson CW, rossi RL. Extended right hepatic lobectomy, left hepatic lobectomy, and skeletonization resection for proximal bile duct cancer. World J Surg 12:52, 1988.
75. Washburn WK, Lewis WD, Jenkins RL. Aggressive surgical resection for cholangiocarcinoma. Arch Surg 130:270, 1995.
76. Baer HU, Stain SC, Dennison AR, Eggers B, Blumgart LH. Improvements in survival by aggressive resections of hilar cholangiocarcinoma. Ann Surg 217:20, 1993.
77. Tsukada K, Yoshida K, Aono T, Koyama S, Shirai Y, Uchida K, Muto T. Major hepatectomy and pancreatoduodenectomy for advanced carcinoma of the biliary tract. Br J Surg 81:108, 1994.
78. Cameron JL, Pitt HA, Zinner MJ, et al. Management of proximal cholangiocarcinomas by surgical resection and radiotherapy. Am J Surg 159:91, 1990.
79. Alexandre JH, Dehni N, Bouillot JL. Stented hepaticojejunostomies after resection for cholangiocarcinoma allow access for subsequent diagnosis and therapy. Am J Surg 169:428, 1995.
80. Ringe B, Wittekind C, Bechstein WO, et al. The role of liver transplantation in hepatobiliary malignancy. Ann Surg 209:88, 1989.
81. O'Grady JG, Polson RJ, Rolles K, et al. Liver transplantation for malignant disease. Ann Surg 207:373, 1988.
82. Funovics JM, Fritsch A, Herbst F, et al. Primary hepatic cancer — the role of limited resection and total hepatectomy with orthotopic liver replacement. Hepatogastroenterology

35:316, 1988.

83. Iwatsuki S, Gordon RD, Shaw BW, Starzl TE. Role of liver transplantation in cancer therapy. Ann Surg 202:401, 1985.

84. Koneru B, Cassavilla A, Bowman J, et al. Liver transplantation for malignant tumors. Gastroenterol Clin North Am 17:177, 1988.

85. Yokoyama I, Todo S, Iwatsuki S, Starzl TE. Liver transplantation in the treatment of primary liver cancer. Hepatogastroenterology 37:188, 1990.

86. Yokoyama I, Sheahan DG, Carr B, et al. Clinicopathologic factors affecting patient survival and tumor recurrence after orthotopic liver transplantation for hepatocellular carcinoma. Transpl Proc 24:2194, 1991.

87. Olthoff KM, Millis JM, Rosove MH, et al. Is liver transplantation justified for the treatment of hepatic malignancies? Arch Surg 125:1261, 1990.

88. Jenkins RL, Pinson CW, Stone MD. Experience with transplantation in the treatment of liver cancer. Cancer Chemother Pharmacol 23(Suppl):104, 1989.

89. Margeiter R. Indications for liver transplantation for primary and secondary liver tumor. Transpl Proc 18(Suppl 3):74, 1986.

90. Angrisano L, Jurewicz WA, Clements DG, et al. Liver transplantation for liver cancer. Transpl Proc 18:1218, 1986.

91. Ismail T, Agnrisani L, Gunson BK, et al. Primary hepatic malignancy: The role of liver transplantation. Br J Surg 77:983, 1990.

92. Van Thiel DH, Carr B, Iwatsuki S, et al. Liver transplantation for alcoholic liver disease, viral hepatitis, and hepatic neoplasms. Transpl Proc 23:1917, 1991.

93. Langer JC, Langer B, Taylor BR, et al. Carcinoma of the extrahepatic bile ducts: Results of an aggressive surgical approach. Surgery 98:752, 1985.

94. Lameris S, Stoker J, Dees J, et al. Non-surgical palliative treatment of patients with malignant biliary obstruction — the place of endoscopic and percutaneous drainage. Clin Radiol 38:603, 1987.

95. Huibregtse K, Tytgat GN. Palliative treatment of obstructive jaundice by transpapillary introduction of large bore bile duct endoprosthesis. Gut 23:371, 1982.

96. O'Brien S, Hatfield ARW, Carig PI, Williams SP. A three year follow-up of self expanding metal stents in the endoscopic palliation of long-term survivors with malignant biliary obstruction. Gut 36:618, 1995.

97. Mueller PR, van Sonnenberg E, Ferrucci JT, Jr. Percutaneous biliary drainage: Technical and catheter-related problems in 200 procedures. AJR 138:17, 1982.

98. Kerlan RK Jr, Pogany AC, Goldberg HI, Ring EJ. Percutaneous biliary drainage in the management of cholangiocarcinoma. AJR 141:1295, 1983.

99. Dooley JS, Dick R, George P, et al. Percutaneous transhepatic endoprosthesis for bile duct obstruction. Gastroenterology 86:905, 1984.

100. Lai ECS, Tompkins RK, Roslyn JJ, et al. Proximal bile duct cancer: Quality of survival. Ann Surg 205:111, 1987.

101. Malangoni MA, McCoy DM, Richardson JD, Flint LM. Effective palliation of malignant biliary duct obstruction. Ann Surg 201:554, 1985.

102. Nordaback IH, Pitt HA, Coleman J, Venbrux AC, et al. Unresectable hilar cholangiocarcinoma: Percutaneous versus operative palliation. Surgery 115:597, 1994.

103. Guthrie CM, Banting SW, Garden OJ, Carter DC. Segment III cholangiojejunostomy for palliation of malignant hilar obstruction. Br J Surg 81:1639, 1994.

104. Farley DR, Weaver AL, Nagorney DM. 'Natural history' of unresected cholangiocarcinoma: Patient outcome after noncurative intervention. Mayo Clin Proc 70:425, 1995.

105. Oberfield RA, Rossi RL. The role of chemotherapy in the treatment of bile duct cancer. World J Surg 12:105, 1988.

106. Curley SA, Cameron JL. Hilar bile duct cancer: A diagnostic and therapeutic challenge. Cancer Bull 44:309, 1992.

107. Meyers WC, Jones RS. Internal radiation for bile duct cancer. World J Surg 12:99, 1988.

108. Karani J, Fletcher M, Brinkley D, et al. Internal biliary drainage and local radiotherapy with iridium-192 wire in treatment of hilar cholangiocarcinoma. Clin Radiol 36:603, 1985.

109. Johnson DW, Safai C, Goffinet DR. Malignant obstructive jaundice: Treatment with external-beam and intracavitary radiotherapy. Int J Radiat Oncol Biol Phys 11:411, 1985.

110. Mornex F, Ardiet JM, Bret P, et al. Radiotherapy of high bile duct carcinoma using intracatheter iridium 192 wire. Cancer 54:2069, 1984.

111. Hishikawa Y, Shinada T, Miura T, et al. Radiation therapy of carcinoma of the extrahepatic bile ducts. Radiology 146:787, 1983.

112. Busse PM, Stone MD, Sheldon TA, et al. Intraoperative radiation therapy for biliary tract carcinoma: Results of a 5-year experience. Surgery 105:724, 1989.

113. Iwasaki Y, Todoroki T, Fukao K, et al. The role of intraoperative radiation therapy in the treatment of bile duct cancer. World J Surg 12:91, 1988.

114. Rich TA. Treatment planning for tumors of the gastrointestinal tract. In Paliwal BR, Griem ML (eds). Syllabus: A Categorical Course in Radiation Therapy Treatment Planning. Illinois: RSNA Division of Editorial and Publishing Services, 1986, p 47.

115. Nunnerley HB. Interventional radiology and internal radiotherapy for bile duct tumors. In Preece PE, Cuschieri A, Rosin RD (eds). Cancer of the Bile Ducts and Pancreas. Philadelphia: W.B. Saunders, 1989, p 93.

116. Rich TA. Intraoperative radiotherapy: A review. Radiother Oncol 6:207, 1986.

117. Deziel DJ, Kiel KD, Kramer TS, et al. Intraoperative radiation therapy in biliary tract cancer. Am Surg 54:402, 1988.

118. Boring CC, Squires TS, Tong T, Montgomery S. Cancer Statistics, 1994. CA Cancer J Clinicians 44:7, 1994.

119. Piehler JM, Crichlow RW. Primary carcinoma of the gallbladder. Surg Gynecol Obstet 147:929, 1978.

120. Aretxabala XD, Roa I, Araya JC, Burgos L, et al. Gallbladder cancer in patients less than 40 years old. Br J Surg 81:111, 1994.

121. Nelson BD, Provaznik J, Benfield JR. Gallbladder disease in southwestern American Indians. Arch Surg 103:41, 1971.

122. Rudolph R, Cohen JJ. Cancer of the gallbladder in an 11-year-old Navajo girl. J Pediatr Surg 7:66, 1972.

123. Mancuso TF, Brennan MJ. Epidemiological considerations of cancer of the gallbladder, bile ducts, and salivary glands in the rubber industry. J Occup Med 12:333, 1970.

124. Enomoto M, Naoe S, Harada M, et al. Carcinogenesis in extrahepatic bile duct and gallbladder; carcinogenic effect of N-hydroxy-2-acetamidofluorene in mice fed a 'gallstone-inducing' diet. Jpn J Exp Med 44:37, 1974.

125. Nagorney DM, McPherson GAD. Carcinoma of the gallbladder and extrahepatic bile ducts. Semin Oncol 15:106, 1988.

126. Diehl AK. Gallstone size and the risk of gallbladder cancer. JAMA 250:2323, 1983.

127. Polk HC. Carcinoma and the calcified gallbaldder. Gastroenterology 50:582, 1966.

128. Berk RN, Armbuster TG, saltz. Carcinoma of the porcelain gallbladder. 2:175, 1973.

129. Csendes A, Becerra M, Burdiles P, et al. Bacteriological studies of bile from the gallbladder in patients with carcinoma of the gallbaldder, cholelithiasis, common bile duct stones and no gallstones disease. Eur J Surg 160:363, 1994.

130. Parkash O. On the relationship of cholelithiasis to carcinoma of the gallbladder and on the sex dependency of the carcinoma of the bile ducts. Digestion 12:129, 1975.

131. Albores-Saavedra J, Acantra-Vazquez A, Cruz-Ortiz H, et al. The precursor lesions of invasive gallbladder carcinoma. Hyperplasia, atypical hyperplasia, and carcinoma in situ. Cancer 45:919, 1980.

132. Black WE. The morphogenesis of gallbladder carcinoma. In Fenoglio CM, Wolff M (eds). Progress in Surgical Pathology. New York: Masson, 1980, p. 207.

133. Kuzuka S, Tsubone M, Yasui A, et al. Relation of adenoma to carcinoma in the gallbladder. Cancer 50:2226, 1982.

304

134. Yukawa M, Fujimori T, Hirayama D, Idei Y, et al. Expression of oncogene products and growth factors in early gallbladder cancer, advanced gallbladder cancer, and chronic cholecystitis. Hum Pathol 24:37, 1993.

135. Sumiyoshi K, Nagai E, Chijiiwa K, Nakayama F. Pathology of carcinoma of the gallbladder. World J Surg 15:315, 1991.

136. Fahim RB, McDonald JR, Richards JC, Ferris DO. Carcinoma of the gallbladder: A study of its modes of spread. Ann Surg 156:114, 1962.

137. Shirai Y, Tsukada K, Ohtani T, Watanabe H, Hatakeyama K. Hepatic metastases from carcinoma of the gallbladder. Cancer 75:2063, 1995.

138. Ito M, Mishima Y, Sato T. An anatomical study of the lymphatic drainage of the gallbladder. Radiol Anat 13:89, 1991.

139. Nevin JE, Moran TJ, Kay S, King R. Carcinoma of the gallbladder. Cancer 37:141, 1976.

140. Japanese Society of Biliary Surgery. The General Rules for Surgical and Pathological Studies on Cancer of Biliary Tract, 2nd ed. Tokyo: Kanehara Syuppan, 1986.

141. Carmo MD, Perpetuo MO, Valdivieso M, et al. Natural history study of gallbladder cancer. Cancer 42:330, 1978.

142. Tashiro S, Konno T, Mochinaga M, et al. Treatment of carcinoma of the gallbladder in Japan. Jpn J Surg 12:98, 1982.

143. Koga A, Yamauchi S, Izumi Y, et al. Ultrasonographic detection of early and curable carcinoma of the gallbladder. Br J Surg 72:728, 1985.

144. Kubota K, Bandai Y, Noie T, Ishizaki V, et al. How should polypoid lesions of the gallbladder be treated in the era of laparoscopic cholecystectomy? Surgery 117:481, 1995.

145. Soiva M, Aro K, Pamilo M, et al. Ultrasonography in carcinoma of the gallbladder. Acta Radiologica 28:711, 1987.

146. Palma LD, Rizzatto G, Pozzi-Mucelli RS, Bazzoccbi M. Gray-scale ultrasonography in the evaluation of the carcinoma of the gallbladder. Br J Radiol 53:662, 1980.

147. Li D, Dong B, Wu Y, Yan K. Image-directed and color Doppler studies of gallbladder tumors. J Clin Ultrasound 22:551, 1994.

148. Itai Y, Araki T, Yoshihawa K, et al. Computed tomography of gallbladder carcinoma. Radiology 137:713, 1980.

149. Chijiiwa K, Yumiyoshi K, Nakayama F. Impact of recent advances in hepatobiliary imaging techniques on the preoperative diagnosis of carcinoma of the gallbladder. World J Surg 15:322, 1991.

150. Thorsen MK, Quiroz F, Lawson TL, et al. Primary biliary carcinoma: CT evaluation. Radiology 152:479, 1984.

151. Hamrick RE, Liner J, Hastings PR, Cohn I. Primary carcinoma of the gallbladder. Ann Surg 195:270, 1982.

152. Klamer TW, Max MH. Carcinoma of the gallbladder. Surg Gynecol Obstet 156:641, 1983.

153. Barr IH. Carcinoma of the gallbladder. Am Surg 50:275, 1984.

154. Gagner M, Rossi RL. Radical operations for carcinoma of the gallbladder: Present status in North America. World J Srug 15:344, 1991.

155. Ogura Y, Mizumoto R, Isaji S, et al. Radical operations for carcinoma of the gallbladder: Present status in Japan. World J Surg 15:337, 1991.

156. Gall FP, Kockerling F, Scheele J, et al. Radical operations for carcinoma of the gallbladder: Present status in Germany. World J Surg 15:328, 1991.

157. Yamaguchi K, Tsuneyoshi M. Subclinical gallbladder carcinoma. Am J Surg 163:382, 1992.

158. Ouchi K, Owada Y, Matsuno S, Sato T. Prognostic factors in the surgical treatment of gallbladder carcinoma. Surgery 101:731, 1987.

159. Bergdahl L. Gallbladder carcinoma first diagnosed at microscopic examination of gallbladders removed for presumed benign disease. Ann Surg 191:19, 1980.

160. Donohoe JH, Nagorney DM, Grant CS, et al. Carcinoma of the gallbladder. Arch Surg 125:237, 1990.

161. Ouchi K, Suzuki M, Tominaga T, Saijo S, Matsuno S. Survival after surgery for cancer of the gallbladder. Br J Surg 81:1655, 1994.

162. Nimura Y, Hayakawa N, Kamiya J, et al. Hepatopancreaticoduodenectomy for advanced carcinoma of the biliary tract. Hepatogastroenterology 38:170, 1991.

163. Alessiani M, Tzakis A, Todo S, Demetris AJ, et al. Assessment of five-year experience with abdominal organ cluster transplantation. J Am Coll Surg 180:1, 1995.

164. Grace PA, Quereshi A, Coleman J, et al. Recuced postoperative hospitalization after laparoscopic cholecystectomy. Br J Surg 78:160, 1991.

165. Fong Y, Brennan MF, Turnbull A, et al. Gallbladder cancer discovered during laparoscopic surgery. Arch Surg 128:1054, 1993.

166. Drouard F, Delamarre J, Capron J. Cutaneous seeding of gallbladder cancer after laparoscopic cholecytectomy. N Engl J Med 325:1316, 1991.

167. Pezet D, Fondrinier E, Rotman N, et al. Pariental seeding of carcinoma of the gallbladder after laparoscopic cholecytectomy. Br J Surg 79:230, 1992.

168. Clair DG, Lautz DB, Brooks DC. Rapid development of umbilical metastases after laparoscopic cholecytectomy for unsuspected gallbladder carcinoma. Surgery 113:355, 1993.

169. Kim HJ, Roy T. Unexpected gallbladder cancer with cutaneous seeding after laparoscopic cholecystectomy. South Med J 87:817, 1994.

170. Jones RS. Palliative operative procedures for carcinoma of the gallbladder. World J Surg 15:348, 1991.

171. Falkson G, MacIntyre JM, Moertel CG. Eastern Cooperative Oncology Group experience with chemotherapy for inoperable gallbladder and bile duct cancer. Cancer 54:965, 1984.

172. Hall SW, Benjamin RS, Murphy WK, et al. Adriamycin, BCNU, FTORAFUR chemotherapy of pancreatic and biliary tract cancer. Cancer 44:2008, 1979.

173. Harvey JH, Smith FP, Schein PS. 5-Fluorouracil, mitomycin, and doxorubicin (FAM) in carcinoma of the biliary tract. J Clin Oncol 2:1245, 1984.

174. Smith GW, Bukowski RM, Hewlett JS, Groppe CW. Heaptic artery infusion of 5-fluorouracil and mitomycin C in cholangiocarcinoma and gallbladder carcinoma. Cancer 54:1513, 1984.

175. Kairaluoma MI, Leinonen A, Niemela R, et al. Superselective intra-arterial chemotherapy with mitomycin C in liver and gallbladder cancer. Eur J Surg Oncol 14:45, 1988.

176. Makela JT, Kairaluoma MI. Superselective intra-artieral chemotherapy with mitomycin for gallbladder cancer. Br J Surg 80:912, 1993.

177. Buskirk SJ, Gunderson LL, Adson MA, et al. Analysis of failure following curative irradiation of gallbladder and extrahepatic bile duct carcinoma. Int J Radia Oncol Biol Phys 10:2013, 1984.

178. Smoron GL. Radiation therapy of carcinoma of gallbladder and biliary tract. Cancer 40:1422, 1977.

179. Pilepich MV, Lambert PM. Radiotherapy of carcinomas of the extrahepatic biliary system. Radiology 127:767, 1978.

180. Kopelson G, Harisiadis L, Tretter P, Chang CH. The role of radiation therapy in cancer of the extra-hepatic biliary system: An analysis of thirteen patients and a review of the literature of the effectiveness of surgery, chemotherapy and radiotherapy. Int J Radia Oncol Biol Phys 2:883, 1977.

181. Martenson JA, Gunderson LL, Buskirk SJ, et al. Hepatic duct stricture after radical radiation therapy for biliary cancer: Recurrence of fibrosis? Mayo Clin Proc 61:530, 1986.

182. Busse PM, Cady B, Bothe A, et al. Intraoperative radiation therapy for carcinoma of the gallbladder. World J Surg 15:352, 1991.

183. Todoroki T, Iwasaki Y, Okamura T, et al. Intraoperative radiotherapy for advanced carcinoma of the biliary system. Cancer 46:2179, 1980.

184. Morrow CE, Sutherland DER, Florack G, et al. Primary gallbladder carcinoma: Significance of subserosal lesions and results of aggressive surgical treatment and adjuvant chemotherapy. Surgery 94:709, 1983.

185. Athlin LEA, Domellof LKH, Bergman FO. Advanced gallbladder carcinoma: A case report and review of the literature. Eur J Surg Oncol 17:449, 1987.
186. Todoroki T, Iwasaki Y, Orii K, et al. Resection combined with intraoperative radiation therapy (IORT) for stage IV (TNM) gallbladder carcinoma. World J Surg 15:357, 1991.

16. Minimally invasive surgery in surgical oncology

Jeffrey W. Milsom, Pierenrico Marchesa, and Andrea Vignali

Introduction

The use of laparoscopy to evaluate the peritoneal cavity by direct vision was first described in 1902 by Kelling [1]. After development of the video endoscope in the 1980s, the success of laparoscopic cholecystectomy procedures stimulated surgical oncologists to consider applying minimally invasive surgical (MIS) techniques broadly to cancer patients.

Minimally invasive therapies for malignant diseases are in their infancy. Therefore, very few current reports represent much more than preliminary ideas or data. Before adapting MIS techniques, most surgeons treating cancer need to see benefits in terms of recurrence and survival rates. In this context, this chapter can serve only as an introduction to the current uses of MIS for diagnostic and staging purposes, for palliative treatment, and for curative treatment of gastrointestinal and other intraabdominal malignancies.

The diagnostic potential of laparoscopy was exploited initially in Europe for the assessment of liver disease and gynecologic problems [2,3]. In particular, gynecologists first explored the feasibility of operative procedures on the adnexa through the laparoscope. However, the absence of adequate instrumentation limited the wider acceptance of MIS until recently. Rapid improvements in optical systems and light sources, combined with the availability of new surgical instruments, such as laparoscopic ultrasonography, have thrust laparoscopy into common usage in nearly every field of abdominal cancer surgery, with novel applications appearing almost daily. Since this field is young, the natural enthusiasm over the use of very fascinating electronic, computer-assisted technology must be tempered with the realization that this technology is expensive, that available health care dollars are decreasing, and in case of curative therapies, very few patients actually will suffer major morbidity because of the incision of conventional surgery.

Diagnostic and staging laparoscopy

Generalities

During the past two decades improvements in both medical and surgical oncology have resulted in a situation in which a variety of therapeutic options

Raphael E. Pollock (ed.), SURGICAL ONCOLOGY. Copyright © 1997. Kluwer Academic Publishers. ISBN 0-7923-9900-5. All rights reserved.

can be offered to the cancer patient, dependent on a precise understanding of the extent of tumor spread. As a result, the most accurate and reliable staging of the tumor with confirmatory tissue biopsies is mandatory. Underestimation of tumor stage could result in an unnecessary exploratory laparotomy when nonoperative management might have been more appropriate [4].

The most common practice for tumor staging has been use of non-invasive imaging studies such as computed tomography (CT), ultrasound (US), and more recently, magnetic resonance imaging (MRI) and immunoscintigraphy with labeled antibodies to tumor-associated antigens. However, these imaging techniques frequently miss lesions under 1 cm in diameter or are lacking in the ability to identify small lesions (seedlings) of the parietal peritoneum or omentum [5].

An emerging alternative to conventional preoperative radiological staging in certain cancer centers has been the use of laparoscopy alone for the assessment of cancer patients. Previous studies in the literature show that laparoscopy and guided biopsy have an 80–90% accuracy in the diagnosis of liver and pancreatic tumors, which is at least comparable with that of noninvasive techniques [4,6]. Among the reported benefits are (1) the possibility to retrieve cytological and histological specimens for diagnostic confirmation of the primary tumor, and (2) demonstration of lymph node spread and hepatic or peritoneal metastasis. Watt et al. demonstrated prospectively that laparoscopy was significantly more sensitive and accurate that ultrasonography or CT with respect to hepatic status in patients with esophageal and gastric cancers [7]. In particular, laparoscopy was the only reliable diagnostic tool for the detection of seedling deposits on the peritoneal surface [8,9].

Currently laparoscopy is considered an ideal complementary modality to noninvasive diagnostic techniques in order to maximize patient benefits and to avoid futile laparotomies, in which the complication rate is still high (23%) compared with 1.8% with no mortality reported in recent series of diagnostic laparoscopies [6]. Many reports in the literature have shown that positive laparoscopic findings, following normal preoperative tests, altered the course of therapy in up to 48% of patients with primary intestinal and pancreatic cancers [5,10,11]. One drawback to laparoscopic staging, solely using the visualization of intraabdominal organs, has been the inability to detect lesions within the solid organs or spread of disease in the retroperitoneum [12]. For example, inability to detect neoplastic infiltration of the portal vein could result in a wrong laparoscopic assessment for resectability of pancreatic cancer [13].

Attempts to overcome similar restrictions often experienced by the surgeon at open operation led to the development of intraoperative contact ultrasonography [14]. The development of a high-frequency linear-array ultra-compact transducer allowed for the development of laparoscopic ultrasonography [15]. The early results of cancer staging by laparoscopy with laparoscopic ultrasonography have been encouraging, providing the surgeon with correct information on both infiltration of primary tumor to the surrounding structures and on whether liver metastases are present or not. In addition, the demonstrated feasibility of laparoscopic pelvic lymphadenectomy has boosted the interest of clinicians to stage both urological and gynecological pelvic cancers using a minimally invasive technique. Additionally, laparoscopic techniques have been demonstrated to be useful for intra-abdominal lymph node sampling in the assessment of patients with lymphomas.

Hepatocellular carcinoma

The laparoscopic technique has been frequently employed in the staging of primary hepatocellular carcinoma (HCC) alone or in combination with ultrasound-guided fine-needle biopsy. This can be done under laparoscopic vision, and potential bleeding from the biopsy site can easily be diagnosed and managed. Very promising early results were reported by Lightdale and Jeffers, who identified, using laparoscopy, multiple tumors and peritoneal metastases in almost all patients of their series who had previously undergone negative preoperative radiographic staging [16,17]. Thus they were able to avoid laparotomy in these patients with a very poor prognosis. These results have been confirmed by the reported experience of several other authors [5,18]. A dissenting view was reported by Gandolfi, who stressed, in a series of 54 patients, the major improvement in the staging of HCC, using ultrasonography, as compared with laparoscopy alone [19]. An additional advantage of the routine use of laparoscopy is its superior ability in identifying cirrhosis, which might preclude resection, as compared with imaging techniques such as ultrasound alone [20]. Hepatic surgeons have long appreciated that, even under direct vision, the differentiation of areas of infiltrating hepatocarcinomas is difficult and routine adoption of laparoscopic ultrasound-guided biopsies has partially solved this problem [21]. Additionally, one of the major criticisms toward the use of laparoscopic evaluation alone (without ultrasonography) is the inability to evaluate for portal vein thrombosis, perilar lymph nodes, and infiltration of retroperitoneal structures, all of which may play a pivotal role in accurate tumor staging [14].

Very promising reports about laparoscopic ultrasonography have appeared in the recent literature. It was first introduced by Okita et al. in 1984 [22] as a means for diagnosing small hepatocellular hepatocarcinomas in chronic liver disease. Many modifications have been made in the probe configuration since this approach has been introduced. In a recent series of 43 patients, laparoscopic ultrasonography provided additional staging information, as compared with that derived from laparoscopic alone, in 18 to 43 patients, leading to an eventual resectability rate of 93% as compared with the 58% obtained in those patients in whom operative assessment was undertaken without laparoscopy [23]. Laparoscopic staging using ultrasonography is rapidly becoming a valued assessment tool.

Pancreatic cancer

The prognosis of most patients with pancreatic cancer remains poor, with only a relatively small (<10%) proportion of patients who benefit from a resective operation. The unheralded presence of metastatic disease at laparotomy in a high percentage of patients has led to major attempts to adequally stage patients before undertaking laparotomy. Accurate preoperative staging is critical in these patients to avoid futile surgical explorations.

The use of laparoscopic staging for pancreatic cancer has become widely popular. Laparoscopy also offers the possibility, in advanced pancreatic cancer, to perform laparoscopic bypasses, thus avoiding the need for a second operation [23–25]. Laparoscopy for staging has been reported to be able to identify intrabdominal spreading of pancreatic cancer in 39–73% patients [8,9]. Warshaw and coworkers discovered liver and peritoneal metastases in 41% of patients who had previously negative CT scans [11]. The most interesting data in this series were that the laparoscopic method has achieved a sensitivity rate of 93%.

The introduction of laparoscopy ultrasound has also increased the diagnostic field even further, leading to a positive predictive value of 97%, which represents an improvement over the 89% value derived from the combination of CT and mesenteric angiography reported by previous series [26,27]. Despite the relative paucity of reports on large clinical series using laparoscopy in pancreatic staging, laparoscopic staging for pancreatic cancer is becoming the new standard of therapy.

Gastrointestinal cancer

Carcinomas of the esophagus and esophagogastric junction usually manifest themselves in an advanced stage in the majority of patients, leading to a very low 5-year survival rate, even when complete (R_0) surgical resection is performed. Laparoscopic staging for this cancer may be attractive in many patients because it may allow them to avoid an unnecessary laparotomy.

Recent reports in the literature stress that laparoscopy is probably more sensitive than ultrasound and CT in assessing nodal involvement [10,28]. Watt et al. reported an overall accuracy rate using laparoscopy of 72%, compared with 52% and 57% for ultrasound and CT, respectively [7]. A 87% sensitivity rate was also reported by Possik et al. in his large series of 360 patients studied laparoscopically [29]. There is also only a 4% false-positive rate for laparoscopic staging [30]. The combination of laparoscopic and laparoscopic ultrasound has further improved the overall staging of gastrointestinal tumors when compared with combined CT scan and endoscopic ultrasonography, which at the present time are considered the most accurate modalities to stage gastric adenocarcinoma [31].

A criticism among surgeons toward the use of laparoscopic staging is that laparoscopic procedures, eventually undertaken for palliation of unresectable gastric cancers, can technically be more difficult and have a higher morbidity than conventional modalities and can be performed only in selected centers [32].

Gynecological cancers

Traditionally the treatment of patients with gynecologic malignancies has involved a laparotomy to acquire the necessary staging information, including primary tumor spread to pelvic and para-aortic lymph nodes, and to the general peritoneal cavity. Gynecologists, familiar with laparoscopic techniques for the treatment of benign diseases, began to perform, surgical-pathological neoplastic staging with a minimal invasive approach in the late 1980s [33].

The technique for laparoscopic pelvic lymphadenectomy was independently developed by Dargent and Querleu in 1991, using the retroperitoneal or transperitoneal approach, respectively, for staging patients with early cervical carcinoma [34,35]. Since then, a growing number of reports in the literature describe the use of laparoscopic procedures in patients with gynecological malignancies.

Recently published series have demonstrated that laparoscopic lymphadenectomy was performed successfully in 94% of 29 endometrial cancer patients [36], and only a single patient out of a combined series of 30 with early cervical cancer had a positive (microscopic) node, identified at laparotomy, that was not removed at laparoscopy [35,37]. Few complications were reported and the procedures were performed in an acceptable length of time. Although the adequacy of the procedure appears to be comparable with that of conventional staging, large prospective controlled studies are necessary to justify laparoscopic lymphadenectomy as an alternative to the laparotomy traditionally offered to cervical cancer patients.

The role of laparoscopy in patients with ovarian cancer is even less defined and is centered around two areas: (1) evaluation of stage I ovarian carcinoma and (2) second-look laparoscopies.

Reich was the first author who reported, in 1990, a complete staging of early ovarian cancer using laparoscopy [38]. The obvious concerns were the possibility for missing extraovarian disease and the risk for tumor cell spillage if uneventful tumor rupture occurred. Further investigations in small series of patients demonstrated the relative safety and oncologic adequacy of the technique. Eight of 14 patients with presumed initial carcinoma were diagnosed with metastatic disease, and a median of eight aortic and six pelvic nodes were obtained on each homolateral chain in 10 patients [39,40].

The possibility of performing a detailed exploration of the peritoneal surface suggested the role for laparoscopy as a modality to reevaluate patients with advanced ovarian cancer who had been surgically debulked and had received platinum-based chemotherapy. The first experiences in 1980 resulted in a false-negative rate of 36% [41]. However, these reports were criticized because para-aortic lymphadenectomies and random multiple biopsies, considered mandatory in a conventional second-look operation, were not performed [42]. Querleu and LeBlanc reported in 1994 a complete oncological in restaging ovarian cancer following adjuvant therapy [43]. More recently, second-look laparoscopy in patients with clinically complete remission in treatment of advanced ovarian cancer were able to detect residual disease in up to 56% of patients, comparable with results reported conventional staging by laparotomy [40]. The role laparoscopy will play in ovarian cancers remains undefined, but further investigations into the validity of this approach are warranted.

Prostatic carcinoma

Pelvic lymph node dissection for staging prostate cancer is probably the most frequent application of laparoscopy in adult urology. However, the diffusion of transrectal ultrasound and evidence for the prognostic value of prostate-specific antigen (PSA) serum concentration have allowed the urologist to detect prostate cancer at a clinically earlier stage. The growing reliability of the noninvasive staging technique parallels the decrease for the need of surgical staging. Laparoscopic pelvic lymphadenectomy has been demonstrated to be as adequate as the open procedure in several studies [44,45]. Both transperitoneal and extraperitoneal laparoscopic approaches have been applied to prostate cancer staging with similar results [46].

To date, laparoscopic staging is limited to patients who are considered to be at high risk for nodal metastases in whom confirmation of nodal disease would preclude radical prostatectomy [47]. In leading centers, patients should meet the following criteria: PSA concentration >40 ng/ml; Gleason grade 8 or more; clinical stage B2, C, or DO; or negative CT-guided fine-needle biopsy of pelvic lymph nodes. No mortality is reported to be associated with this procedure, and the overall complication rate was 15% in a large review of 500 patients [48].

Lymphomas

Accurate evaluation of the liver and abdominal node harvest are the rationale for laparotomy as a staging procedure in systemic lymphoma, while the need for splenectomy is controversial. Laparoscopic staging in patients with Hodgkin's and non-Hodgkin's lymphomas has been demonstrated to be feasible, even though early studies reported a high false-negative rate, especially in patients with non-Hodgkin's lymphoma [49,50]. Few studies have been published in which a complete laparoscopic staging seems to provide as much information as the standard staging laparotomy, although there have not been any comparative studies between the two [51–53].

314

Palliative treatment

The laparoscopic approach has many attractive features for palliative treatment of patients with inoperable malignancies. The favorable impact of laparoscopic techniques on postoperative recovery, with avoidance of the discomfort and debilitation of laparotomy, is desirable in such patients, who by the nature of their disease would gain most from the resulting reduced hospitalization and shorter convalescence. In conventional surgery, when the neoplasia is assessed to be unresectable in the preoperative period, palliative operations are usually performed through small laparotomies in order to minimize the postoperative stress response. The overall advantage of laparoscopic methods with palliative intent is to permit a complete inspection of the abdominal cavity with the potential for a precisely defined intraoperative diagnosis. Furthermore, additional problems can be assessed and other procedures (e.g., feeding tubes) can be performed at the same time.

Different laparoscopic palliative procedures have been described, including diverting and feeding enterostomies, and more complex operations such as enteral or biliary bypasses and segmental bowel resections. Patients with extensive pharingo-esophageal tumors, preventing the passage of the gastroscope for performing a percutaneous endoscopic gastrostomy (PEG), are ideal candidates for laparoscopic feeding gastrostomy or jejunostomy [54–56]. Morbidity and mortality rate are reported to be lower and the mean operative time significantly shorter than comparable open procedures, although results are only preliminary.

A variety of bypass procedures are possible with a laparoscopic approach. Patients with duodenal obstruction secondary to inoperable pancreatic or duodenal neoplasms have been successfully palliated by laparoscopic gastroenterostomy [57–59]. The procedure is relatively easy to perform using laparoscopic stapling devices, and postoperative complications have been relatively low and unrelated to the surgical procedure. Nagy et al. reported 2 conversions to conventional surgery out of 10 patients [57]. Laparoscopic bilioenteric bypass may be an effective alternative in patients with obstructive jaundice due to unresectable carcinoma of the pancreas or the distal bile duct [58,59]. A mechanical anastomosis is performed between the gallbladder and the proximal jejunum if the cystic duct is demonstrated to be patent. Otherwise, a choledoco-jejunostomy (technically more challenging) may be necessary. This new approach has resulted in the abolition of episodes of cholangitis frequently associated with endoscopic stenting. However, endoscopic stenting is indicated in patients with large advanced lesions and metastatic spread, resulting in short life expectancy, whereas laparoscopic treatment is more appropriate in patients who are likely to survive several months. More recently, a combination of laparoscopic biliary and gastric bypass has been proposed to overcome the obstruction of both intestinal and biliary transit [56]. The procedure is indicated when duodenal obstruction results, along with a failed stenting of the biliary tree, or when peritoneal or liver metastasis is found at laparoscopy.

Patients with obstructing locally advanced tumors of the large intestine can be palliated by either diverting end colostomies or loop ileostomies. Safe and effective laparoscopic diversion techniques have been described by several cancer centers [60–62]. The surgical technique is relatively simple and allows the surgeons to precisely identify the appropriate segment of bowel and to pull it to the stoma site with the proper orientation, avoiding the worrisome complications that are possible after conventional 'blind' stoma formation. Most patients resume normal bowel function and are able to restart the oral nutrition 24–48 hours after surgery.

Laparoscopic-assisted segmental colon resection with either intracorporeal or extracorporeal division of feeding vessels can be a reasonable palliative procedure for patients with colon cancer and secondary hepatic or pulmonary metastatic spread not suitable for surgical ablation [63,64]. Removal of a short intestinal segment bearing the primary tumor with clear margins is often readily accomplished using laparoscopic techniques. Nevertheless, if the primary tumor is too bulky and/or infiltrating the surrounding tissues, the surgery should be converted to an 'open' procedure, or a bypass without resection performed.

Curative therapy in gastrointestinal cancers

Because MIS has only been applied to the management of patients with potentially curable abdominal malignancies in the last 3–5 years, there are relatively little data on whether or not it is as effective as conventional surgery in eliminating disease. There is almost no question that every part of the gastrointestinal tract is removable using minimally invasive surgical methods, yet there has been a natural reluctance on the part of most surgeons to proceed with curative therapy using MIS because of the lack of data supporting its use and the difficulty of removing after a bulky lesion that cannot be directly palpated, and that often must be removed through a large incision just to accommodate its size. In this section we attempt to review the available data on curative minimally invasive surgery for each area of the gastrointestinal tract, commenting on the concerns and current foci of interest for each area.

Esophageal cancers

There are few reports on the use of MIS techniques for curative purposes in esophageal cancers. In several small series, a thorascopic approach is used to mobilize the esophagus, and then a gastroplasty is carried out by laparotomy. The third stage of the operation entails anastomosis between the cervical esophagus and the gastric pull-up. A number of problems have been noted with this approach, including difficulty in dissecting a bulky lesion, respiratory complications (up to 19% in a series of 29 patients), and the potential risk of parietal seeding, reported recently in one series [65–67]. Currently, it is too early to know if MIS techniques are of benefit in esophageal patients. Esophagectomy using MIS must currently be considered investigational.

Gastric cancers

Although gastric tumors may often be bulky lesions, there are a number of reports from Japan describing the use of MIS techniques for curative purposes in very early gastric cancers. These preliminary reports represent small series of patients undergoing wedge resections of a portion of the stomach. Yamashita et al. reported on seven patients with early gastric cancers (limited to the mucosa) who had lesions ranging from 10 to 21 mm in diameter. The lesions were located by a conventional gasrofiberscope passed transorally; then a laparoscope was used to inspect the abdominal cavity and also to locate the lesion using transillumination by the gastroscope. A 3 cm incision in the upper midline was made for exteriorization of the cancer, and an extracorporeal wedge resection was carried out [68]. After a follow-up ranging from 13 to 28 months, all seven patients were alive without recurrence. Another technique of early gastric cancer resection is the 'lesion lifting' method described by Ohgami et al. [69]. Early gastric cancers have also been removed using trocars passed through both the abdominal and stomach walls (laparoscopic intragastric surgery) [70]. The results of these preliminary series show that these methods are feasible, but acceptance and oncologic results await larger series and longer follow-up.

Hepatopancreaticobiliary cancer

Very little is known about the curative treatment of these cancers using MIS techniques. In liver surgery, when being performed with a curative attempt, these may be an advantage to performing a preliminary laparoscopy with laparoscopic ultrasonography to verify resectability prior to making any major incision, thus avoiding a laparotomy in an incurable situation [23,71].

Liver tumors

Of the many different technologies available to ablate liver tumors (ultrasonic dissector, argon-beam coagulator, electrosurgery), perhaps the most promising is the cryosurgical probe, which can be passed into hepatic tumors using ultrasound guidance. While very little survival data are available, Cuschieri et al. describe its use in 22 patients with primary or secondary liver cancers. Preliminary results describing the feasibility of laparoscopic freezing of tumors were encouraging, with only one death attributable to the procedure [72]. Laparoscopic liver surgery, including cryotherapy, is currently only an investigational procedure.

Using more conventional techniques, several authors have described the use of endoscopic staplers to excise a very peripherally located small lesion on the liver. Obviously, only preliminary data about the use of MIS techniques in liver surgery are currently available; thus, this technique cannot be recommended as anything other than investigational therapy. The success of laparoscopic liver ultrasound imaging should greatly complement the potential success of MIS in treating liver cancers [71].

Pancreatic tumors

While laparoscopic techniques have become more and more important in the staging and biopsy of pancreatic cancers, there is no current role for curative therapy using laparoscopic techniques. A preliminary report on MIS pancreaticoduodenectomy for cancers was published by Gagner and Pomp in 1994 [73]. No survival data are available. The current role of MIS is pancreatic surgery largely rests on staging and palliation [24,25].

Gallbladder and bile duct cancers

Although much interest has focused on proper therapy for gallbladder cancers in the age of laparoscopic cholecystectomy, all experts in this field recommend conversion to conventional surgical techniques if a primary gallbladder tumor is suspected during laparoscopic cholecystectomy. The large number of case reports of cannula site implantation with gallbladder cancer support this policy at the present time [74–76]. Unfortunately, nearly all gallbladder cancers are discovered incidentally after laparoscopic cholecystectomy. There are no known reports on the use of laparoscopic techniques to resect primary bile duct tumors, probably because of their rarity, proximity to many vascular structures, and complexity in treatment.

Splenic tumors

Splenectomy by laparoscopic techniques had become a common procedure used by many surgeons for the curative/ablative therapy in a number of hematologic malignancies, including Hodgkin's disease, hereditary spherocytosis, hairy cell leukemia, and idiopathic thrombocytopenia purpura [77,78]. In nearly all instances, the splenic hilum is approached first, ligated, then the various other vascular and body wall attachments are lysed and ligated, and the organ is placed into an impermeable bag. Thereafter, the spleen may be removed from the bag in small chunks after pulling the mouth of the bag out through an abdominal-wall cannula site [78,79]. This approach has permitted most patients to undergo splenectomy without a major laparotomy and to seemingly recover quickly after surgery. It is likely that use of MIS techniques will increase in splenic disease, given that the spleen is an end organ that can safely be removed after fragmentation in an impermeable bag.

Small bowel malignancies

Because of their relative varity, there are no known reports about the use of laparoscopic techniques for curative removal of these tumors. Theoretically, if the lesion were small and able to be isolated preoperatively, a laparoscopic resection with proximal mesenteric vascular ligation could be feasible.

Large bowel malignancies

Adenocarcinomas of the large intestine represent the most common indication for large bowel surgery in the United States, and accordingly have been the most common indication for laparoscopic large-bowel resection in most series [65,80,81]. This is somewhat suprising because there are almost no data regarding whether there are advantages to laparoscopic bowel surgery compared with conventional surgery. Additionally, lesions are often bulky, the conventional surgical techniques to treat colorectal cancer usually entail removal of a very large section (12–18 inches) of intestine that is filled with bacteria-laden liquid, and major mesenteric blood vessels must be safety exposed and ligated near their origins — a task often made difficult by overlying loops of small intestine that must be retracted to another part of the abdomen.

Common questions about curative laparoscopic colorectal cancer surgery have been (1) What is an adequate extent of resection? (2) Is laparoscopic resection equivalent to conventional resection? (3) Can the surgeon adequately stage the rest of the abdomen during a laparoscopic resection?

Laparoscopic techniques have been successfully applied to cancers that are well localized and do not infiltrate other organs. The main specific contraindications to laparoscopic colorectal cancer resections probably should include:

1. Infiltrating tumors (into adjacent structures)
2. Large and bulky lesions >8 cm
3. Obstructing tumors (because of related bowel distension)

Although all areas of the colon and rectum may be approached using laparoscopic techniques, we currently avoid using laparoscopic techniques on lesions in the transverse colon and splenic flexure, because these areas are difficult to approach laparoscopically. Likewise, in the treatment of midrectal cancers, current technology does not permit accurate anastomotic formation deep in the pelvis, so we avoid using laparoscopy to treat these tumors.

We have demonstrated in fresh cadaver models that an oncologic type of resection is *anatomically* feasible using laparoscopic techniques for right hemicolectomy, proctosigmoidectomy with colorectal anastomosis [82], and abdominoperineal resection [83]. Current laparoscopic studies should be designed to demonstrate whether there are short-term advantages versus conventional surgery in curative colorectal cancer surgery. If clinically relevant short-term advantages are found, then multiinstitutional phase III studies should be pursued evaluating the long-term endpoints, recurrence and survival. Only after these types of studies demonstrate advantages to laparoscopic surgery patients can laparoscopic colorectal surgery with curative intent be widely recommended.

Problems with laparoscopic colorectal surgery

Early local recurrences in cannula sites are of major concern in many gastrointestinal and gynecologic malignancies, and have been reported after gastric [84], gallbladder [65,85], pancreatic [86], ovarian [87], and colorectal [75] malignancies. The precise pathogenesis of these early recurrences (weeks to several months) is not known, but may be attributable to the pneumoperitoneum or direct pressure effect of it, the effect of carbon dioxide, increased exfoliation of tumor cells using laparoscopic techniques, or some other unknown mechanism. Tumor seeding potential may be minimized by careful attention to technical details and placement of the specimen into an impermeable bag as soon as possible before delivery through the abdominal wall. The video recording capabilities of MIS should allow the surgeon to document the important oncologic steps of each operation, and this video documentation may someday become an important component of the medical record.

Current status of laparoscopic colorectal cancer surgery

There have been a variety of case series reporting on the feasibility and safety of MIS of colon cancer surgery [64,80,88]. None of the studies reported to date have proven these are major advantages to curative colorectal cancer surgery using laparoscopic techniques, in part because of the nonrandomized and highly selected nature of most of these series.

In general, since very little local recurrence and survival data are available as yet on MIS used in curative colorectal cancer therapy, most surgeons believe that this type of surgery should only be performed in the context of a prospective randomized trial.

In an attempt to address some of these concerns, a national cooperative National Cancer Institute–funded study is currently underway evaluating whether these are advantages to laparoscopic versus conventional colorectal cancer surgery. This multi-institutional study will address oncologic outcomes after laparoscopic surgery, and will also evaluate some short-term endpoints as well (economic, postoperative pain, and return of normal bowel function) [89].

In our institution, we are also performing a prospective, randomized trial in colorectal cancer patients, looking primarily at short-term outcomes after laparoscopic and conventional surgery. Recovery of pulmonary function, return of gastrointestinal function, amount of pain medicine used, and quality of life are the primary endpoints we are evaluating. Over 100 patients have been enrolled thus far. Preliminary analysis of the data has not been performed, but

18 months into the study we have seen no unusual patterns of recurrence in the laparoscopic group [90]. Conclusions from the study await the accrual of larger numbers of patients, but we hope to publish preliminary results by the end of 1996.

Urological and adrenal neoplasms

The development of techniques for organ entrapment and rapid tissue morcellation led to the performance of the initial laparoscopic transperitoneal nephrectomy in 1990 [91]. Since then, ablative urological laparoscopy has spread worldwide, predominantly for benign disease. Conversely, few centers have pursued the application of laparoscopic techniques for the treatment of urological tumors.

Both total and radical nephrectomies, using minimally invasive techniques, have been performed in patients with renal tumors [44,92]. To date, this approach has been limited to tumors of 6 cm in size or smaller without evidence of renal vein involvement [93]. However, Clayman recently reported removing an 8 cm tumor as well as a stage III tumor via laparoscopic radical nephrectomy [94]. Although there have been no deaths associated with laparoscopic nephrectomy, the reported complication rate in different studies is more than 30%, suggesting careful evaluation is necessary prior to popularizing this procedure [95].

Because of the potential for tumor seeding at trocar ports or secondary intraabdominal spillage of tumor cells during laparoscopic dissection or morcellation, alternative laparoscopic modalities have been investigated [96]. Gasless laparoscopic-assisted nephrectomy for renal carcinoma was demonstrated to be feasible without major adverse complications in seven patients [97]. The small number of patients in this series reflects a preliminary evaluation that does not allow for significant conclusions.

Laparoscopic nephro-ureterectomy has been described for treatment of midproximal ureteral or renal pelvic transitional cell carcinoma [98]. The reported results on only a few case reports, showing significant morbidity rate and excessive operating time, confine this technique to an investigational modality [99].

Schuessler has proposed a technique for laparoscopic radical prostatectomy with clinical experience in two patients [2]. To date it should be consider a clinically difficult procedure in need of significant technological breakthroughs.

The small size of the adrenal gland and the benign nature of most adrenal tumors made the laparoscopic resection of this gland attractive. The initial results of laparoscopic adrenalectomy, first described in 1992, seemed to be favorable [100–102]. Laparoscopic removal of both cortical and medullary hormone-producing benign tumors has been attempted with success in the past few years, while invasive malignancy is still considered a contraindication. Use of MIS techniques (transperitoneal vs. intraperitoneal) in adrenal surgery is controversial due to the small number of patients in the reported series [103–105]. Comparisons of the endoscopic versus conventional access to adrenalectomy are difficult to make. Postoperative morbidity rate appears to be similar, with the advantages over the standard open procedure being the same as those of other laparoscopic operations, especially in terms of rapid postoperative recovery favorable outcome [106].

In conclusion, the use of laparoscopic surgery in patients with malignancies of the kidney and ureter remains controversial. Refinement of techniques and long-term follow-up are mandatory to confirm the efficacy in a clinical setting. The laparoscopic approach for benign hormone-producing tumors of the adrenal glands may be effective, but long-term results and multi-institutional studies are advisable before there is wider acceptance of this technique.

Gynecological neoplasms

The need for a complete surgical staging in order to individualize the treatment in patients with gynecological malignancies has become clear in the last decade. The first reports on performance of laparoscopic pelvic node sampling and dissection demonstrated this technique to be less morbid and expensive than the traditional open techniques, but some early technical problems arose in the attempt to evaluate the para-aortic lymph nodes [35,107]. With the availability of new instrumentation, some groups provided evidence of adequate nodal sampling by MIS techniques and proposed them as a complementary procedure to vaginal hysterectomy for patients with endometrial cancer [36,108]. A number of different techniques for performing laparoscopic hysterectomy have been proposed [109]. Among them laparoscopic-assisted vaginal hysterectomy (LAVH) has been considered to provide an excellent opportunity for combining radicality with the advantages of the vaginal approach [110,111]. Recent prospective randomized studies have shown that the laparoscopic approach can be considered a substitute for abdominal hysterectomy in benign diseases, while comparisons between vaginal and laparoscopic techniques are still a matter of debate [112]. The role of operative laparoscopy in gynecological oncology is still in its infancy, but there appear to be several malignancies in which it will be used routinely in the future.

The use of laparoscopic pelvic and para-aortic lymphadenectomy in patients with gynecological malignancies, compared with a conventional radical treatment and staging, is rapidly gaining acceptance, and numerous accounts of the use of these techniques have recently been published [35,43,113]. However, this approach needs to be justified by prospective randomized trials, several of which are currently underway.

The application of laparoscopic 'radical' gynecologic surgery has been confined to centers with experienced surgeons and under certain research protocols. Both total laparoscopic hysterectomy and LAVH have been proposed for the treatment of early cervical carcinoma [114]. Patients with stage I_A-I_B-II_A cervical carcinoma with negative nodes are considered candidates for the laparoscopic approach, while the presence of positive nodes makes this approach controversial.

The number of reports on the role of laparoscopic radical surgery in endometrial cancer is even smaller and, consequently, less clear [36]. This approach is limited to patients with negative intra-peritoneal disease, assessed laparoscopically. Laparoscopic-assisted vaginal hysterectomy is possible in patients with well-differentiated adenocarcinoma lesions and is followed by lymphadenectomy only in the presence of myometrial invasion greater than 50%. Patients with grade 2 or 3 lesions should undergo lymphadenectomy prior to the hysterectomy [114].

Since malignant ovarian neoplasms are considered a contraindication for the laparoscopic approach, a critical issue is the preoperative prediction as to whether the lesion is benign or malignant [115]. Laparoscopic staging of early ovarian cancer has been proposed as an alternative to traditional surgical staging [33,39,40]. The major criticism regards the risk of rupture of an early malignancy, leading to tumor spill. This concern is supported by reports of peritoneal and port-site seeding following laparoscopic biopsy of borderline ovarian neoplasms. Nevertheless, controlled but limited series have considered this staging procedure to be safe and effective [40,43].

In conclusion, laparoscopic radical surgery in the management of gynecological neoplasms is also still in its earliest stages. Survival data for gynecologic patients with malignancies managed using laparoscopy in lieu of laparotomy are lacking. It is imperative that cooperative trials demonstrate the merits of laparoscopy in these settings.

Conclusions

The possibility of performing minimally invasive surgery for the diagnosis, palliation, and potential cure of patients afflicted with cancer has increasingly tantalized the surgical oncologic community over the past 5 years. If this 'minimal invasion' can prove to allow cancer patients to recover quickly, to potentially have less suppression of their immune system, and to improve their quality of life, then this will represent a major advance in cancer therapy.

Diagnostically, MIS is unquestionably a valued tool in nearly all fields of

Table 1. Value of diagnostic/staging laparoscopy in surgical oncology

Definite	Possible
Esophageal	Lymphomas
Stomach	Certain colorectal cancers
Pancreas	Unexplained ascites or weight loss
Hepatobilism	Undiagnosed mass lesion
Gynecologic	Urologic

intraabdominal malignancies (Table 1). The recent development of 10 mm laparoscopic ultrasound probes capable of flexing and extending at their tip has added great potential for evaluation of solid organs and for ultrasound-guided biopsies.

Indications for palliative therapies using MIS are also rapidly expanding as well. The possibility of performing feeding tube insertions, bypass procedures, limited resections, and diversions without a major laparotomy will almost certainly be demonstrated to be a major advantage to cancer patients over the next several years.

The most controversial use of MIS techniques centers around curative therapy. Are the potential short-term advantages of MIS important enough to avoid a laparotomy in a patient with surgically curable disease? Are laparoscopic techniques 'radical' enough to justify their use? Is the risk of surgical dissemination actually increased using MIS techniques? These oncologic questions are unanswered, as are the important economic questions that may eventually help justify MIS techniques (shorter hospitalization, faster recovery, and return to work). Many of these issues must continue to be studied in animal experiments and controlled clinical trials in the next several years.

This is a rapidly expanding and dynamic field of oncologic surgery, with many advantages to offer patients in need of diagnosis, accurate staging, or palliation of malignant disease. Curative therapies will likely be proven to be feasible and advantageous using minimally invasive techniques, as well, but the concerted efforts of surgical oncologists and their research colleagues will be required to prove this in well-constructed future trials.

References

1. Kelling G. Ueber Oesophagoskopie, Gastroskopie und Kölioskopie. Münch Med Wochenschr 49:21–24, 1902.
2. Kalk H, Bruhl W. Leitfaden der laparoskopie. Stutgart: Thieme, 1951.
3. Orndoff BH. The peritoneoscope in diagnosis of diseases of the abdomen. J Radiol 1:307–325, 1920.
4. Lightdale CJ. Laparoscopy for cancer staging. Adv Surg Oncol 24:682–686, 1992.
5. Brady PG, Peebles M, Goldschmid S. Role of laparoscopy in the evaluation of patients with susected hepatic or peritoneal malignancy. Gastrointest Endosc 37:27–30, 1991.
6. Hemming AW, Nagy AG, Scudamore CH, Edelmann K. Laparoscopic staging of intraabdominal malignancy. Surg Endosc 9:325–328, 1995.
7. Watt I, Stewart I, Anderson D, Bell G, Anderson JR. Laparoscopy, ultrasound and computed tomography in cancer of the oesophagus and gastric cardia: A prospective comparison for detecting intra-abdominal metastases. Br J Surg 76:1036–1039, 1989.
8. Ishida H. Peritoneoscopy and pancreas biopsy in the diagnosis of pancreatic diseases. Gastrointest Endosc 29:211–218, 1983.
9. Cuschieri A, Hall AW, Clark J. Value of laparoscopy in the diagnosis and management of pancreatic carcinoma. Gut 19:672–677, 1978.
10. Kriplani AK, Kapur BM. Laparoscopy for pre-operative staging and assessment of operabil-

ity in gastric carcinoma. Gastrointest Endosc 37:441–443, 1991.

11. Warshaw AL, Gu ZY, Wittenberg J, Waltman AC. Preoperative staging and assessment of resectability of pancreatic cancer. Arch Surg 125:230–233, 1990.

12. John TG, Garden OJ. Laparoscopic ultrasonography: Extending the scope of diagnostic laparoscopy. Br J Surg 81:5–6, 1994.

13. Cuschieri A. Laparoscopy for pancreatic cancer: Does it benefit the patient? Eur J Surg Oncol 14:41–44, 1988.

14. Bismuth H, Castaing D, Garden OJ. The use of operative ultrasound in surgery of primary liver tumors. World J Surg 11:610–614, 1987.

15. John TG, Garden OJ. Clinical experience with sector scan and linear array ultrasound probes in laparoscopic surgery. Endosc Surg Allied Technol 2:134–142, 1994.

16. Jeffers L, Spieglman G, Reddy R, et al. Laparoscopically directed fine needle aspiration for the diagnosis of hepatocellular carcinoma: A safe and accurate technique. Gastrointest Endosc 34:235–237, 1988.

17. Lightdale CJ. Laparoscopy and biopsy in malignant liver disease. Cancer 50:2672–2675, 1982.

18. Schrenk P, Woisetschlager R, Wayand WU, Rieger R, Sulzbacher H. Diagnostic laparoscopy: A survey of 92 patients. Am J Surg 168:348–351, 1994.

19. Gandolfi L, Muratori R, Solmi L, Rossi A, Leo P. Laparoscopy compared with ultrasonography in the diagnosis of hepatocellular carcinoma. Gastrointest Endosc 35:508–511, 1989.

20. Herrera JL, Brewer TG, Peura DA. Diagnostic laparoscopy: A prospective review of 100 cases. Am J Gastroenterol 84:1051–1054, 1989.

21. Boyce HW. Diagnostic laparoscopy in liver and biliary disease. Endoscopy 24:676–681, 1992.

22. Okita K, Kodama T, Oda M, Takemoto T. Laparoscopic ultrasonography. Diagnosis of liver and pancreatic cancer. Scand J Gastroenterol 94:91–100, 1984.

23. John TG, Greig JD, Crosbie JL, Miles WF, Garden OJ. Superior staging of liver tumors with laparoscopy and laparoscopic ultrasound. Ann Surg 220:711–719, 1994.

24. Fernandez-del Castillo C, Rattner DW, Warshaw AL. Further experience with laparoscopy and peritoneal cytology in the staging of pancreatic cancer. Br J Surg 82:1127–1129, 1995.

25. Moossa AR, Gamagami RA. Diagnosis and staging of pancreatic neoplasms. Surg Clin North Am 75:871–890, 1995.

26. John TG, Greig JD, Carter DC, Garden OJ. Carcinoma of the pancreatic head and periampullary region. Tumor staging with laparoscopy and laparoscopic ultrasonography. Ann Surg 221:156–164, 1995.

27. Bemelman WA, de Wit LT, van Delden OM, et al. Diagnostic laparoscopy combined with laparoscopic ultrasonography in staging of cancer of the pancreatic head region. Br J Surg 82:820–824, 1995.

28. Hunerbein M, Rau B, Schlag PM. Laparoscopy and laparoscopic ultrasound for staging of upper gastrointestinal tumours. Eur J Surg Oncol 21:50–55, 1995.

29. Possik RA, Franco EL, Pires DR, Wohnrath DR, Ferreira EB. Sensitivity, specificity, and predictive value of laparoscopy for the staging of gastric cancer and for the detection of liver metastases. Cancer 58:1–6, 1986.

30. Vander Velpen GC, Shimi SM, Cuschieri A. Diagnostic yield and management benefit of laparoscopy: A prospective audit. Gut 35:1617–1621, 1994.

31. Bartlett DL, Conlon KC, Gerdes H, Karpeh MS, Jr. Laparoscopic ultrasonography: The best pretreatment staging modality in gastric adenocarcinoma? Case report. Surgery 118:562–566, 1995.

32. Irvin TT, Bridger JE. Gastric cancer: An audit of 122 consecutive cases and the results or R1 gastrectomy. Br J Surg 75:106–109, 1988.

33. Dargent D. A new future for Schauta's operation through a pre-surgical retroperitoneal pelviscopy. Eur J Gynaecol Oncol 8:292–296, 1987.

34. Dargent D, Mathevet P. Hysterectomie elargie laparoscopico-vaginale. J Gynecol Obstet Biol Reprod (Paris) 21:709–710, 1992.

35. Querleu D, Leblanc E, Castelain B. Laparoscopic pelvic lymphadenectomy in the staging of early carcinoma of the cervix. Am J Obstet Gynecol 164:579–581, 1991.
36. Childers JM, Brzechffa PR, Hatch KD, Surwit EA. Laparoscopically assisted surgical staging (LASS) of endometrial cancer. Gynecol Oncol 51:33–38, 1993.
37. Fowler JM, Carter JR, Carlson JW, et al. Lymph node yield from laparoscopic lymphadenectomy in cervical cancer: A comparative study. Gynecol Oncol 51:187–192, 1993.
38. Reich H, McGlynn F, Wilkie W. Laparoscopic management of stage I ovarian carcinoma. A case report. J Gynecol Surg 35:601–604, 1990.
39. Pomel C, Provencher D, Dauplat J, et al. Laparoscopic staging of early ovarian cancer. Gynecol Oncol 58:301–306, 1995.
40. Childers JM, Lang J, Surwit EA, Hatch KD. Laparoscopic surgical staging of ovarian cancer. Gynecol Oncol 59:25–33, 1995.
41. Quinn MA, Bishop GJ, Campbell JJ, Rodgerson J, Pepperell RJ. Laparoscopic follow-up of patients with ovarian carcinoma. Br J Obstet Gynaecol 87:1132–1139, 1980.
42. Mangioni C, Bolis G, Molteni P, Belloni C. Indications, advantages, and limits of laparoscopy in ovarian cancer. Gynecol Oncol 7:47–55, 1979.
43. Querleu D, LeBlanc E. Laparoscopic infrarenal paraaortic lymph node dissection for restaging of carcinoma of the ovary or fallopian tube. Cancer 73:1467–1471, 1994.
44. Eraky I, el-Kappany H, Shamaa MA, Ghoneim MA. Laparoscopic nephrectomy: An established routine procedure. J Endourol 8:275–278, 1994.
45. Kerbl K, Clayman RV, Petros JA, Chandhoke PS, Gill IS. Staging pelvic lymphadenectomy for prostate cancer: A comparison of laparoscopic and open techniques. J Urol 150:396–399, 1993.
46. Etwaru D, Raboy A, Ferzli G, Albert P. Extraperitoneal endoscopic gasless pelvic lymph node dissection. J Laparoendosc Surg 4:113, 1994.
47. Danella JF, deKernion JB, Smith RB, Steckel J. The contemporary incidence of lymph node metastases in prostate cancer: Implications for laparoscopic lymph node dissection. J Urol 149:1488–1491, 1993.
48. Gill IS, Clayman RV. Laparoscopic pelvic lymphadenectomy. Surg Oncol Clin North Am 3:323, 1994.
49. Veronesi U, Spinelli P, Bonadonna G, et al. Laparoscopy and laparotomy in staging Hodgkin's and non-Hodgkin's lymphoma. Am J Roentgenol 127:501–503, 1976.
50. Coleman M, Lightdale CJ, Vinciguerra VP, et al. Peritoneoscopy in Hodgkin disease. Confirmation of results by laparotomy. JAMA 236:2634–2636, 1976.
51. Childers JM, Balserak JC, Kent T, Surwit EA. Laparoscopic staging of Hodgkin's lymphoma. J Laparoendosc Surg 3:495–499, 1993.
52. Lefor AT, Flowers JL, Heyman MR. Laparoscopic staging of Hodgkin's disease. Surg Oncol 2:217–220, 1993.
53. Beretta G, Spinelli P, Rilke F, et al. Sequential laparoscopy and laparotomy combined with bone marrow biopsy in staging Hodgkin's disease. Cancer Treat Rep 60:1231–1237, 1976.
54. Arnaud JP, Casa C, Manunta A. Laparoscopic continent gastrostomy. Am J Surg 169:629–630, 1995.
55. Eltringham WK, Roe AM, Galloway SW, Mountford RA, Espiner HJ. A laparoscopic technique for full thickness intestinal biopsy and feeding jejunostomy. Gut 34:122–124, 1993.
56. Rhodes M, Nathanson L, Fielding G. Laparoscopic biliary and gastric bypass: A useful adjunct in the treatment of carcinoma of the pancreas. Gut 36:778–780, 1995.
57. Nagy A, Brosseuk D, Hemming A, Scudamore C, Mamazza J. Laparoscopic gastroenterostomy for duodenal obstruction. Am J Surg 169:539–542, 1995.
58. Wilson RG, Varma JS. Laparoscopic gastroenterostomy for malignant duodenal obstruction. Br J Surg 79:1348, 1992.
59. Sosa JL, Zalewski M, Puente I. Laparoscopic gastrojejunostomy technique: Case report. J Laparendosc Surg 4:215–220, 1994.
60. Lyerly HK, Mault JR. Laparoscopic ileostomy and colostomy. Ann Surg 219:317–322, 1994.

61. Fuhrman GM, Ota DM. Laparoscopic intestinal stomas. Dis Colon Rectum 37:444–449, 1994.
62. Ludwig KA, Milsom JW, Garcia-Ruiz A, Fazio VW. Laparoscopic techniques for fecal diversion. Dis Colon Rectum 1996, in press.
63. Elftmann TD, Nelson H, Ota DM, Pemberton JH, Beart RW, Jr. Laparoscopic-assisted segmental colectomy: Surgical techniques. Mayo Clin Proc 69:825–833, 1994.
64. Milson JW, Hammerhofer KA. Role of laparoscopic techniques in colorectal cancer surgery. Oncology 9:393–399, 1940.
65. Walsh DCA, Wattchow DA, Wilson TG. Subcutaneous metastases after laparoscopic resection of malignancy. Aust J Obstet Gynecol 63:563–565, 1993.
66. Cushieri A. Thoracoscopic subtotal oesophagectomy. Endosc Surg Allied Technol 21:21–25, 1994.
67. Segalin A, Bonavina L, Rosati R, Bettazza S. Parietal seeding of oesophageal caner after thoracoscopic resection. Dis Esophagus 7:64–65, 1994.
68. Yamashita Y, Kurohiji T, Kakegawa T, Bekki F, Ogata M. Laparoscopy-guided extracorporeal resection of early gastric carcinoma. Endoscopy 27:248–252, 1995.
69. Ohgami M, Kumai K, Otani Y, Wakabayashi G, Kubota T, Kitajima M. Laparoscopic wedge resection of the stomach for early gastric cancer using a lesion-lifting method. Dig Surg 11:64–67, 1994.
70. Ohashi S. Laparoscopic intraluminal (intragastric) surgery for early gastirc cancer. A new concept in laparoscopic surgery. Surg Endosc 9:169–171, 1995.
71. Eubanks S. The role of laparoscopy in diagnosis and treatment of primary or metastatic liver cancer. Semin Surg Oncol 10:404–410, 1994.
72. Cuschieri A, Crosthwaite G, Shimi S, et al. Hepatic cryotherpay for liver tumors. Development and clinical evaluation of a high-efficiency insulated multineedle probe system for open and laparoscopic use. Surg Endosc 9:483–489, 1995.
73. Gagner M, Pomp A. Laparoscopic pylorus-preserving pancreatoduodenectomy. Surg Endosc 8:408–410, 1994.
74. Sailer M, Debus K, Fuchs KH, Thiede A. Peritoneal seeding of gallbladder cancer after laparoscopic cholecystectomy. Surg Endosc 9:1298–1300, 1995.
75. Wexner SD, Cohen SM. Port site metastases after laparoscopic colorectal surgery for cure of malignancy. Br J Surg 82:295–298, 1995.
76. Drouard F, Delamarre J, Capron JP. Cutaneous seeding of gallbladder cancer after laparoscopic cholecystectomy. N Eng J Med 325:1316, 1991.
77. Robles AE, Andrews HG, Garberolgio C. Laparoscopic splenectomy: Present status and future outlook. Int Surg 79:332–334, 1994.
78. Emmermann A, Zornig C, Peiper M, Web HJ, Broelsch CE. Laparoscopic splenectomy: Technique and results in a series of 27 cases. Surg Endosc 9:924–927, 1995.
79. Poulin E, Thibault C, Mamazza J, Girotti M, Cote G, Renaud A. Laparoscopic splenectomy: Clinical experience and the role of preoperative splenic artery embolization. Surg Laparosc Endosc 3:445–450, 1993.
80. Ambroze WL, Jr., Orangio GR, Armstrong D, Schertzer M, Lucas G. Laparoscopic surgery for colorectal neoplasms. Semin Surg Oncol 10:398–403, 1994.
81. Milson JW, Bohm B. Indications and contraindications: Common indications — colorectal tumors. In Laparoscopic Colorectal Surgery. New York: Springer-Verlag, 1996, pp 88–92.
82. Milsom JW, Bohm B, Decanini C, Fazio VW. Laparoscopic oncologic proctosigmoidectomy with low colorectal anastomosis in a cadaver model. Surg Endosc 8:1117–1123, 1994.
83. Decanini C, Milsom JW, Bohm B, Fazio VW. Laparoscopic oncologic abdominoperineal resection. Dis Colon Rectum 37:552–558, 1994.
84. Cava A, Roman J, Gonzalez-Quintela A, Martin F, Aramburo P. Subcutaneous metastasis following laparoscopy in gastric adenocarcinoma. Eur J Surg Oncol 16:63–67, 1990.
85. Clair DG, Lautz DB, Brooks DC. Rapid development of umbilical metastases after

laparoscopic cholecystectomy for unsuspected gallbladder carcinoma. Surgery 113:355–358, 1993.

86. Landen SM. Laparoscopic surgery and tumor seeding. Surgery 114:131–132, 1993.

87. Miralles RM, Petit J, Gine L, Balaguero L. Metastatic cancer spread at the laparoscopic puncture site. Report of a case in a patient with carcinoma of the ovary. Case report. Eur J Gynaecol Oncol 10:442–444, 1989.

88. Franklin ME, Jr., Ramos R, Rosenthal D, Schussler W. Laparoscopic colonic procedures. World J Surg 17:51–56, 1993.

89. Nelson H. Principal Investigator for Intergroup Protocol #0146. A phase III prospective randomized trial comparing laparoscopic-assisted colectomy versus open colectomy for colon cancer. (Study) 1995.

90. Milsom JW. Principal Investigator for Cleveland Clinic Research Program's Committee #4237. Laparoscopic versus conventional oncologic large bowel resection is patients with colorectal cancer. (Study) 1995.

91. Clayman RV, Kavoussi LR, Soper NJ, et al. Laparoscopic nephrectomy: Initial case report. J Urol 146:278–282, 1991.

92. Kavoussi LR, Kerbl K, Capelouto CC, McDougall EM, Clayman RV. Laparoscopic nephrectomy for renal neoplasms. Urology 42:603–609, 1993.

93. McDougall EM, Clayman RV, Fadden PT. Retroperitoneoscopy: The Washington University Medical School experience. Urology 43:446–452, 1994.

94. Gill IS, Clayman RV, McDougall EM. Advances in urological laparoscopy. J Urol 154:1275–1294, 1995.

95. Gill IS, Kavoussi LR, Clayman RV, et al. Complications of laparoscopic nephrectomy in 185 patients: A multi-institutional review. J Urol 154:479–483, 1995.

96. Ono Y, Katoh N, Kinukawa T, Sahashi M, Ohshima S. Laparoscopic nephrectomy, radical nephrectomy and adrenalectomy: Nagoya experience. J Urol 152:1962–1966, 1994.

97. Suzuki K, Masuda H, Ushiyama T, Hata M, Fujita K, Kawabe K. Gasless laparoscopy-assisted nephrectomy without tissue morcellation for renal carcinoma. J Urol 154:1685–1687, 1995.

98. Kerbl K, Clayman RV, McDougall EM, Urban DA, Gill I, Kavoussi LR. Laparoscopic nephroureterectomy: Evaluation of first clinical series. Eur Urol 23:431, 1993.

99. McDougall EM, Clayman RV, Elashry O. Laparoscopic nephroureterectomy for upper tract transitional cell cancer: The Washington University experience. J Urol 154:975–980, 1995.

100. Deans GT, Kappadia R, Wedgewood K, Royston CM, Brough WA. Laparoscopic adrenalectomy. Br J Surg 82:994–995, 1995.

101. Schlinkert RT, van Heerden JA, Grant CS, Thompson GB, Segura JW. Laparoscopic left adrenalectomy for aldosteronoma: Early Mayo Clinic experience. Mayo Clin Proc 70:844–846, 1995.

102. Gagner M, Lacroix A, Prinz RA, et al. Early experience with laparoscopic approach for adrenalectomy. Surgery 114:1120–1125, 1993.

103. Nakagawa K, Murai M, Deguchi N, et al. Laparoscopic adrenalectomy: Clinical results in 25 patients. J Endourol 9:265–267, 1995.

104. Suzuki K, Kageyama S, Ueda D, et al. Laparoscopic adrenalectomy: Clinical experience with 12 cases. J Urol 150:1099–1102, 1993.

105. Gagner M, Lacroix A, Bolte E, Pomp A. Laparoscopic adrenalectomy. The importance of a flank approach in the lateral decubitus position. Surg Endosc 8:135–138, 1994.

106. Guazzoni G, Montorsi F, Bocciardi A, et al. Transperitoneal laparoscopic versus open adrenalectomy for benign hyperfunctioning adrenal tumors: A comparative study. J Urol 153:1597–1600, 1995.

107. Herd J, Fowler JM, Shenson D, Lacy S, Montz FJ. Laparoscopic para-aortic lymph node sampling: Development of a technique. Gynecol Oncol 44:271–276, 1992.

108. Querleu D. Laparoscopically assisted radical vaginal hysterectomy. Gynecol Oncol 51:248–254, 1993.

109. Reich H, Maher PJ, Wood C. Laparoscopic hysterectomy. Clin Obstet Gynaecol 8:799–815, 1994.

110. Massi G, Savino L, Susini T. Schauta-Amreich vaginal hysterectomy and Wertheim-Meigs abdominal hysterectomy in the treatment of cervical cancer: A retrospective analysis Am J Obstet Gynecol 168:928–934, 1993.

111. Nezhat CR, Burrell MO, Nezhat FR, Benigno BB, Welander CE. Laparoscopic radical hysterectomy with paraaortic and pelvic node dissection. Am J Obstet Gynecol 166:864–865, 1992.

112. Raju KS, Auld BJ. A randomised prospective study of laparoscopic vaginal hysterectomy versus abdominal hysterectomy each with bilateral salpingo-oophorectomy. Br J Obstet Gynaecol 101:1068–1071, 1994.

113. Childers JM, Hatch KD, Tran AN, Surwit EA. Laparoscopic para-aortic lymphadenectomy in gynecologic malignancies. Obstet Gynecol 82:741–747, 1993.

114. Childers JM. Operative laparoscopy in gynaecological oncology. Clin Obstet Gynaecol 8:831–849, 1994.

115. Trimbos JB, Zola P. The present role of laparoscopy in gynaecological oncology; the EORTC point of view. Eur J Cancer 31A:803–805, 1995.

17. Prognostic factors in surgical resection for hepatocellular carcinoma

Barry J. Roseman and Mark S. Roh

Introduction

Although a variety of new treatment modalities for hepatocellular carcinoma (HCC) have been explored in the past few years, the fact remains that surgical resection provides the only chance for long-term survival in this aggressive disease. Five-year survival rates after curative surgery average 18–36%. In general, a resectable tumor must be (1) confined to the liver (absence of vascular invasion or distant metastases) and (2) entirely encompassed by local excision with an adequate margin. In order to be a candidate for resection, the patient must also have adequate liver reserve. Only 10–15% of patients with primary liver cancer meet these requirements. Unfortunately, the majority of these patients develop recurrence and do not benefit from further resection.

Obviously, other factors are present that impact on the outcome. Recently, multiple prognostic indicators have been identified that can be used to predict the outcome after surgical treatment of hepatoma. These indicators are classified as *patient factors* (correlated with perioperative morbidity and mortality), *tumor factors* (predict recurrence or metastasis), and *surgeon factors* (impact on recurrence and survival in surgical patients). This chapter reviews how traditional prognostic factors and newer methodologies can be used to help select appropriate patients for surgical treatment.

Patient factors

The first factor in evaluating the outcome of surgery for HCC is perioperative morbidity and mortality. Age, while previously thought to have an impact on perioperative morbidity and mortality, is not an independent predictor of these complications. Chen et al. found that resection of HCC in patients over 60 years old was associated with slightly higher operative morbidity and mortality than with younger patients, but the risks were not significant enough to deny surgery to selected patients in this age group [1]. Two subsequent studies showed that in patients over 70 years of age there were equivalent post-

Raphael E. Pollock (ed.), SURGICAL ONCOLOGY. Copyright © 1997. Kluwer Academic Publishers. ISBN 0-7923-9900-5. All rights reserved.

operative complication rates, long-term survival, and disease-free survival in these patients compared with a younger cohort [2,3,6].

Comorbid diseases, poor nutritional status, and low serum albumin level [4] are associated with increased complications after major abdominal surgery. In a retrospective study of 114 patients with cirrhosis who underwent resection for HCC, PTT elevation was the only factor by multivariate analysis independently associated with operative mortality [5], suggesting that impaired coagulative status will put the patient at increased risk for perioperative and postoperative bleeding and mortality [5].

Child's classification has a predictive value in prognosis for surgically treated HCC. For example, Nagasue et al. found that in a group of 32 patients over 70 years of age who underwent resection for HCC, 5-year survival was 17.6%, but patients with Child's class A disease had a 5-year survival of 30%, with a similarly lower incidence of perioperative morbidity and mortality [2]. Regardless of the patient's underlying medical condition, however, careful intraoperative monitoring and aggressive postoperative medical care are clearly essential in preventing postoperative complications.

The most important determinant of perioperative morbidity and mortality in hepatoma patients undergoing liver resection appears to be the functional status of the patient's remaining liver tissue. The ability of the surgeon to perform large resections is predicated on the potential of the liver to regenerate, in order to restore adequate liver mass for the patient's body. Liver reserve closely predicts the risk of postoperative hepatic failure [86].

Several objective criteria can be used to estimate the hepatic reserve in a patient being considered for hepatic resection. History, physical examination, blood chemistries, volumetric analysis of CT scans, use of the trimethadione (TMO) tolerance test, glucose tolerance, and the ^{14}C-aminopyrine breath test are all valuable tests in determining the functional status of a patient's liver [7–10].

The indocyanine green (ICG) retention test has been shown in several studies to be an accurate indicator of hepatic reserve, with retention of indocyanine green of more than 10–15% at 15 minutes after injection correlating with a poor operative outcome [10–12]. For example, in a study of 54 cirrhotic patients who underwent major hepatectomy for HCC, Fan et al. found that preoperative ICG retention was the only measurement that could predict hospital mortality in the patients with cirrhosis, and an ICG retention of 14% at 15 minutes was the level that could maximally separate the patients with and without hospital mortality [11].

Taken together, these data utilizing preoperative assessment tests emphasize the importance of establishing objective criteria to determine which patients can safely withstand the substantial reduction in liver parenchyma associated with hepatic resection. If these parameters are not satisfactorily met, the patient should not undergo resection because the risk of postoperative liver failure is prohibitively high.

The fibrosis associated with chronic hepatitis and cirrhosis severely limits liver regeneration. In these patients, after large resections there is little growth and restoration of liver mass, often resulting in liver failure and death. Extensive literature exists documenting the detrimental effects of cirrhosis on the postoperative course in liver resection [13–17], and the increased risk of tumor recurrence in patients with cirrhosis (see Tumor Factors, later). Cirrhotic patients tend to have many other preop risk factors (e.g., malnutrition, coagulopathy), which puts them at even higher operative risk for major hepatic resection.

Tumor factors

HCC recurrences generally result from one of several mechanisms. First, the cancer may be inadequately resected, often due to unsuspected infiltration of the tumor into the liver parenchyma or vessels. Second, unsuspected small tumors and micrometastases, unable to be detected by current techniques, may be present within other areas of the liver at the time of surgery, resulting in subsequent intrahepatic recurrence. Third, metachronous hepatic recurrences may represent areas of unresected liver that subsequently develop de novo foci of cancer, particularly in patients with cirrhosis or chronic hepatitis.

One biological characteristic of HCC that correlates with recurrence is histopathologic type. In contrast to the nodular and diffuse variety, the fibrolamellar variant distinguishes itself with a much better prognosis than other histopathologic types [18,19], with higher resectability rates of up to 75% and also prolonged survival time after resection [87]. This variety usually occurs in a younger age group (average 25 years) and is not associated with elevated serum AFP levels, chronic hepatitis B virus infection, or cirrhosis.

These characteristics often lend the tumor a favorable resection outcome with 5-year survival datas of 40–60% [19,20], compared with reported 5-year survivals of 15–30% in most HCC series. Ringe et al. found that in 20 consecutive patients with fibrolamellar carcinoma who underwent either curative resection or transplantation, the 5-year survival rate was 36.6%, with a median survival of 44.5 months for partial hepatic resection and 28.5 months for transplantation [20].

Many studies have shown tumor size to be one of the most important predictors of recurrence and long-term survival in HCC [12,14,22–24], probably due to the low frequency of satellite lesions, multicentricity, and vascular invasion found with smaller tumors. On the other hand, tumors greater than 5 cm are generally associated with a worse prognosis. For example, in a series of 47 patients with resected HCC, Belghiti et al. found that the cumulative intrahepatic recurrence rate at 3 years was 81%, significantly higher in 19 patients patients with tumor ≥5 cm compared with 28 patients whose tumors were <5 cm [25].

In a series of 106 patients who underwent hepatic resection for HCC,

Vauthey et al. used univariate analysis to show that survival was greater in association with tumors ≤5 cm [26]. Zhou et al. studied a group of 508 patients who underwent resection with a 5-year survival of 45.5% and a 10-year survival of 32.6%. In a subgroup of 210 patients with small HCC (≤5 cm), 5-year survival was 63.8% and 10-year survival was 43.5% [27].

Lai et al. reported that size had little influence on prognosis; however, in their studies tumors <5 cm in diameter had less venous invasion and more frequent encapsulation, two factors independently associated with improved outcome [28,29]. Kawarada et al. reported a series of 149 resected cases of HCC with a cumulative 5-year survival of 39.4%. However, in a subgroup of 15 patients with a solitary tumor of 2 cm or less, all patients were alive with a 5-year survival rate of 100% [32]. Zhou et al. reported 14 patients with clinical stage I HCC (T1NOMO) as detected by AFP elevation and/or ultrasound screening who underwent radical resection, with a 5-year survival of 100% [30].

The recent advent of screening high-risk patients by AFP levels and liver ultrasound should promote the early diagnosis of HCC. Because small tumors are associated with a particularly good prognosis [30–34], this practice should lead to an increased number of resections for small HCCs, and correspondingly improved survival results.

The location of HCC within the parenchyma has been shown to be an important predictor of disease-free survival in some studies [31,35]. Shirabe et al. found that in a group of 50 patients who underwent resection for small HCC (<3 cm), tumor location was a significant risk factor for recurrence in stepwise regression analysis, perhaps because deeper tumors are more likely to infiltrate and cause vascular invasion than those near the liver surface [31]. Tumors located in the caudate lobe will lead to higher surgical risk, more frequent postoperative complications, and a higher rate of early recurrence [36]. Centrally located large HCC require extended hepatectomy [37], with the likelihood of increased blood loss and sacrifice of extensive liver parenchyma, which may put some patients at high risk for liver failure.

The presence of a tumor capsule has been shown to be an important predictor of survival in several studies [6,35,38]. Encapsulated tumors tend to be smaller with infrequent occurrence of intrahepatic metastases. Non-encapsulation has been shown to be independently associated with histological spread of tumor [29]. While difficult to determine preoperatively, the finding of a discrete tumor capsule at exploration predicts a greater chance of removing all of the disease at the initial operation, with an increased likelihood of a clear margin of resection on permanent histopathology.

Vascular invasion is probably the most important predictor of poor outcome in patients with HCC. Tumor thrombus in the portal or hepatic vein implies microscopic spread of tumor within the vascular system, and it is unlikely that a surgeon can ever adequately remove all of the tumor that has grown along the vascular endothelium in these cases. Preoperative or intraoperative ultrasound are probably the best radiographic tests to evaluate the presence of vascular invasion in hepatoma patients [39]. If present, vascular invasion is a major contraindication to resection.

Many studies demonstrate the importance of vascular invasion in outcome, often as the only factor or the most important factor by multivariate or univariate analysis [40–42]. The presence of vascular invasion in itself correlates with tumor size, the presence of tumor capsule, capsular invasion, vascular invasion, and intrahepatic metastasis [6,12,16,21,23,26,29,31,33,43] and is therefore an important predictor in most large series.

Liver invasion, or the presence of intrahepatic metastasis, is an equally forboding prognostic factor in patients undergoing surgical resection for HCC [4,21,24,31,42]. Tumor invasiveness, defined by the presence of vascular invasion and/or intrahepatic metastases, is a major prognostic factor for early recurrence in patients treated with curative resection [12,41]. It is likely that the presence of intrahepatic metastases is a marker of locally advanced disease, and that in such cases complete resection of all macroscopically or radiographically detectable disease will still be inadequate to remove all of the patient's HCC cells.

Hepatocellular carcinoma is multifocal in nature. Particularly for larger tumors, the evidence from liver transplantation indicates that there are often multiple small tumors present in the liver at a considerable distance from the primary lesion. While CT angiography and intraoperative ultrasound have greatly improved the detection of smaller lesions compared with past techniques, microscopic foci several centimeters from the known tumor may still be present that are not diagnosed operatively, and yet that lead to ultimate local failure and diminished overall prognosis.

Multicentricity is clearly a poor prognositic indicater in HCC. Multiple and multinodular tumors are associated with histologic spread [29], significant increases in recurrence [23], and markedly decreased survival [21,26,38,44]. Several studies show that patients with satellite nodules have a high incidence of recurrence [6,45].

Harada et al. studied 118 patients who underwent hepatic resection for primary HCC and found that while 9 of 20 patients without satellite nodues recurred at a mean of 13.4 months postoperatively, 11 of 13 patients with satellite nodules recurred at a mean of 10.5 months [45]. All of the patients with satellite lesions found in a separate lobe of the liver recurred, despite what was initially thought to be curative surgery. As is the case with intrahepatic metastases, patients with satellite lesions are likely to harbor undetectable micrometastases and are thus at excessive risk for subsequent intrahepatic recurrence.

Direct invasion to or other organs, on the other hand, does not appear to be a particularly bad prognostic factor. Jeng et al. found that in cases of large HCC with local invasion to neighboring organs, after appropriate patient selection (solitary tumor, no vascular invasion, no metastases) aggressive en-bloc resection resulted in morbidity, mortality, survival, and disease-free interval comparable with matched HCC patients with no involvement of neighboring organs [46]. Similarly, Lau et al. found no difference in outcome in patients with or without diaphragmatic invasion [47].

Many recent articles stress that the principal cause of either recurrence or new tumors in the remnant liver after hepatectomy is the state of the underlying liver parenchyma. For example, in cirrhosis, in which all of the liver tissue has potentially premalignant or dysplastic changes, it is predictable that new primary HCCs will develop in unresected cirrhotic nodules. Major hepatic resection is a potent growth stimulus for these residual microscopic foci and nodules, resulting in subsequent accelerated growth and the development of new cancers.

Cirrhosis from almost any cause (e.g., alcoholism, hemochromatosis, α1-antitrypsim deficiency) is associated with an increased risk of hepatocellular carcinoma. Several studies demonstrate the presence of cirrhosis as an independent predictive factor for poor prognosis [13,14,16,48] and accelerated recurrence [17]. While cirrhosis is generally associated with poor liver function, inadequate hepatic reserve, and a variety of associated comorbid medical problems, cirrhotic patients with HCC and adequate liver function may be suitable for major hepatectomy. Two studies have demonstrated similar mortality rates in selected cirrhotic patients as in patients with normal livers [11,50]. Capussotti et al. found a group of 31 cirrhotics undergoing major hepatectomy for hepatocellular carcinoma with Childs A status. Operative mortality was 3% and 3-year survival was 37%, only slightly lower than historical controls [50]. Fan et al. found that in cirrhotic patients with adequate hepatic reserve, demonstrated by ICG retention of 14% or less at 15 minutes, the hospital mortality rate was not different from the rate for patients with normal livers [11].

Chronic hepatitis B virus (HBV) infection is the principal etiologic factor for HCC worldwide. Patients chronically seropositive for HBsAg constitute a high-risk group for the development of hepatoma, which in some cases may be detected early by screening for serum alpha-fetoprotein levels. Several studies have demonstrated that HBsAg-positive patients with HCC have a high mortality compared with HBsAg-negative patients, probably because of the association with cirrhosis in this group of patients. For example, Chou et al. studied 84 patients with HCC who underwent surgical resection. Hepatitis B surface antigen was positive in 83% of the patients. Multivariate analysis of multiple factors showed that the only factor that predicted better survival was negative hepatitis B surface antigen [49].

On the other hand, hepatitis C carrier status does not appear to negatively influence survival. One study shows that 3- and 5-year survival rates after hepatectomy were similar in anti-hepatitis C virus–positive patients compared with a similar group who were anti-hepatitis C virus negative [51].

Active inflammation in the nontumoros portion of HCC patients' livers is a marker of a premalignant state. For example, using a bromodeoxyuridin labeling index, Tarao et al. found a significant correlation between DNA synthesis of hepatocytes from the cirrhotic tissue of HCC patients and that of their tumor cells [52]. DNA synthetic activity of hepatocytes from noncancerous cirrhotic tissue could actually predict the survival of 30 patients with HCC who had undergone hepatectomy [52].

Similarly, using DNA flow cytometry and cell-cycle analysis of the nontumor parts of resected HCC specimens, a markedly increased proliferative capacity in the nontumor portions ($\geq318\%$) was significantly linked to tumor recurrence after liver resection for HCC [53]. In another study, Adachi et al. demonstrated that in 102 patients with small (<3 cm) HCC, a high proliferating cell nuclear antigen labeling index (>23.2% in the nontumorous portion of resected HCC specimens) was a significant risk factor for recurrence [54].

Alpha-fetoprotein is a globulin normally present only in the fetal circulation but is present in high concentration in the serum of about 80% of patients with primary hepatomas. It is also elevated to a lesser degree in chronic active hepatitis and acute viral and alcoholic hepatitis, where it seems to reflect the extent of liver regeneration. Belghiti et al. showed that out of a group of 47 patients, 55% with alpha-fetoprotein levels less than 100 ng/ml had a cumulative intrahepatic recurrence rate at 3 years that was higher than the 45% of patients with preoperative AFP levels above 100 ng/ml [25].

Preoperative AFP levels significantly inflence the recurrence rate in HCC [55]. In a group of 25 patients who underwent surgical resection of HCC, the 5-year cumulative survival was 72.7% in patients with preop AFP levels of <200 µg/l but was only 25% in those patients with AFP levels of >200 µg/l [55]. In another study, Chen et al. found that preoperative AFP levels were directly related to the length of time to recurrence. In a group of 149 patients with surgically treated HCC, the cumulative intrahepatic recurrence rate after resection was 85% in those patients with preoperative AFP levels >400 µg/l, and 60% had recurred at 1 year. However, the recurrence rate was 55% in those with preoperative AFP levels of <10 µg/l, and only 25% had recurred at the first year [56]. Since changes in AFP levels in patients with hepatoma correlate with growth activity of the tumor, AFP can be also be used postoperatively as an index of the succes of hepatic resection, with lack of AFP normalization after resection a poor prognostic variable [33].

Features of the tumor cells in resected specimens, such as differentiation [35] and DNA ploidy [16,22,32], correlate with recurrence and long-term survival. Kawaii et al. evaluated several morphometric indices in 84 resected HCC patients to determine their relation to survival. Mean survival time was 58 months in cases with a nucleo-cytoplasmic (N/C) area ratio of less than 0.28, significantly higher than the 38-month mean survival in cases with a N/C ratio of less than 0.28. This variable correlated closely with intrahepatic metastases and vascular invasion as well.

Kawaii et al. also found that the mean survival was 71 months for those cases for which the coefficient of variance of the nuclear form factor (NCV) was less than 5.5%, significantly longer than the mean survival of 33 months for cases with a NCV of more than 5.5% [57]. These differences held up when patients were subclassified according to disease stage. These findings suggest a possible role for these and other genetic and molecular markers in predicting outcome after surgery for HCC.

Surgeon factors

Careful patient selection, early detection, improved operative techniques, effective treatment of recurrences, and advances in postoperative critical care have all helped to decrease postoperative complications and have contributed to the improved prognosis of surgically resected HCC patients in the past decade. Kim and Kion compared the incidence of complications and operative mortality in patients undergoing HCC resection from 1980 to 1990, and found a decrease in both of these parameters over the decade [58]. In a separate study, Lai et al. found that patients with HCC who were resected between 1992 and 1995 had better resectability rate, reduced morbidity and mortality, and better survival compared with patients resected prior to 1987 or during the period of 1987–1992 [59]. The above-mentioned factors, such as early detection of small tumors, improved perioperative and postoperative care, and aggressive treatment of recurrences, were implicated in these findings.

Several specific resection techniques may account for this improvement. For example, intraopertive ultrasonography (IOUS) is useful in surgery for HCC in that it can identify inoperable tumors, can define a tumor's relation to locoregional vascular structures, and can elucidate appropriate parenchymal transaction planes with the least chance of tumor infiltration in the resected margin [60–63]. IOUS is also useful in assisting in inablative therapies such as cryosurgery for isolated intrahepatic metastases [64].

The optimal margin of resection in HCC is controversial, although most studies show that it has a significant impact on recurrence and survival. For example, in one study of 205 patients, resected margins <1 cm had relatively higher recurrence rates than those with resected margins of >1 cm in diameter [56]. A similar study showed 74% 3-year survival in patients with a greater than 1 cm free surgical margin, compared with 21% 3-year survival in those having complete resection of the tumor with a <1 cm free surgical margin [43].

Lai et al. attempted to determine the necessary resection margin for cure during hepatectomy for HCC. A >0.5 cm macroscopic margin was associated with less residual histological disease, whereas a postive histologic margin was associated with an increased risk of microsatellites and multiple tumor nodules [28]. Based on these studies and others, a 1 cm macroscopic resection margin is probably adequate to ensure complete histological disease clearance.

On the contrary, surgical margin was not a significant factor in the resection of HCC >2 cm in one study [65], and in other reports the width of resection margin did not affect recurrence [66] or overall prognosis [41]. Many large and small tumors have either microsatellites and/or histologic venous permeation found beyond 1 cm from the lesion. Lai et al. found that in the presence of either microsatellites or histologic venous permeation, no distance could ensure a complete disease clearance [29].

A significant decrease in recurrence and increase in survival has been found in patients undergoing subsegmental or segmental resection for HCC [67], perhaps because of the theoretically improved efficacy of segmental resection over nonanatomic resection in treating microscopic satellitosis or vascular invasion. In another study, extent of hepatic resection, not macroscopic surgical margin, correlated with long-term prognosis in patients with solitary HCC [35]. These authors postulated that one explanation for this result is that patients undergoing a larger resection are selected on the basis of their improved hepatic functional reserve, and that the functional reserve of the liver may be the factor influencing survival.

Several studies strongly suggest that perioperative blood transfusion substantially promotes the recurrence of HCC after hepatectomy, possibly due to immunosuppressive effects [4,17]. Operative mortality and postoperative hepatic failure are higher when there has been significant blood loss, compared with other cases [14]. In one study, the incidence of operative mortality (47%) and postoperative hepatic failure (73%) was markedly higher when there had been massive operative blood loss ($\geq 4.0 l$) and/or persistent postoperative hemorrhage, compared with 0% and 24%, respectively, in cases without massive perioperative bleeding [68].

The use of specific vascular techniques may help to minimize blood loss. Total hepatic vascular exclution used for up to 85 minutes reduced blood loss significantly and had no effect on morbidity, mortality, or postoperative liver function [37,69]. The use of autologous blood transfusion yielded superior results when compared with homologous transfusion for hepatectomy patients with cirrhosis [70]. Postoperative hematocrit recovered more quickly, and serum bilirubin concentrations were significantly lower. Erythropoetin administration minimized the typical presurgical decreases in hemoglobin caused by autologous blood donation [70]. Based on these data, it appears to be advantagous to arrange for autologous blood donation in patients with HCC that are surgically resectable.

Surgery for recurrent disease prolongs survival in several studies, justifying an aggressive approach to selected patients. Long-term survivors resulted from rehepatectomy in several studies [71,72]. Repeat hepatectomy, with indications the same as for the first operation, has been shown to be beneficial for recurrent tumors in patients whose liver functional status has been relatively stable since the first hepatic resection [73–76].

Although secondary recurrence after resection of metasases in HCC develops more commonly in the liver than in extrahepatic organs, Lo et al. reported that 12 of 36 patients with recurrence confined to extrahepatic organs underwent surgical resection [77]. The 1-, 2-, and 5-year survival rates for these 12 patients after resection were 92%, 52%, and 26% respectively, and were better than those of 24 patients who did not undergo resection for recurrence. Thus, in selected patients with isolated extrahepatic recurrence of HCC, surgery is effective in controlling extrahepatic disease and offers the only opportunity for long-term survival [77].

Surgical innovations, such as cryosurgery and percutaneous alcohol injection, have not yet been shown to offer any survival advantage. Transplantation for HCC provides an additional surgical technique to deal with extensive hepatic malignancies, those lesions associated with cirrhosis, or centrally located tumors. The reported 3-year survival of patients undergoing liver transplantation for HCC ranges from 20% to 50% percent [78–80], with overall 5-year survival of 15–20% [81].

Appropriately selected patients undergoing liver transplantation for hepatocellular carcinoma show results similar to those from resection when evaluated by stage of disease. For example, Bismuth and Chiche compared 3-year survival with and without recurrence in 60 patients who underwent resection and 60 who underwent transplantation [80]. Resection and transplantation had the same survival rates at 3 years (50% vs. 47%), with less recurrence in the transplantation group. As with resection, those patients with small tumors (<3 cm) had the most favorable recurrence-free survival [80]. McPeake et al. studied 87 patients who underwent liver transplantation for HCC [78]. Of the 62 patients who survived more than 90 days, 5-years survival was 57.1% for patients with single tumors <4 cm, 44.4% for patients with lesions 4–8 cm, and 11.1% in those with tumors >8 cm or multifocal tumors, comparable with the results of resection [78].

Regardless of tumor stage, the major complication of liver transplantation for malignancy is recurrence (40–65%), and most deaths after transplantation for tumor are directly attrributable to tumor recurrence. A particularly high risk of recurrence after transplantation is found in patients with larger tumors, multiple tumors, and the presence of portal vein thrombus – similar risk factors as for resection [79,81]. Even advocates of liver transplantation concede that patients must be carefully selected to optimize the results of transplantation, given the limited donor organs and expenditure of resources required for this treatment.

Adjuvant therapy

Conventional chemotherapy is ineffective in HCC. Modifications of chemotherapy, including intra-arterial infusion, chemoembolization, lipiodol, styrene-maleic acid-ceocarzinostatin, and isolated hepatic perfusion have led to improved tumor responses, but have not substantially affected patient outcome [82]. However, given the high rate of recurrence and subsequent death after surgery for HCC, it is clear that effective adjuvant chemotherapy is needed for selected patients following surgical resection. While there are an abundance of experimental regimens showing effects of chemotherapy on recurrence and survival [83–85], no agents to date have proven to be effective in prospective randomized trials.

340

Conclusions

Careful patient selection is clearly the goal in optimizing the results for the operative management of hepatoma. Operative morbidity and mortality are influenced primarily by the patient's general medical condition and the functional reserve of the patient's noncancerous liver. Recurrences typically are due to the biologic characteristics of the tumor, although several operative factors were identified that may help to decrease this risk.

Understanding the principal prognostic factors in the outcome of surgically resected HCC patients is important in determining which patients are at highest risk for postoperative complications and recurrence of disease. As our understanding of the molecular basis for HCC continues to develop, so does our chance of having an impact on long-term survival for patients with this disease.

Systematic screening for AFP and intensive use of noninvasive imaging techniques has led to an increase in the early detection for HCC and is necessary to give patients optimal chance for long-term survival. A multidisciplinary approach with adjuvant therapy (hepatic artery chemo-embolization and radiation therapy, postoperative systemic chemotherapy, and immunotherapy) in association with liver transplantation is a sensible direction for the surgical treatment of HCC in the future.

References

1. Chen MF, Hwang TLC, Jenny YY, Wang CS. Influence of age on results of resection of hepatocellular carcinoma. Eur J Surg 157:591–593, 1991.
2. Nagasue N, Chang YC, Takemoto Y, Taniura H, Kohno H, Nakamura T. Liver resection in the aged (seventy years or older) with hepatocellular carcinoma. Surgery 113:148–154, 1993.
3. Takenaka K, Shimada M, Higashi H, Adachi E, Nishizaki T, Yanaga K, Matsumata T, Ikeda T, Sugimachi K. Liver resection for hepatocellular carcinoma in the elderly. Arch Surg 129:846–850, 1994.
4. Matsumata T, Ikeda Y, Hayashi H, Kamakura T, Taketomi A, Surimachi K. The association between transfusion and cancer-free survival after curative resection for hepatocellular carcinoma. Cancer 72:1866–1871, 1993.
5. Bernardi M, Grazi GL, Colantoni A, Sica G, Mazziotti A, Trevisant F, Gozzetti G, Gasbarrini G. Prognostic indicators in patients with cirrhosis and hepatocellular carcinoma undergoing surgical resection. J Surg Oncol 3(Suppl):67–69, 1993.
6. Nagasue N, Uchida M, Makino Y, Takemoto Y, Yamanoi A, Hayashi T, Chang YC, Kohno H, Nakamura T, Yukaya H. Incidence and factors associated with intrahepatic recurrence following resection of hepatocellular carcinoma. Gastroenterology 105:488–494, 1993.
7. Demers ML, Ellis LM, Roh MS. Surgical management of hepatoma. Cancer Treat Res 69:277–290, 1994.
8. Uchida K, Jikko A, Yamato T, Kamiyama Y, Ozawa K. Relationship of glucose intolerance and indocyanine green clearance to respiratory enzyme levels in human cirrhotic liver. Am J Med Sci 290:19–27, 1985.
9. Yamanaka N, Okamoto E, Oriyama T, Fujimoto J, Furukawa K, Kawamura E, Tanaka T, Tomada F. A prediction scoring system to select the surgical treament of liver cancer. Futher refinement based on 10 years of use. Ann Surg 219:342–346, 1994.

10. Ishikawa A, Fukao K, Tsuji K, Osada A, Yamamoto Y, Ohtsuka M, Tanaka E. Trimethadione tolerance tests for the assessment of feasible size of hepatic resection in patients with heaptocellular carcinoma. J Gastroenterol Hepatol 8:426–432, 1993.
11. Fan ST, Lai EC, Lo CM, Ng IO, Wong J. Hospital mortality of major hepatectomy for hepatocellular carcinoma associated with cirrhosis. Arch Surg 130:198–203, 1995.
12. Yamanaka N, Okamoto E, Toyosaka A, Mitunobu M, Fujihara S, Kato T, fujimoto J, Oriyama T, Furukawa K, Kawamura E. Prognostic factors after hepatectomy for hepatocellular carcinomas. Cancer 65:1104–1110, 1990.
13. Nagao T, Nagashima I, Inoue S, Omori Y, Kawano N, Morioka Y. Hepatic resection for minute hepatocellular carcinoma. Surg Today 22:110–114, 1992.
14. Nagasue N, Kohno H, Chang YC, Taniura H, Yamanoi A, Uchida M, Kimoto T, Takemoto Y, Nakamura T, Yukaya H. Liver resection for hepatocellular carcinoma. Results of 229 consecutive patients during 11 years. Ann Surg 217:375–384, 1993.
15. Nagasue N, Kohno H, Chang YC, Taniura H, Yamanoi A, Uchida M, Kimoto T, Takemoto Y, Nakamura T, Yukaya H. Liver resection for hepatocellular carcinoma. Results of 229 coansecutive patients during 11 years. Ann Surg 217:375–384, 1993.
16. Okada S, Shimada K, Yamamoto J, Takayama T, Kosuge T, Yamasaki S, Sakamoto M, Hirohashi S. Predictive factors for postoperative recurrence of hepatocellular carcinoma. Gastroenterology 106:1618–1624, 1994.
17. Yamamoto J, Kosuge T, Takayama T, Shimada K, Yamasaki S, Ozaki H, Yamaguchi N, Mizuno S, Makuuchi M. Perioperative blood transfusion promotes recurrence of hepatocellular carcinoma after hepatectomy. Surgery 115:303–309, 1994.
18. Ringe B, Pichlmayr R, Wittekind C, Tusch G. Surgical treatment of hepatocellular carcinoma: Experience with liver resection and transplantation in 198 patients. World J Surg 15:270–285, 1991.
19. Soreide O, Czerniak A, Bradpiece H, Bloom S, Blumgart L. Characteristics of fibrolamellar hepatocellular carcinoma. A study of nine cases and review of the literature. Am J Surgery 151:518–523, 1986.
20. Ringe B, Wittekind C, Weimann A, Tusch G, Pichimayr R. Results of hepatic resection and transplantation for fibrolamellar carcinoma. Surg Gynecol Obstet 175:299–305, 1992.
21. Makuuchi M, Kosuge T, Takayamas T, Yamazaki S, Kakazu T, Miyagawa S, Kawasaki S. Surgery for small liver cancers. Semin Surg Oncol 9:298–304, 1993.
22. Jwo SC, Chiu JH, Chau GY, Loong CC, Lui WY. Risk factors linked to tumor recurrence of human hepatocellular carcinoma after hepatic resection. Hepatology 16:1367–1371, 1992.
23. Suenaga M, Nakao A, Harada A, Nonami T, Okada Y, Surgiura H, Uehara S, Takagi H. Hepatic resection for hepatocellular carcinoma. World J Surg 16:97–105, 1992.
24. Sugioka A, Tsuzuki T, Kanai T. Postresection prognosis of patients with hepatocellular carcinoma. Surgery 113:612–618, 1993.
25. Belghiti J, Panis Y, Farges O, Benhamou JP, Fekete F. Intrahepatic recurrence after resection of hepatocellular carcinoma complicating cirrhosis. Ann Surg 214:114, 1991.
26. Vauthey JN, Kimstra D, Franceschi D, Tao Y, Fortner J, Blumgart L, Brennan M. Factors affecting long-term outcome after hepatic resection for hepatocellular carcinoma. Am J Surg 169:28–34; discussion pp 34–35, 1995.
27. Zhou X, Yu Y, Tang Z. Advances in surgery for hepatocellular carcinoma. Asian J Surg 17:34–39, 1994.
28. Lai E, Ng I, You K, Choi T, Fan S, Mok F, Wong J. Hepatectomy for large hepatocellular carcinoma: The optimal resection margin. World J Surg 15:141–145, 1991.
29. Lai EC, You KT, Ng IO, Shek TW. The pathological basis of resection margin for hepatocellular carcinoma. World J Surg 17:786–791, 1993.
30. Zhou X, Tang A, Yu Y, Ma Z, Yang B, Lu J, Lin Z, Wang J. Solitary minute hepatocellular carcinoma. A study of 14 patients. Cancer 67:2855–2858, 1991.
31. Shirabe K, Kanematsu T, Matsumata T, Adachi T, Adachi E, Akazawa K, Sugimachi K. Factors linked to early recurrence of small hepatocellular carcinoma after hepatectomy: Univariate and multivariate analyses. Hepatology 14:802–805, 1991.

342

32. Kawarada Y, Ito F, Sakurai H, Tanigawa K, Iwata M, Imai T, Yokoi H, Noguchi T, Mizumoto R. Surgical treatment of heaptocellular carcinoma. Cancer Chemother Pharmacol 33(Suppl): S12–S17, 1994.
33. Zhou XD, Tang ZY, Yu YQ, Ma ZC, Yang BH, Lu JZ, Lin ZY, Tang CL. Prognostic factors or primary liver cancer: Report of 83 patients surviving 5 years of more compared with 811 patients surviving less than 5 years. J Exp Clin Cancer Res 10:81, 1991.
34. Bruix J, Cireral I, Calvet X, Fuster J, Bru C, Ayuso C, Vilana R, Boix L, Visa J, Rodes J. Surgical resection and survival in Western patients with hepatocellular carcinoma. J Hepatol 15:350–355, 1992.
35. Torii A, Nonami T, Harada A, Yasui M, Nakao A, Takagi H. Extent of hepatic resection as a prognostic factor for small, solitary hepatocellular carcinomas. J Surg Oncol 54:13–17, 1993.
36. Shimada M, Matsumata T, Maeda T, Yanaga K, Taketomi A, Sugimachi K. Characteristics of hepatocellular carcinoma originating in the caudate lobe. Hepatology 19:911–915, 1994.
37. Wu CC, Hwang CJ, Yang MD, Liu TJ. Preliminary results of hepatic for centrally located large hepatocellular carcinoma. Austral N Z Surgery 63:525–529, 1993.
38. Zhou X, Yu Y, Tang Z, Ma Z. Results of liver resection for primary liver cancer. J Hep Bil Cancer Surg 2:118–122, 1994.
39. LaBerge L, Laing F, Federle M, Jeffrey R, Lim R. Hepatocellular carcinoma: Assessment of resectability by computed tomography and ultrasound. Radiology 152:485–490, 1984.
40. Izumi R, Shimizu K, Ii T, Yagi M, Matsui O, Nonomura A, Miyazaki I. Prognostic factors of hepatocellular carcinoma in patients undergoing hepatic resection. Gastroenterology 106:720–727, 1994.
41. Kosuge T, Makuuchi M, Takayama T, Yamamoto J, Shimada K, Yamasaki S. Long-term results after resection of hepatocellular carcinoma: Experience of 480 cases. Hepatogastroenterology 40:328–332, 1993.
42. Kawasaki S, Makuuchi M, Miyagawa S, Kakazu T, Hayashi K, Kasai H, Miwa S, Hui AM, Nishimaki K. Results of hepatic resection for hepatocellular carcinoma. World J Surg 19:31–34, 1995.
43. Ozawa K, Takayasu T, Kumada K, Yamaoka Y, Tanaka K, Kobayashi N, Inamoto T, Shimahara Y, Mori K, Honda K, Asonuma K. Experience with 225 hepatic resection for hepatocellular carcinoma over a 4-year period. Am J Surg 161:677, 1991.
44. Harada T, Shigemura T, Kodama S, Higuchi T, Ikeda S, Okazaki M. Hepatic resection is not enough for hepatcellular carcinoma. A follow-up study of 92 patients. J Clin Gastroenterol 14:245–250, 1992.
45. HaradaT, Kodama S, Matsuo K, Higuchi T, Nagai T, Ikeda S, Okazaki M. Surgical management of large hepatocellular carcinomas: Criteria for curative hepatectomy. Int Surg 78:284–287, 1993.
46. Jeng KS, Chen BF, Lin HJ. En bloc resection for extensive hepatocellular carcinoma: Is it advisable? World J Surg 18:834–839, 1994.
47. Lau WY, Leung KL, Leung TW, Liew CT. Resection of hepatocellular carcinoma with diaphragmatic invasion. Br J Surg 82:264–266, 1995.
48. Sasaki Y, Imaoka S, Masutani S, Ohashi I, Ishikawa O, Koyama H, Iwanaga T. Influence of coexisting cirrhosis on long-term pognosis after surgery in patients with hepatocellular carcinoma. Surgery 112:515–521, 1992.
49. Chou FF, Sheen-Chen SM, Chen CL, Chen YS, Chen MJ. Prognostic factors after hepatectomy for hepatocellular carcinoma. Hepatogastroenterology 41:419–423, 1994.
50. Capussotti L, Borgonovo G, Bouzari H, Smudge C, Grange D, Franc D. Results of major hepatectomy for large primary liver cancer in patients with cirrhosis. Br J Surg 81:427–431, 1994.
51. Takeda S, Nagafuchi Y, Tashiro H, Abe Y, Fukushige H, Komori H, Okamoto K, Ohsato K, Haratake J. Antihepatitis C virus status in hepatocellular carcinoma and the influence on clinicopathological findings and operative results. Br J Surg 79:1195–1198, 1992.
52. Tarao K, Ohkawa S, Shimizu A, et al. DNA synthesis activities of hepatocytes from noncancerous cirrhotic tissue and of hepatocellular carcinoma (HCC) cells from cancerous tissue can

predict the survival of hepatectomized patients with HCC. Cancer 71:3859–3863, 1993.

53. Chiu JH, Wu LH, Kao HL, Chang HM, Tsay SH, Loong CC, Chau GY, Lui WY. Can determination of the proliferative capacity of the nontumor portion predict the risk of tumor recurrence in the liver remnant after resection of human hepatocellular carcinoma? Hepatology 18:96–102, 1993. [published erratum appears in Hepatology 18:1292, 1993.]

54. Adachi E, Maeda T, Matsumata T, Shirabe K, Kinukawa N, Sugimachi K, Tsuneyoshi M. Risk factors for interhepatic recurrence in human small hepatocellular carcinoma. Gastroenterology 108:768–775, 1995.

55. Chen MF, Hwang TL, Jeng LB. Hepatic resection for 28 patients with small hepatocellular carcinoma. Int Surg 77:72–76, 1992.

56. Chen MF, Hwang TL, Jeng LB, Wang CS, Jan YY, Chen SC. Postoperative recurrence of hepatocellular carcinoma. Two hundred five consecutive patients who underwent hepatic resection in 15 years. Arch Surg 129:738–742, 1994.

57. Kawai Y, Takeshige K, Nunome M, Kuroda H, Suzuki H, Banno K, Koide T, Kobayashi H, Owa Y, Koike A. Prognosis after hepatic resection in patients with hepatocellular carcinoma, estimated on the basis of the morphometric indices. Cancer Chemother Pharmacol 33(Suppl):S24–S28, 1994.

58. Kim ST, Kim KP. Hepatic resections for primary liver cancer. Cancer Chemother Pharmacol 33(Suppl):S18–S23, 1994.

59. Lai EC, Fan ST, Lo CM, Chu KM, Liu CL, Wong J. Hepatic resection for hepatocellular carcinoma. An audit of 343 patients. Ann Surg 221:291–298, 1995.

60. Gouillat C, Manganas D, Berard P. Ultrasonically guided hepatic tumorectomy. J Am Coll Surg 180:616–618, 1995.

61. Lau WY, Leung KL, Lee TW, Li AK. Ultrasonography during liver resection for hepatocellular carcinoma. Br J Surg 80:493–494, 1993.

62. Lygidakis NJ, Makuuchi M. Clinical application of preoperative ultrasonography in liver surgery. Hepatogastroenterology, 39:232–236, 1992.

63. Wu CC, Yang MD, Liu TJ. Improvements in hepatocellular carcinoma resection by intraoperative ultrasonography and intermittent hepatic inflow blood occusion. Jpn J Clin Oncol 22:107–112, 1992.

64. Ravikumar TS, Buenaventura S, Salem RR, D'Andrea B. Intraoperative ultrasonagraphy of liver: Detection of occult liver tumors and treatment by cryosurgery. Cancer Detect Prev 18:131–138, 1994.

65. Masutani S, Sasaki Y, Imaoka S, et al. The prognostic significance of surgical margin in liver resection of patients with hepatocellular carcinoma. Arch Surg 129:1025–1030, 1994.

66. Ouchi K, Matsubara S, Fukuhara K, Tominaga T, Matsuno S. Recurrence of hepatocellular carcinoma in the liver remnant after hepatic resection. Am J Sur 166:270, 1993.

67. Hamazaki K, Mimura H, Orita K, Lygidakis NJ. Surgical treatment for hepatocellular carcinoma (HCC) 3 cm or less than 3 cm in diameter. Hepatogastroenterology 39:574–576, 1992.

68. Tjandra JJ, Fan ST, Wong J. Peri-operative mortality in hepatic resection. Austal N Z J Surg 61:201–206, 1991.

69. Huguet C, Gavelli A, Chieco PA, Bona S, Harb J, Joseph JM, Jobard J, Garmaglia M, Lasserre M. Liver ischemia for hepatic reseaction: Where is the limit? Surgery 111:251–259, 1992.

70. Kajikawa M, Nonami T, Kurokawa T, Hashimoto S, Harada A, Nakao A, Takagi H. Autologous blood transfusion for hepatectomy in patients with cirrhosis and hepatocellur carcinoma: Use of recombinant human erythropoietin. Surgery 115:727–734, 1994.

71. Bismuth H, Chiche L, Castaing D. Surgical treatment of hepatocellular carcinomas in noncirrhotic liver: Experience with 68 liver resections. World J Surg 19:35–41, 1995.

72. Kakazu T, Makuuchi M, Kawasaki S, Miyagawa S, Hashikura Y, Kosuge T, Takayama T, Yamamoto J. Repeat hepatic resection for recurrent hepatocellular carcinoma. Hepatogastroenterology 40:337–341, 1993.

73. Nakajima Y, Ohmura T, Kimura J, Shimamura T, Misawa K, Matsushita M, Sato N, Une Y, Uchino J. Role of surgical treatment for recurrenct hepatocellular carcinoma after hepatic

resection. World J Surg 17:792–795, 1993.

74. Shimada M, Matsumata T, Taketomi A, Yamamoto K, Itasaka H, Sugimachi K. Repeat hepatectomy for recurrent hepatocellular carcinoma. Surgery 115:703–706, 1994.

75. Suenaga M, Surgiura H, Kokuba S, Kurumiya T. Repeated hepatic resection of recurrent hepatocellular carcinoma in eighteen cases. Sugery 115:452–457, 1994.

76. Zhou X, Tang Z, Yu Y, Yang B, Lin Z, Lu J, Ma Z, Tang C. Long-term survivors after resection for primary liver cancer. Clinical analysis of 19 patients surviving more than ten years. Cancer 63:2201–2206, 1989.

77. Lo CM, Lai EC, Fan ST, Choi TK, Wong J. Resection for extrahepatic recurrence of hepatocellular carcinoma. Br J Surg 81:1019–1021, 1994.

78. McPeake JR, O'Grady JG, Zaman S, Portmann B, Wight DG, Tan KC. Calne RY, Williams R. Liver transplantation for primary hepatocellular carcinoma: Tumor size and number determine outcome. J Hepatol 18:226–234, 1993.

79. Bismuth H, Chiche L, Adam R, Castaing D, Diamond T, Dennison A. Liver resection versus transplantation for hepatocellular carcinoma in cirrhotic patients. Ann Surg 218:145–151, 1993.

80. Bismuth H, Chiche L. Comparison of hepatic resection and transplantation in the treatment of liver cancer. Semin Surg Oncol 9:341–345, 1993.

81. Caine R, Yamanoi A, Oura S, Kawamura M. Liver transplantation for hepatocarcinoma. Surg Today 23:1–3, 1993.

82. Venook AP. Treatment of hepatocellular carcinoma: Too many options? J Clin Oncol 12:1323–1334, 1994.

83. Lygidakis NJ, Konstantinidou T, Pothoulakis J. Pre- and post-operative adjuvant targeting locoregional chemotherapy combined with locoregional targeting immunostimulation and surgical resection for hepatocellular carcinoma. A new promising alternative. Anticancer Res 14:1351–1355, 1994.

84. Gururangan S, O'Meara A, MacMahon C, Guiney EJ, O'Donnell B, Fitzgerald RJ, Breatnach F. Primary hepatic tumors in children: A 26-year review J Surg Oncol 50:30–36, 1992.

85. Harada A, Nonami T, Kishimoto W, Nakao A, Takagi H. Results of hepatic resection and postoperative arterial chemotherapy for hepatocellular carcinoma. Cancer Chemother Pharmacol 31(Suppl):S35–S37, 1992.

86. Tsuzuki T, Sugioka A, Ueda M, Iida S, Kanai T, Yoshii H, Nakayau K. Hepatic resection for hepatocellular carcinoma. Surgery 107:511–520, 1990.

87. Nagorney DM, Adson MA, Weiland LH. Fibrolamellar hepatoma. Am J Surgery 149:113–119, 1985.

18. Colon cancer

David M. Ota

Introduction

The primary treatment of localized colon adenocarcinoma is surgical resection, and the operative procedures have been designed to maximize the chance of cure. Miles' theory was that wide excision and regional lymphadenectomy would result in the highest cure rate from the locally invasive and regional metastatic aspects of colon carcinoma [1]. Therefore, the operative techniques have focused on the regional arterial blood supply of the colon. The regional artery has defined the extent of mesenteric, lymphatic, and colonic resection. Other intraoperative considerations that may influence survival include the no-touch technique and intraluminal spread of exfoliated tumor cells, and have been reviewed [1]. There are two recent advances in colon cancer management that influence the surgeon's approach to this disease. First, effective postoperative adjuvant chemotherapy is available for patients who are at high risk for developing recurrent disease. Second is the development of new laparoscopic instruments and techniques that permit colonic resections through small incisions, reducing postoperative pain, stress, and recovery time. These new aspects of colon carcinoma management re-emphasize the significance and rationale of adequate excision and lymphadenectomy, and warrant this review.

No-touch technique

The theory of the 'no-touch technique' was that intraoperative manipulation of the primary tumor during dissection of the colon and mesentery could dislodge tumor cells into the venous circulation and disseminate disease to distant organs. Thus, the first step in the no-touch technique was to ligate the regional arterial and venous blood supply before the colon and mesentery were mobilized. Turnbull theorized that the no-touch technique would reduce the risk of systemic and intraperitoneal dissemination, thus improving survival [3]. Other investigators have argued that his results could be attributed to patient selection and similar results could be obtained with extended resection and lymphadenectomy [4,5].

Raphael E. Pollock (ed.), SURGICAL ONCOLOGY. Copyright © 1997. Kluwer Academic Publishers. ISBN 0-7923-9900-5. All rights reserved.

A major limitation of Turnbull's theory was the absence of prospective randomized data. In 1988 Wiggers et al. reported the survival data of a prospective randomized trial that compared the no-touch isolation technique with a conventional resection technique [5]. Patients were registered and randomized preoperatively. Eligibility and exclusion criteria were judged reasonable. There were 117 patients in the no-touch group and 119 patients in the control arm. This group observed that complications were equal in both groups, but survival was not significantly different among the two treatment groups. The final conclusion was that the no-touch technique did not statistically improve survival.

Intraluminal spread

Intraluminal exfoliation of tumor cells and implantation on the anastomotic site, giving rise to so-called suture line recurrence, is another potential problem. Suture line recurrence rates have ranged from 10% to 35%, with a higher incidence noted in distal colon carcinomas [6]. These recurrences may be related to (1) implantation of exfoliated tumor cells at the suture line, (2) proximity of the tumor to the anastomosis, and (3) extraluminal residual disease growing into suture line. Recurrence can theoretically be avoided by (1) isolation of the colon with constricting tapes, (2) painting the anastomotic site with alcohol solutions, and (3) chemical lavage of the colon lumen. However, it should be pointed out that there have been no randomized trials comparing these precautionary techniques. Nonetheless, some investigators have pointed out that these maneuvers are simple and do not contribute to morbidity or operating time. Adequate distal and proximal luminal resection (10 cm) should also be observed to prevent suture line recurrence.

Extent of colonic resection

The extent of colonic resection and lymphadenectomy has been debated since Miles put forth his rationale for the abdomino-perineal resection [1]. The theory of extended lymphadenectomy is that if a wider dissection removes more lymph nodes with potential metastatic deposits, the chance for cure should increase with an extended lymphadenectomy. Although the early studies by Gabriel et al. showed that lymphatic metastases advanced in an orderly fashion from proximal to more distant nodes [7], the concept of the 'skip' lymph node metastases was proposed to explain nodal metastases far from the primary tumor without involvement of adjacent lymph nodes. This was attributed to unusual lymphatic drainage or clogging of lymphatic vessels, resulting in retrograde lymphatic flow and the development of lymph node metastases far from the primary tumor [8].

Sugarbaker and Corlow analyzed the results of lymphadenectomy from several studies that retrospectively compared extended regional hemicolectomy with a regional colectomy [6]. An extended regional hemicolectomy included the regional arterial blood supply and periaortic node dissection. The definition of a regional hemicolectomy was a colon resection with removal of the regional arterial blood supply. They concluded that the extended regional hemicolectomy resulted in a theoretical 5% survival advantage over regional hemicolectomy, and no statistical significance was found in the studies that were reviewed. The controversy regarding segmental versus radical hemicolectomy has persisted for many years. Recently, the French Association for Surgical Research reported the results of a randomized trial that compared segmental hemicolectomy with radical hemicolectomy for carcinomas in either the left or sigmoid colon [9]. The radical hemicolectomy included the inferior mesenteric artery in the mesenteric resection, while the segmental colectomy took either the left colic or superior rectal artery in the mesenteric resection. The authors found no difference in survival rates between the two groups, indicating wider mesenteric lymphadenectomy offers no survival benefit.

The current recommendation is that a colectomy should be performed with at least 10 cm of proximal and distal luminal margins, and the regional arterial blood supply should be taken at its origin, thus ensuring an adequate mesenteric resection. Thus, a lesion in the right colon requires a colonic resection with ileocolic-right colic artery and the right branch of the middle colic artery. A transverse colon cancer should include the middle colic artery. For left colonic carcinomas, the colonic resection should include the left colic artery, while a resection of a sigmoid tumor would include the superior rectal artery.

Although the extent of lymphadenectomy may not necessarily influence survival, important prognostic information is available in the regional lymph nodes of the resected mesentery. Cady has put forth the evolving concept that regional lymph nodes are not 'governors' but are 'indicators' of survival [10]. For solid tumors, such as breast and prostate, bladder, and cervix, removal of regional lymph nodes provides important staging information and may not add to survival. The surgical treatment of colon adenocarcinomas may evolve in a similar direction when more data become available.

There is another reason to perform an adequate node dissection for colon cancer. Postoperative adjuvant systemic chemotherapy improves survival in patients with node-positive tumors ($T_{any}N_1M_0$ stage, stage III or Astler-Coller classification Dukes' C tumors), while no benefit was seen with node-negative tumors ($T_{1-3}N_0M_0$, stage II, Dukes' B tumors) [11]. Therefore, an adequate lymph node sampling during a curative colonic resection is necessary in order to stage the disease and to select those patients who will benefit from postoperative adjuvant chemotherapy. Resecting colon and mesentery according to the regional arterial blood supply will provide sufficient node sampling for pathologic assessment and for adjuvant chemotherapy.

Controversy over laparoscopic colectomy for colon cancer

The primary treatment of localized colon adenocarcinoma is surgical resection, and the objective of operative procedures is to obtain sufficient distal and proximal luminal margins and a regional lymphadenectomy. Recently, there has been tremendous interest in developing minimally invasive surgical techniques to treat inflammatory and neoplastic diseases of the gastrointestinal tract. The laparoscopic cholecystectomy procedure rapidly became the standard treatment for cholelithiasis and laparoscopic appendectomy, and Nissen fundoplication may also replace the open laparotomy technique. Laparoscopic surgery is being developed for gastrointestinal cancer surgery, and there are several reports that describe a series of patients who have had a laparoscopic-assisted colectomy for resectable malignant disease [12–18]. While the procedure is feasible, it is not clear if laparoscopic colectomy is equivalent to open colectomy. Issues such as compromised cancer control, complications, quality of life, and health care costs must be considered.

Laparoscopic colectomy

Laparoscopic surgery is rapidly evolving. A number of procedures have been developed for benign diseases, and cholecystectomy, appendectomy, and hysterectomy are becoming the standards of care. Advances in laparoscopic instrumentation have resulted in new procedures, such as colon resections for polyps or malignant disease. T_1, T_2, and T_3 colonic tumors are amenable to laparoscopic resection, while T_4 tumors (invasion of adjacent organs) require open laparotomy. Lesions located in the ascending, descending, and sigmoid colon are amenable to laparoscopic colectomy. At the present time, the transverse colon is difficult to resect because of its greater omentum. Another indication for laparoscopic colectomy is a near-obstructing colonic lesion with unresectable metastatic disease. Significant palliation can be achieved with a laparoscopic segmental colectomy, resulting in faster recovery and better quality of life. Ondrula et al. have described the significant comorbid diseases processes that increase the morbidity of colorectal resections [19]. Those patients with significant congestive heart failure, a history of myocardial infarction, and severe chronic obstructive pulmonary disease can benefit from minimal access surgery that reduces postoperative stress and pain.

Experience with laparoscopic colectomy for colonic neoplasms is increasing, but there are now data detailing the benefits and risks of these procedures. Prospective trials are underway, and they will determine (1) learning time, (2) factors that contribute to open laparotomy, (3) operative time, (4) complications, (5) hospital of hospital stay, and (6) pathologic assessment of the resected specimen. Published reports indicate that the benefits of laparoscopic colectomy include less postoperative pain, shorter hospital stay, and earlier return to work [12–18]. Despite these encouraging observations, there are several questions that remain to be answered regarding this technique.

Presently, laparoscopic colectomy for resectable colon carcinomas is investigational. As with all new treatment modalities, comparison with traditional open colectomy is necessary and a multiinstitutional trial randomized trial is needed. Such a trial should compare extent of node sampling, proximal and distal luminal margins, conversion rates, hospitalization/operating room costs, and patterns of recurrence and survival. Until these issues are resolved, laparoscopic colectomy should be done under an institutional review board–approved protocol in order to monitor complications, extent of resection, conversion rates, and hospitalization time.

The objective of laparoscopic colon resections is to resect at least 10 cm of proximal and distal colon with a regional lymphadenectomy. The lymphadenectomy requires that the major arterial blood supply be taken with the resected specimen. The steps to this procedure include (1) port placement, (2) inspection of the abdominal cavity, (3) mobilization of the colon and mesentery, (4) dissection of the mesentery and securing the regional arterial and venous blood vessels, (5) transection of the bowel and specimen removal, and (6) anastomosis. At all times, the surgeon should be aware of reasons for converting a laparoscopic procedure to an open laparotomy. These include (1) poor exposure because of adhesions, extensive tumor, or obesity; (2) bleeding; (3) injury to other organs; and (4) lack of progress after 1 hour.

Both operative technique and instrumentation for laparoscopic surgery have undergone significant changes recently. Laparoscopic and ultrasound probes are now available in order to evaluate the liver for occult metastasis. Recent studies indicate that intraoperative liver ultrasonography is equivalent to CT scanning for staging purposes and is considerably less costly. Video technology will continue to improve and progress to three-dimensional imaging, virtual reality imaging, and split-screen technology. Instrumentation has also improved with reliable reusable laparoscopic instruments, and this will help to reduce operating room costs. The surgeon's goal in either an open or laparoscopic colectomy procedure is to obtain adequate luminal margins and adequate lymph node sampling. If new surgical technology can be applied cost effectively while maintaining standards of anatomical resection, then minimally invasive surgery will be a welcome advance.

Cancer control

There are several important cancer control issues regarding laparoscopic colectomy. These include (1) the extent of lymph node dissection, (2) tumor implantation at port sites, and (3) adequacy of intraperitoneal staging. The role of lymphadenectomy in colorectal resections has been controversial for many years. It is possible that a laparoscopic colectomy results in a lesser lymphadenectomy. Several reports suggest that lymph node counts in laparoscopic-assisted colectomy specimens are similar to open colectomy specimens [12–18]. However, these studies had a considerable mix of proximal and distal colorectal carcinomas, and, because there is considerable variability in node counts from proximal to distal colon, these analyses of nodal counts that do not consider this variation may be misleading. A recent study of 14 laparoscopic-assisted right hemicolectomies found that the mean nodal count was 8.8 ± 5.4 ($\pm$SD), and this was significantly less than what was observed in the historical right colon resections shown in Table 1 ($p < 0.05$). Vayer et al. made a similar finding. They also compared laparoscopic right colectomies with open laparotomy right colon resections during a similar time period [20]. The mean node count for the laparoscopic group was 6.6, and this was significantly less than the 9.6 nodes found in the open colectomy group.

It is not clear if significant differences in nodal counts between laparoscopic-assisted and open colectomy are clinically meaningful. There is significant prognostic information in resected lymph nodes. Systemic adjuvant chemotherapy has been shown to be effective in increasing the survival of colon cancer patients who are node positive [11]. If laparoscopic colectomy results in fewer lymph nodes compared with open colectomy, then the potential for understaging this disease exists. This could lead to withholding postoperative systemic adjuvant chemotherapy from patients who might otherwise benefit from it, resulting in lower survival. Another important consideration is whether a lesser lymphadenectomy will affect locoregional control of disease. Only a randomized trial comparing laparoscopic with open colectomy will resolve all these issues.

Tumor implantation at either a port site or the specimen wound is another cancer control issue. There are several reports that have described tumor implantation at port sites for a variety of abdominal malignancies of gallbladder, stomach, pancreas, and ovary origin [20–24]. Similar reports regarding tumor implantation at wound or port sites after laparoscopic colectomy have now appeared in the literature [25–27]. Such reports point out that new operative technology, while having short-term benefits such as shorter hospitalization, can have long-term consequences on cancer contro. Wound recurrence is uncommon with open colectomy, but the true incidence of port-site recurrence with laparoscopic colectomy will never be known until a large prospective study is done. The potential mechanism of port-site recurrence is the shedding of malignant cells during the procedure. From a technical standpoint, the laparoscopic surgeon should avoid grasping the colonic wall near the

Table 1. Number of lymph nodes in resected right colectomy specimens for Astler-Coller Dukes' B and C colon carcinomas

Procedure	n^1	Mean nodes $\pm$ S.D.
Open	101	18.8 ± 11.2
Laparoscopic	14	8.8 ± 5.4

tumor. Laparoscopic Babcock clamps are now available and should be used carefully.

Intraperitoneal staging is another limitation of laparoscopic colectomy. The surgeon is no longer able to palpate the liver for metastases, although the surface of the liver can be seen. Preoperative staging with either ultrasound or CT scan may be necessary. As mentioned earlier, laparoscopic ultrasound probes are now available and can be used effectively to assess for liver metastases. Intraperitoneal metastases to the ovaries, pelvic cul-de-sac, or paracolic gutters can be missed. The incidence of such understaging is unknown and hopefully is low enough to avoid entering patients into systemic adjuvant chemotherapy trials now underway.

Complications

During the early stages of laparoscopic cholecystectomy, unusual complications, such as common bile duct injury, cystic duct leakage, and stones scattered throughout the peritoneal cavity, were reported. The laparoscopic approach to colon resection has also resulted in unusual complications. Ureteral injury is rare with open laparotomy, but such injuries have been observed with the laparoscopic technique. Some surgeons routinely place lighted ureteral stents prior to the procedure in order to visualize the structure, but this obviously increases the cost. Inadvertent and undetected small bowel perforation is another significant injury. This presumably occurs because the grasping instruments can traumatize the bowel wall or cauterizing instruments can injure the bowel outside the range of laparoscope view. Other injuries include uncontrolled hemorrhage, bladder injury, and hypercapnia-induced cardiac arrhythmias or decompensation.

Cost analysis and quality of life

Advocates of laparoscopic surgery point out that this new technology results in faster patient recovery, lower health care costs, and better quality of life compared with open laparotomy [28,29]. Shorter hospitalization time and fewer postoperative complications should reduce costs. Less postoperative pain and faster return to normal activity may result in improved quality of life. While many surgeons would agree with these impressions, attempts to quantify these parameters have been very difficult. Under the pressure of growing concern over spiraling medical costs, economic analysts have developed new tools that make it possible to conduct rational analyses of the economic and quality-of-life effects of new medical interventions [30]. These studies have been applied to several cancer therapies with intriguing results and conclusions [31].

The goal of a randomized laparoscopic colectomy trial for resectable disease is to determine whether it is equivalent to open colectomy in terms of disease-free and overall survival. If laparoscopic colectomy does not meet that test, then the issues of cost and quality of life are irrelevant because the standard open colectomy has minimum morbidity and mortality (less than 1%). If this procedure does not compromise survival, then the choice between laparoscopic and open procedures should be guided by costs and quality of life. Because laparoscopic technology is new and seemingly less traumatic, one should not assume that it is better. Tate et al. recently reported their randomized trial of laparoscopic versus open appendectomy [32]. They found that hospitalization time and return to work were similar, while operating room time was greater with the laparoscopic approach. Their conclusion is that the procedures are equivalent and, therefore, they question whether the laparoscopic approach is better. A prospective study comparing open versus laparoscopic colectomy is necessary in order to resolve the issues of outcome, cost, and quality of life before the new procedure is accepted as standard of therapy.

Conclusions

Laparoscopic surgery has the potential to have a significant impact on abdominal surgery. Minimal invasive techniques may have an important role in palliating the symptoms of advanced disease, but its application in treating potentially curable colon carcinoma is controversial. The surgeon's goal is to obtain adequate luminal margins and adequate lymph node sampling. If new surgical technology can be applied cost effectively while maintaining standards of anatomical resection, then minimally invasive surgery will be a welcome advance. Before laparoscopic colectomy can replace open colectomy, a prospective randomized clinical trial comparing disease control, complications, costs, and quality of life must be done.

Acknowledgment

The author wishes to thank Mrs. Dianna Staab for her diligence and patience in the preparation of this manuscript.

References

1. Miles EE. A method of performing abdomino-perineal excision for carcinoma of the rectum and of the terminal portion of the pelvic colon. Lancet 2:1812–1813, 1908.
2. Turnbull RB, Jr., Kyle K, et al. Cancer of the colon: The influence of the no-touch isolation technic on survival rates. Ann Surg 166:420–427, 1967.
3. Stearns MW, Schottenfeld D. Techniques for the surgical management of colon cancer. Cancer 28:165–169, 1971.

4. Enker WE, Laffer UT, Block GE. Enhanced survival of patients with colon and rectal cancer is based upon wide anatomic resection. Ann Surg 190:350–360, 1979.
5. Wiggers T, Jeekel J, Arends JW, et al. No-touch isolation technique in colon cancer: A controlled prospective trial. Br J Surg 75:409–415, 1988.
6. Sugarbaker PH, Corlew S. Influence of surgical techniques on survival in patients with colorectal cancer: A review. Dis Colon Rectum 25:545–557, 1982.
7. Gabriel WB, Dukes C, Bussy HJ. Lymphatic spread in cancer of the rectum. Br J Surg 23:395–413, 1935.
8. Grinnell RS. Lymphatic block with atypical and retrograde lymphatic metastasis and spread in carcinoma of the colon and rectum. Ann Surg 163:272–280, 1966.
9. The French Association for Surgical Research. Curative resection for left colonic carcinoma: Hemicolectomy vs. segmental colectomy. Dis Colon Rectum 37:651–659, 1994.
10. Cady B. Lymph node metastasis: Indicators but not governors of survival. Arch Surg 119:1067–1072, 1984.
11. Steele G. Adjuvant therapy for patients with colon and rectal cancer: Clinical indications for multimodality therapy in high-risk groups and specific surgical questions for future multimodality trials. Surgery 112:847–849, 1992.
12. Jacobs M, Verdeja JC, Goldstein HS. Minimally invasive colon resection (laparoscopic colectomy). Surg Laparosc Endosc 1:144–150, 1991.
13. Fowler DL, White SA. Laparoscopy-assisted sigmoid resection. Surg Laparosc Endosc 1:183–188, 1991.
14. Schlinkert RT. Laparoscopic-asisted right hemicolectomy. Dis Colon Rectum 34:1030–1031, 1991.
15. Phillips EH, Franklin M, Carroll BJ, Fallas MJ, Ramos R, Rosenthal D. Laparoscopic colectomy. Ann Surg 216:703–707, 1992.
16. Falk PM, Beart RW, Wexner SD, Thorson AG, Jagelman DG, Lavery IC, Johansen OB, Fitzgibbons RJ, Jr. Laparoscopic colectomy: A critical appraisal. Dis Colon Rectum 36:28–34, 1993.
17. Scoggin SD, Frazee RC, Snyder SK, Hendricks JC, Roberts JW, Symmonds RE, Smith RW. Laparoscopic-assisted bowel surgery. Dis Colon Rectum 36:747–750, 1993.
18. Peters WR, Bartels TL. Minimally invasive colectomy – are the potential benefits realized? Dis Colon Rectum 36:751–756, 1993.
19. Ondrula DP, Nelson RL, Prasad ML, et al. Multifactorial index of preoperative risk factors in colon resections. Dis Colon Rectum 35:117–122, 1992.
20. Vayer AJ, Larach SW, Williamson PR, Ferrara A, Salomow M. Cost effectiveness of laparoscopic assisted colectomy. Proc Am Soc Colon/Rectal Surgeons, 92nd Annual Meeting, 1993, p 37.
21. Cava A, Ronian J, Gonzalez Quintala A, Martin F, Aramburo P. Subcutaneous metastasis following laparoscopy in gastric adenocarcinoma. Eur J Surg Oncol 16:63–67, 1990.
22. Clair DG, Lautz DB, Brooks DC. Rapid development of umbilical metastases after laparoscopic cholecystectomy for unsuspected gallbladder carcinoma. Surgery 113:355–358, 1993.
23. Fong Y, Brennan MF, Turnbull A, Colt DG, Blumgart LH. Gallbladder cancer discovered during laparoscopic surgery: Potential for iatrogenic tumor dissemination. Arch Surg 128:1028–1032, 1993.
24. Gleeson NC, Nicosia SV, Mark JE, Hoffman MS, Cavanagh D. Abdominal wall metastases from ovarian cancer after laparoscopy. Am J Obstet Gynecol 169:522–523, 1993.
25. Delcastillo CF, Warshaw L. Peritoneal metastases in pancreatic carcinoma. Hepatogastroenterology 40:430–432, 1993.
26. Walsh DCA, Wattchow DA, Wilson TG. Subcutaneous metastases after laparoscopic resection of malignancy. Aust N Z J Surg 63:563–565, 1993.
27. O'Rourke N, Price PM, Kelly S, Sikora K. Tumor inoculation during laparoscopy. Lancet 342:368, 1993.

28. Fusco MA, Paluzzi MW. Abdominal wall recurrence after laparoscopic-assisted colectomy for adenocarcinoma of the colon. Dis Colon Rectum 36:858–861, 1993.
29. Fritts LL, Orlando R, Thompson WR, May GA, Hight DW, Touloukian RJ. Laparoscopic appendectomy – a safety and cost analysis. Arch Surg 128:521–525, 1993.
30. Bass EB, Pitt HA, Lillemoe KD. Cost-effectiveness of laparoscopic cholecystectomy versus open cholecystectomy. Am J Surg 165:466–471, 1993.
31. Detsky AS, Naglie I. A clinician's guide to cost-effective analysis. Ann Intern Med 113:147–154, 1990.
32. Smith TJ, Hillner BE, Desch CE. Efficacy and cost-effectiveness of cancer treatment: Rational allocation of resources based on decision analysis. J Natl Cancer Inst 85:1460–1474, 1993.
33. Tate JJT, Dawson JW, Chung SCS, Lau WY, Li AKC. Laparoscopic versus open appendectomy – prospective randomized trial. Lancet 342:633–637, 1993.

Index

Mesorectal excision, 34–36. *See also*
    Rectal cancer, mesorectal excision
Meta-analysis, in soft tissue sarcoma,
    98–99
Metastases
    in biliary tract cancer, 275
    in gallbladder carcinoma, 290–291
    in gastric carcinoma, 242–243, 247–
        248
    in gastrointestinal neuroendocrine
        tumors, 231–232
    intrahepatic, 335
    in melanoma, 3–4
    in pancreatic cancer, 115
    in rectal cancer, 31–32, 34, 36, 45–46
    in thyroid carcinoma, medullary,
        162–163
Methotrexate, 96
Minimally invasive surgery, 309–324
    in adrenal neoplasms, 321–322
    in colorectal cancer, 320–321
    diagnostic value of, 323–324
    in esophageal cancer, 316–317
    in gallbladder and bile duct cancer,
        318
    in gastric cancer, 317
    in gastrointestinal cancers, 316–324
    in gynecological neoplasms, 322–323
    in hepatopancreaticobiliary cancer,
        317
    laparoscopy in, 309–324 (*See also*
        Laparoscopy)
    in large bowel malignancies, 318
    in liver tumors, 317–318
    palliative treatment of, 315–316
    in pancreatic tumors, 318
    in small bowel malignancies, 319–320
    in splenic tumors, 318
    in urological neoplasms, 321–322
Mitomycin C, 285
MRI, 173–174
Mucosa-associated lymphoid tissue
    (MALT)
    gastric carcinoma and, 248
    in non-Hodgkin's lymphoma, 206–
        208
Multimodality therapy
    in cholangiocarcinoma, Hilar bile
        duct, 283–284
    in pancreatic cancer, 114–117
    in rectal cancer, 34–41 (*See also*
        Rectal cancer, multimodality
        treatment)
Multiple endocrine neoplasia (MEN),
    213–223
    familial medullary thyroid
        carcinoma, 214, 218–223 (*See also*
        Multiple endocrine neoplasia
        (MEN), type IIa and IIb)
    type I, 213–218 (*See also* Multiple
        endocrine neoplasia (MEN), type
        I)
    type IIa and IIb, 218–223 (*See also*
        Multiple endocrine neoplasia
        (MEN), type IIa and IIb)
Multiple endocrine neoplasia (MEN),
    type I, 213–218. *See also* Multiple
    endocrine neoplasia (MEN), type
    IIa and IIb
    familial medullary thyroid cancer in,
        214
    genetics of, 214–215
    glucagonomas in, 216
    history of, 213–214
    hyperparathyroidism in, primary,
        215, 217
    imaging in, 216–217
    insulinomas in, 216, 217
    oncogenesis in, 214–215
    pancreaticoduodenal disease in, 216–
        217 (*See also* Pancreaticoduodenal
        disease)
    parathyroid disease in, 215
    parathyroidectomy in, 215
    pituitary tumors in, 217–218 (*See
        also* Pituitary tumors)
    screening for, 215
    somatostatin scintigraphy in, 216–217
    syndromes of, 214
    Wermer's syndrome in, 214
    Zollinger-Ellison syndrome (ZES)
        in, 216
Multiple endocrine neoplasia (MEN),
    type IIa and IIb, 218–223. *See also*
    Multiple endocrine neoplasia
    (MEN), type I
    chromosome 10 in, 219
    definition of, 218
    familial medullary thyroid carcinoma
        vs., 218
    gastrointestinal disease in, 223
    genetics of, 219–220
    Hirschsprung's disease in, 223
    history of, 219
    medullary thyroid cancer in,
        diagnosis of, 220–221
    medullary thyroid cancer in,
        incidence of, 220

364

medullary thyroid cancer in,
  presentation of, 220
medullary thyroid cancer in,
  treatment of, 221–222
parathyroid disease in, 223
pheochromocytoma in, 222–223
RET protooncogene in, 219
thyroidectomy in, 221
urine test in, 222
Muscle flaps, 139
Myelosuppression, 100

N
Neoplasia, multiple endocrine. *See*
  Multiple endocrine neoplasia
  (MEN)
Nephrectomy, 321
Neuroblastoma, 61–64
  diagnosis of, 61–62
  incidence of, 61
  molecular genetics of, 62
  neuronal markers in, 63
  new therapies for, 64
  oncogene in, 62
  screening of, 62
  staging of, 63
  treatment of, 63–64
Non-Hodgkin's lymphoma, 203–210
  anthracycline for, 209
  antimicrobial therapy for, 208
  B-cell neoplasms, 204
  bone marrow transplant in, 209–210
  chemotherapy response rates of, 205,
    209
  cisplatin for, 209
  classification of, 203–205
  cytarabine (DHAP) for, 209–210
  dexamethasone for, 209
  doxorubicin for, 209
  fine-needle aspiration (FNA) biopsy
    of, 204, 208
  future trends in, 210
  Heliobacter pylori in, 207–208
  histology of, 204
  international index of, 205
  mantle cell, 208–209
  Mediterranean, 207
  mucosa-associated lymphoid tissue
    (MALT) in, 206–208
  prognostic factors in, 205–206
  surgery *vs.* chemotherapy for, 208
  survival rates of, 205, 209
  survival rates of, mantle cell, 208–

209
T-cell neoplasms, 204
transplant *vs.* standard treatment,
  209–210
tumor progression in, 207
tumor score in, 206

O
Octreotide, 234
Oncogenes
  in thyroid carcinoma, medullary, 160
  in thyroid carcinoma, well-
    differentiated, 151, 152–153
Orchiectomy, 60
Osteoconduction, 139
Osteogenesis, 140–141

P
Pancreatectomy, 230
Pancreatic cancer, 109–121
  angiogenesis in, 121
  chemoradiation for, 114
  chemoradiation for, preoperative,
    116
  diagnostic imaging for, 109–114 (*See
    also* Pancreatic cancer, diagnostic
    imaging in)
  external-beam radiation therapy
    (EBRT) for, 114
  5-fluorouracil (FU) chemotherapy
    for, 114
  gemcitabine (Gemzar) for, 118–119
  genetic alterations in, 120
  Kocher maneuver in, 110
  K-*ras* oncogene in, 120
  liver disease and, 121
  metastases in, 115
  multimodality therapy for, 114–117
  palpation in, intraoperative, 110
  pancreaticoduodenectomy in, 110
  p51 gene in, 120
  positive margin in, 112
  research on, 120–121
  resectibility of, 110–111
  resectibility of, criteria for, 111
  survival rates in, 109–110, 115, 119
  systemic therapy for, 118–119
  testosterone in, 119
  tumor control in, locoregional, 116
  vascular endothelial growth factor
    (VEGF) in, 121
  vascular resection in, 117–118

103
salvage rate in, 103
tumor necrosis factor in, 102
Soft tissue sarcoma, prognostic factors
   for, 91–95
  high-risk profile in, 93
  histopathology in, 93
  leiomyosarcoma in, 93
  liposarcoma in, 93
  multivariate analyses of, 92
  prospective *vs.* retrospective data in,
   93
  sample size in, 92
  staging systems and, 94-95
Somatostatin
  in gastrointestinal neuroendocrine
   tumor, 229
  in scintigraphy, 216–217
Somatostatinoma, 216
Staging, surgical
  accuracy in, 12
  of colon cancer, 353
  of early breast cancer, 171–172
  of gallbladder carcinoma, 291–292
  of gastrointestinal neuroendocrine
   tumors, 229–231
  of melanoma, 12–24
  of neuroblastoma, 63
  of rhabdomyosarcoma, 57
  of soft tissue sarcoma, 94–95
  of Wilm's tumor, 52–53
Stereotactic core needle biopsy
  (SCNB), 176–177
Streptozotocin, 234
Surgery, minimally invasive, 309–324.
  See also Minimally invasive
  surgery
Surgery, plastic, 71–88. *See also*
  Reconstruction
Survival rates
  in bone sarcoma reconstruction, 138
  in cholangiocarcinoma, Hilar bile
   duct, 282
  in hepatocellular carcinoma, 331
  in melanoma, 3, 14–15, 18–19
  in non-Hodgkin's lymphoma, 205,
   208–209, 209
  in pancreatic cancer, 109–110, 115,
   119
  in pediatric tumors, 51
  in rectal cancer, 31–32, 37, 42
  in rectal cancer, coloanal
   anastomosis, 37
  in rectal cancer, local excision, 31–

32, 35
  in rectal cancer, mesorectal excision,
   35
  in thyroid carcinoma, 28150
  in Wilm's tumor, 51

T
Tamoxifen, 182, 190
T-cell neoplasms, in non-Hodgkin's
  lymphoma, 204
Testosterone, 119
Thyroid carcinoma, 149–165
  cytogenetics of, 150–152 (*See also*
   Thyroid carcinoma, cytogenetics
   of)
  etiology of, 149–150
  medullary, 159–164 (*See also*
   Thyroid carcinoma, medullary)
  well-differentiated, 149–159 (*See also*
   Thyroid carcinoma, well-
   differentiated)
Thyroid carcinoma, cytogenetics of,
  150–152
  follicular, 151
  oncogenes in, 151
  papillary, 151
Thyroid carcinoma, medullary, 159–
  164
  anaplastic, 163–164
  calcitonin in, 160, 162–163
  carcinoembryonic antigen (CEA) in,
   160, 162
  chemotherapy for, 162
  diagnosis of, 159–160
  external-beam radiation therapy
   (XRT) in, 161–162
  fine-needle aspiration of, 159
  markers for, 160–161
  occult metastatic, 162–163
  oncogenes in, 160
  prognosis of, 160–161
  RET gene, 160
  thyroidectomy for, 161
  treatment of, 161–162
Thyroid carcinoma, well-differentiated,
  149–159
  antibodies in, 155
  carcinogenesis of, 150
  contralateral lobes in, 157
  cytogenetics of, 150–152 (*See also*
   Thyroid carcinoma, cytogenetics
   of)
  diagnosis of, 154–156

369

incision in, transperitoneal, 53
metastic, 55
nephrectomy in, 53–54
nonmetastic, 54
Société Internationale d'Oncologie
    Pédiatrique (SIOP) in, 54

staging of, 53
vincristine in, 53

Z
Zollinger-Ellison syndrome (ZES), 216